Nutritional Issues in Cancer Care

Edited by

Valerie J. Kogut, MA, RD, LDN
Sandra L. Luthringer, RD, LDN

Oncology Nursing Society
Pittsburgh, PA

ONS Publishing Division
Publisher: Leonard Mafrica, MBA, CAE
Director, Commercial Publishing: Barbara Sigler, RN, MNEd
Production Manager: Lisa M. George, BA
Technical Editor: Angela Klimaszewski, RN, MSN
Staff Editor: Lori Wilson, BA
Copy Editor: Amy Nicoletti, BA
Graphic Designer: Dany Sjoen

Nutritional Issues in Cancer Care

Library of Congress Control Number: 2005929989

ISBN 1-890504-54-8

Publisher's Note

This book is published by the Oncology Nursing Society (ONS). ONS neither represents nor guarantees that the practices described herein will, if followed, ensure safe and effective patient care. The recommendations contained in this book reflect ONS's judgment regarding the state of general knowledge and practice in the field as of the date of publication. The recommendations may not be appropriate for use in all circumstances. Those who use this book should make their own determinations regarding specific safe and appropriate patient-care practices, taking into account the personnel, equipment, and practices available at the hospital or other facility at which they are located. The editors and publisher cannot be held responsible for any liability incurred as a consequence from the use or application of any of the contents of this book. Figures and tables are used as examples only. They are not meant to be all-inclusive, nor do they represent endorsement of any particular institution by ONS. Mention of specific products and opinions related to those products do not indicate or imply endorsement by ONS.

ONS publications are originally published in English. Permission has been granted by the ONS Board of Directors for foreign translation. (Individual tables and figures that are reprinted or adapted require additional permission from the original source.) However, because translations from English may not always be accurate or precise, ONS disclaims any responsibility for inaccuracies in words or meaning that may occur as a result of the translation. Readers relying on precise information should check the original English version.

Printed in the United States of America

Oncology Nursing Society
Integrity • Innovation • Stewardship • Advocacy • Excellence • Inclusiveness

Contributors

Editors

Valerie J. Kogut, MA, RD, LDN
Oncology Nutritionist
Department of Otolaryngology
University of Pittsburgh Medical
    Center
Pittsburgh, Pennsylvania

Sandra L. Luthringer, RD, LDN
Clinical Dietitian
The Regional Cancer Center
Erie, Pennsylvania

Authors

Kristen Baileys, MSN, CRNP, OCN®
Education Associate
Oncology Nursing Society
Pittsburgh, Pennsylvania
Chapter 13. Lymphoma

Marion S. Bragdon, RN, BSN, MEd,
    OCN®
Oncology Information and Educa-
    tion Specialist
University of Pittsburgh Medical
    Center Cancer Centers
University of Pittsburgh Cancer
    Institute
Pittsburgh, Pennsylvania
Chapter 1. Cancer Prevention

Mary Reilly Burgunder, RN, BSN,
    MS, OCN®
Infusion and Oncology Specialty
    Clinician
University of Pittsburgh Medical
    Center/South Hills Health Sys-
    tem, Home Health, LP
Pittsburgh, Pennsylvania
*Chapter 16. Hematopoietic Stem Cell
Transplantation*

Tinrin Chew, RD
Oncology Dietitian
Alta Bates Comprehensive Cancer
    Center
Berkeley, California
Consulting Dietitian
Hospice and Palliative Care of
    Contra Costa
Concord, California
Chapter 14. Multiple Myeloma, Melanoma, and Sarcoma

Susan Anne Churma, RD, LD
Clinical Dietitian
University of Pittsburgh Medical
    Center—McKeesport
McKeesport, Pennsylvania
Chapter 4. Esophageal and Gastric Cancers

Joyce G. Diacopoulos, RD, LDN,
    CNSD
Nutrition Coordinator
The Hillman Cancer Center
University of Pittsburgh Medical
    Center
Pittsburgh, Pennsylvania
Chapter 20. Resources and References

Barbara J. Dickson, RD, MS, CD
Clinical Dietitian
Veterans Affairs—Puget Sound
    Health Care System
Seattle, Washington
Chapter 16. Hematopoietic Stem Cell Transplantation

Erin Dummert, RD, CD
Director of Nutritional Services
Oncology Alliance, S.C.
Milwaukee, Wisconsin
Chapter 5. Genitourinary Cancers

Bernadette Festa, MS, RD
Nutrition Services Coordinator
Alta Bates Comprehensive Cancer
    Center
Berkeley, California
Chapter 14. Multiple Myeloma, Melanoma, and Sarcoma

Diane M. Fletcher, RN, MA, BSN,
    OCN®
Executive Director, Pennsylvania
    Cancer Control Consortium
    (PAC3)
Assistant Director, Cancer Control
    and Population Sciences
University of Pittsburgh Cancer
    Institute
Pittsburgh, Pennsylvania
Chapter 2. Breast Cancer

Colleen A. Gill, MS, RD
Clinical Dietitian, Oncology
    Services
Anschutz Cancer Center
University of Colorado Hospital
Aurora, Colorado
Chapter 18. Immunonutrition: The Role of Specialized Nutritional Support for Patients With Cancer

Jennifer L. Guy, BS, RN, OCN®
Self-Employed Oncology Consultant/Medical Writer
Columbus, Ohio
Chapter 10. Pancreatic Cancer

Kathryn Hamilton, MA, RD, CDN
Outpatient Clinical Oncology
    Dietitian
Morristown Memorial Hospital
Morristown, New Jersey
Chapter 6. Gynecologic Cancers

Ria G. Hawks, RN, MS, CNS, CPNP
Nurse Practitioner
Division of Pediatric Hematology
and Blood and Marrow Trans-
plantation
Columbia University
New York, New York
Chapter 15. Pediatric Cancers

Michele C. Hayward, RD, LDN
Senior Research Manager
University of Pittsburgh Cancer
Institute
Pittsburgh, Pennsylvania
Chapter 2. Breast Cancer

Cindy Jo Horrell, MS, CRNP, AOCN®
Oncology Nurse Practitioner
The Regional Cancer Center
Erie, Pennsylvania
*Chapter 4. Esophageal and Gastric
Cancers*

Helen C. James, MS, APRN, BC,
OCN®
Oncology Nurse Practitioner
Baystate Medical Center
Springfield, Massachusetts
Chapter 8. Hepatobiliary Cancer

Gayle S. Jameson, RN, MSN, CRNP,
AOCN®
Nurse Practitioner
Allegheny Hematology/Oncology
Associates
Pittsburgh, Pennsylvania
Chapter 12. Adult Leukemia

Sarah H. Kagan, PhD, RN, APRN,
BC, AOCN®
Associate Professor of Gerontologi-
cal Nursing
University of Pennsylvania
Philadelphia, Pennsylvania
Chapter 7. Head and Neck Cancers

Anne Z. Kisak, RN, MBA, BSN
Division Administrator—Cancer
Control and Population Sciences
University of Pittsburgh Cancer
Institute
Pittsburgh, Pennsylvania
Chapter 9. Lung Cancer

Lesley B. Klein, MS, RD, LD
Clinical Dietitian—Oncology
Comprehensive Cancer Center
John F. Kennedy Medical Center
Lake Worth, Florida
Chapter 9. Lung Cancer

Karen P. Kulakowski, MA, RD, LDN
Senior Oncology Dietitian
Baystate Medical Center
Springfield, Massachusetts
Chapter 8. Hepatobiliary Cancer

Elena J. Ladas, MS, RD
Director, Integrative Therapies Pro-
gram for Children With Cancer
Columbia University
New York, New York
Chapter 15. Pediatric Cancers

Natalie Lagomarcino Ledesma,
MS, RD
Oncology Dietitian
University of California, San Fran-
cisco Comprehensive Cancer
Center
San Francisco, California
Chapter 11. Prostate Cancer

Karen Masino, MS, CNP, APRN-BC,
OCN®, RD, LDN, CNSD
Advanced Practice Nurse
Bone Marrow Transplant
Northwestern Memorial Hospital
Chicago, Illinois
Chapter 3. Colorectal Cancer

Eileen Milakovic, MA, BSN, RN, OCN®, CHPN
Program Manager, Professional Education
University of Pittsburgh Medical Center Cancer Centers
Pittsburgh, Pennsylvania
Chapter 5. Genitourinary Cancers

Kathleen Murphy-Ende, RN, PhD, AOCNP
Nurse Practitioner and Clinical Assistant Professor
University of Wisconsin Hospitals and Clinics
University of Wisconsin School of Nursing
Madison, Wisconsin
Chapter 18. Immunonutrition: The Role of Specialized Nutritional Support for Patients With Cancer

Jamie S. Myers, RN, MN, AOCN®
Regional Scientific Associate Director
Novartis Oncology Scientific Operations
Edwardsville, Kansas
Chapter 11. Prostate Cancer

Marcia Nahikian-Nelms, PhD, RD, LD
Professor, Director of Didactic Program in Dietetics
Southeast Missouri State University
Cape Girardeau, Missouri
Chapter 13. Lymphoma

Carolyn D. Nunnally, RN, MN
Clinical Nurse Specialist—Cancer Information and Referral Service
University of Pittsburgh Medical Center Cancer Centers
Pittsburgh, Pennsylvania
Chapter 20. Resources and References

Maryellen O'Leary, RN
Practice Nurse
Alta Bates Comprehensive Cancer Center
Berkeley, California
Chapter 14. Multiple Myeloma, Melanoma, and Sarcoma

Maria Petzel, RD, LD, CNSD
Senior Clinical Dietitian
The University of Texas M.D. Anderson Cancer Center
Houston, Texas
Chapter 12. Adult Leukemia

Jill Place, MA, RD
The Supplement Savvy RD
Nutritional Counselor
A Transformation Celebration™
Consultant, Author, and Motivational Speaker
Los Angeles, California
Chapter 17. Complementary and Alternative Medicine in Cancer Care

Susan M. Roche, CRNP, MSN, OCN®, APRN-BC
Nurse Practitioner
The Regional Cancer Center
Erie, Pennsylvania
Chapter 6. Gynecologic Cancers

Clara Schneider, MS, RD, RN, LD, CDE
Consulting Dietitian and Nurse
American Institute for Cancer Research
American Diabetes Association
Diabetes Specialist
Virginia Hospital Center
Arlington, Virginia
Chapter 19. Palliative Care and Hospice

Sally Scroggs, MS, RD, LD
Senior Health Education Specialist
Cancer Prevention Center
The University of Texas M.D. Anderson Cancer Center
Houston, Texas
Chapter 1. Cancer Prevention

Tracy R. Smith, PhD, RD, LD
Senior Scientist
Ross Products Division of Abbott Labs
Columbus, Ohio
Chapter 10. Pancreatic Cancer

Ellen Sweeney-Cordes, MS, RD, LDN
Clinical Dietitian Specialist
Abramson Cancer Center—University of Pennsylvania
Philadelphia, Pennsylvania
Chapter 7. Head and Neck Cancers

About the Editors

Valerie J. Kogut, MA, RD, LDN

Valerie is chairman of the Oncology Nutrition Dietetic Practice Group, a subgroup of the American Dietetic Association (ADA). She has more than 10 years of experience as an oncology dietitian. She has worked in medical and surgical oncology as well as working in bone marrow transplant. She is currently the oncology nutritionist for the University of Pittsburgh Medical Center in the Department of Otolaryngology in Pittsburgh, Pennsylvania. In her position at the University of Pittsburgh Medical Center, she is responsible for nutrition education and evaluation of outpatients with head and neck cancer. She develops, implements, and coordinates all aspects of nutritional services for the University Ear, Nose, and Throat Specialists. Val has a strong enthusiasm for oncology nutrition and especially for teaching healthcare professionals and patients. She is also a member of the Oncology Nursing Society.

Sandra L. Luthringer, RD, LDN

Sandra is a founding member and former chairman of the Oncology Nutrition Dietetic Practice Group, a subgroup of the American Dietetic Association (ADA). As a registered dietitian at the Regional Cancer Center in Erie, Pennsylvania, she brings more than 20 years of clinical experience to this project. She has written numerous chapters for oncology-related textbooks, journals, and other publications and has spoken to many professional groups on a variety of nutrition and oncology topics. Nationally, Sandra serves on the ADA research team (oncology work group), which currently is developing protocols for medical nutrition therapy in the cancer population, and she is a member of the National Cancer Institute's PDQ® Supportive Care Editorial Board.

Table of Contents

Preface

The concept of the healthcare team reaches its fundamental significance in the management of patients with cancer. The nutritional care of patients with cancer can be very complex and must be individualized. It is the collaboration between oncology nurses and dietitians that will provide the best nutritional care to each patient. This book has been very exciting for us to organize and prepare and will provide the reader with general information on most of the common cancers as well as their nutritional consequences. The book is unique in that oncology nurses as well as dietitians combined their expertise to provide first-hand suggestions for the many problems, frustrations, and difficulties they have had in managing the nutritional needs of patients with cancer during and after treatments. It is our hope that healthcare providers, those both new to the field of oncology as well as seasoned professionals, will open this book and learn how to effectively manage the nutritional needs of their patients. We are grateful to all of our patients and their families who have been our best teachers.

Valerie and Sandra

Acknowledgments

We would like to gratefully acknowledge the generous contributions of all of the oncology dietitians and nurses who provided the "nuts and bolts" for this book, and to all healthcare professionals who work with patients, as well as their families affected by cancer. Our jobs as caregivers can only pale to the jobs that our patients and their families have 24/7. They do not get to take lunch breaks or punch out at the end of each day.

The editors would also like to thank their parents, Stanley and Ann Kogut who have been a constant source of love and support for Val, and Nick and Julie DeDad, who courageously fought cancer and showed the true meaning of care-giving while Sandra worked on this project. A special thanks also to Jeff, Corey, and Julia Luthringer for their encouragement and patience. You are all so very special to us!

CHAPTER 1

Cancer Prevention

Marion S. Bragdon, RN, BSN, MEd, OCN®
Sally Scroggs, MS, RD, LD

Overview

Perhaps no subject is more confusing or emotionally charged than food, as it influences our well-being. Eating and taking pleasure in food are central to health (Weil, 2000). The word "cancer," in contrast, connotes pain, suffering, and death. Cancer causes fear and panic and offers no immunity. Food is our nourishment, associated with comfort and pleasure. Food also is a cancer mediator and deserves closer study.

Michael Sporn, cancer researcher at Dartmouth Medical School, said, "People are obsessed with cures . . . and the (elusive) miraculous cure. They are being . . . selfish by ignoring what could be done in terms of prevention" (Leaf, 2004, p. 88). Andy von Eschenbach, director of the National Cancer Institute (NCI) and a cancer survivor, said we must be on a "mission to prevent the (cancer) process" from occurring at all (Leaf, p. 90). Our society can promote specific behaviors to reduce the risk of cancers. One of the greatest cancer preventions is acting on the knowledge of the benefits and detriments of nutrition.

Early in the 1930s, laboratory studies were conducted that found a correlation between diet and carcinogenesis (Kiple & Ornelas, 2000). Later, human epidemiologic studies were conducted that did not support the relationship. The United States, because of its large number of immigrants, was unique in allowing such an observation to occur. Immigrants showed a variation in cancer incidence compared to U.S.-born citizens. Factors could be genetic makeup, ethnic persona, and specific diets and lifestyles. These ethnic factors gave a control to the studies conducted in the 1930s (Clifford & McDonald, 2001; Weil, 2000; World Cancer Research Fund [WCRF] & American Institute for Cancer Research [AICR], 1997).

Current scientific evidence relates diet and nutrition to cancer risk (WCRF & AICR, 1997). Although factors other than diet can play a role in the development of cancer, health experts know that paying attention to diet and related factors, including weight and exercise, is a proven way to reduce cancer risk.

Research is ongoing, and scientists are beginning to sort out the complex relationships between specific food components and their effects on health. Health and research agencies, such as the American Cancer Society (ACS) and AICR, attempt to summarize the current research in the form of recommendations that are frequently updated as more data are gathered. A landmark report by Doll and Peto (1981) estimated that 10%–70% of cancer deaths in the United States could be attributed to diet. They concluded that dietary factors could account for 35% of all cancer deaths. The Commission on Life Sciences (1982) reported convincing evidence that diet plays a role in human cancer and included guidelines for risk reduction. Several years later, Willett and Trichopoulos (1996) estimated that one-third of cancers could be completely avoided if specific dietary guidelines were followed. Expert advisory committees used this research as a basis for ACS's revised nutrition guidelines advocating a plant-based diet with the addition of physical activity (ACS, 1996). More recently, these guidelines were reviewed and revised (Byers et al., 2002). Referenced in these guidelines is the most comprehensive review to date from WCRF and AICR (1997). AICR estimated that 30%–40% of all cancers could be prevented with a healthier diet and exercise. The joint report included 15 specific guidelines for public health goals and advice to individuals. An AICR panel convened in 2003 with the mission of reviewing 10,000 reports from 1997–2003 to further refine the guidelines. The revisions of these guidelines will be completed in 2006. Recommendations of ACS (Byers et al.) and WCRF and AICR (1997) include a plant-based diet to reduce the risk of certain types of cancer.

Diet's Protective Influence

The Role of Whole Foods Versus Dietary Supplements

Nutrients from whole foods are more beneficial than those obtained from supplements. A single fruit or vegetable contains many nutrients and protective chemicals. These chemicals act together to provide a better defense against disease (Cataldo, DeBruyne, & Whitney, 2003). It is not likely that a person would receive dangerously high doses of any single plant chemical if obtained from food sources rather than a pill. Certain dietary supplements can increase cancer risk, and megadosing of some vitamins and minerals can pose unique or unsafe risks from side effects. However, because of the suggestion that plant ingredients might protect against cancer and other diseases, many people are turning to vitamin and mineral supplements or to special diets. Polunin (1999) demonstrated that supplements of beta-carotene and vitamin C showed no protective effect, but eating the actual antioxidant-rich foods had a protective effect on cells. Willett

(1999) noted that at least 200 epidemiologic studies suggested that people who consistently consume large amounts of fruits and vegetables have a reduced risk of developing cancer at a number of sites. In a review by Block, Patterson, and Subar (1992) of 156 studies, 82% showed that adequate fruit and vegetable consumption had a protective effect against epithelial types of cancer, including all gastrointestinal, laryngeal, and lung and some skin cancers. WCRF and AICR (1997) reported that vegetable intake decreases one's risk of cancer at 16 cancer sites, and fruits decrease cancer risk at 12 sites, yet the National Health and Nutrition Examination Survey (Patterson, Block, Rosenberger, Pee, & Kahle, 1990) indicated that only 1 in 11 Americans met the guidelines for eating at least three servings of vegetables and two servings of fruit a day.

The Role of Food Components in Carcinogenesis

The cancer process involves three stages: initiation, promotion, and progression (Ruoslahti, 1996). Nutrients and phytochemicals are influences in all stages. Dietary factors influence carcinogenesis directly and indirectly. Nutrients and phytochemicals can inhibit enzymes that activate carcinogens and induce enzymes that detoxify them. Phytochemicals protect plants from insects, disease, and harsh environmental conditions. Research shows that some phytochemicals and nutrients play a role in protecting human cells from cancer. Phytochemicals are non-nutrient chemicals in plant foods that provide pigment and flavor; they give onions and garlic their pungent taste and aroma and other fruits and vegetables their bright and varied colors (Boik, 2001).

In initiation, the procarcinogens enter the cell. Nutrients and phytochemicals can inhibit or block the chemical change by enzyme-driven mechanisms. Vitamin C, for example, inhibits enzymatic activation of chemicals that prevents nitrates from being changed into carcinogenic nitrosamines associated with gastric cancer. Other enzymes induced by phytochemicals, such as glutathione S-transferase, can detoxify and remove potential carcinogens (Health Science Institute, 1997b). If the potential carcinogen compound is not deactivated at this point, it can enter the cell's nucleus, where its DNA can be altered. Once initiation has occurred, the damaged cell cannot be repaired (Health Science Institute, 1997b).

In promotion and progression, latent initiated cells can be transformed into differentiated cells that progress into a tumor (Health Science Institute, 1997a, 1997b). This is a relatively prolonged process that can take several years. Unlike initiation, the processes of promotion and progression can be reversed. Food components can play a vital role in this reversal. For example, certain types of dietary fats act as promoters, and animal research has shown removing fat from the diet can slow the progression of a tumor (Wang et al., 1995).

Phytochemicals and Nutrients

Phytochemicals have the ability to act as antioxidants. Antioxidants work in a variety of ways to stabilize, deactivate, or transform oxygen free radicals

(AICR, 1999a). Studies suggested these protective molecules work at all stages of carcinogenesis (Caragay, 1992). Any single fruit or vegetable may contain hundreds or more of the thousands of known phytochemicals (AICR, 1999b). Isolating single phytochemicals does not always demonstrate the same protection as in a combination found in whole food. Chemoprevention trials (Alpha-Tocopherol, Beta Carotene Cancer Prevention Study Group, 1994; Goodman et al., 1993) found that synthetic beta-carotene supplements might increase the risk for lung cancer in a high-risk group of cigarette smokers. Moss (2000) expressed concern over supplementation of carotenoids: "Giving too much of one carotenoid decreases the others, and may paradoxically lower one's resistance to cancer" (p. 32).

Similar to the evidence that some nutrients are dependent on others for completeness of metabolism and function, the same holds true for phytochemicals. Finding the correct phytochemical that offers protection at a specific cancer site is a tedious process. Several phytochemicals currently are being studied to determine how they influence the cancer process. Some of the phytochemicals of interest and their proposed mechanism of action are listed in Table 1-1.

Table 1-1. Phytochemicals, Food Sources, and Their Proposed Mechanisms of Action

Phytochemical	Food	Proposed Mechanism(s) of Action
Allicin, diallyl sulfide, and S-allyl-L-cys-teine	Garlic and onions	Inhibit phase I enzymes that activate carcinogens; induce phase II enzymes that detoxify carcinogens
Catechins	Tea: green and black	Antioxidant; prevent lipid peroxidation by inhibiting lipoxygenase enzymes; inhibit cyclooxygenase enzymes
Ellagic acid	Strawberries and grapes	Antioxidant
Flavonoids		
Citrus: diosmin and hesperidin	Grapefruit and orange juice	Decrease polyamine levels that have a role in cell growth and proliferation
Noncitrus: genistein and daidzein (phy-toestrogens)	Soy, red grapes, and apples	Antioxidant; compete with and block estrogens/androgens from binding to their receptors, which retard cell proliferation
Indoles	Cabbage and turnips	Increase conversion of estrogens to inactive forms; induce phase II enzymes (glutathione S-transferase) to increase carcinogen detoxification

(Continued on next page)

Table 1-1. Phytochemicals, Food Sources, and Their Proposed Mechanisms of Action *(Continued)*

Phytochemical	Food	Proposed Mechanism(s) of Action
Isothiocyanates	Cruciferous vegetables (broccoli, brussels sprouts, cauliflower)	Inhibit phase I enzymes that activate carcinogens; induce phase II enzymes that detoxify carcinogens (Note: phase II enzymes include glutathione S-transferases and NADPH: quinone reductase)
Lignans	Flaxseed and grains	Prevent estrogens and prostaglandins from binding to their receptors, which retard cell proliferation
Lycopene	Tomatoes and watermelon	Antioxidant
Monoterpenes Limonene	Lemon and orange peel	Decrease cell proliferation by decreasing ornithine decarboxylase activity, which is important to the induction of carcinogenesis; decrease activity of growth-promoting *ras* proteins; increase latent period as inhibitor of promotion; prevent oncogene expression; induce phase II carcinogen detoxification enzymes
Phenols	Turmeric, mustard, tea, berries, grapes, and sesame seeds	Antioxidant; inhibit activity of lipoxygenase and cyclooxygenase enzymes; inhibit formation of carcinogens such as nitrosamines; induce phase II enzymes that detoxify carcinogens
Phytate	Soybeans, grains, nuts, and seeds	Inhibits cell proliferation and metastasis
Polyphenols	Artichokes	Antioxidant; induce phase II enzymes that detoxify carcinogens
Protease inhibitors	Soybeans, dried beans, and lentils	Antioxidant; inhibit malignant cell transformation; inhibit gene amplification; inhibit estrogen- and glucocorticoid-receptor binding; inhibit c-*myc* oncogene expression and cell proliferation
Saponins	Soy foods, legumes, herbs, and vegetables	Inhibit proliferation of malignant cells
Sulforaphane	Broccoli	Induces phase II enzymes that detoxify carcinogens

Note. Based on information from "Beyond Vitamins," 1999; Gollman & Pierce, 1998; Health Science Institute, 1997a, 1997b.

Fiber

Fiber has been associated with a possible decreased risk for colorectal, pancreatic, and breast cancers (WCRF & AICR, 1997). Proposed mechanisms for fiber in colon cancer reduction include lowering the colonic pH, diluting and binding genotoxic agents, and increasing short chain fatty acids to help to slow cell proliferation (Kiple & Ornelas, 2000; Willett, 1999). Fiber increases the bulk of the intestinal contents, which stimulates intestinal peristalsis and speeds food through the colon for reduced contact time. However, in large prospective studies, total fiber intake has not been shown to reduce the risk of colon cancer (Willett, 1999). Confounding issues include the interactions of nutrients and other phytochemicals in foods that contain fiber. Even though evidence is inconclusive, ACS recommends consumption of high-fiber foods (Byers et al., 2002). The National Academy of Sciences (Hermann, 2002) did not set an upper limit for individuals because of the likelihood that consumption is self-limiting, but specific fiber amounts related to gender and age have been determined. For example, the current guidelines recommend 14 grams per 1,000 calories of adult food intake. More trials are needed to explore the connection between the interaction of nutrients and phytochemicals in foods that contain fiber and the interaction of fat consumption and fiber.

Physical Activity's Protective Influence

In 2001, the World Health Organization reviewed the role of physical activity for cancer risk reduction. This work group reported recent research studies that indicated moderate to vigorous activity decreases the risk of colon and breast cancers independent of an individual's weight (Vainio & Bianchini, 2002). That same work group reported limited evidence suggesting a preventive effect of physical activity on endometrial and prostate cancers. Exact amounts for duration and frequency of exercise still are being studied. ACS currently recommends moderate to vigorous activity for 45 minutes five or more days per week to further reduce the risk of breast and colon cancers. The benefit is cumulative, but 20 or more minutes per session are suggested (Courneya, 2002). Physical activity affects different mechanisms that may play a role in cancer risk reduction. It can help with achieving and maintaining a healthy body weight. A healthy body weight could lead to less adipose tissue, which would decrease the exposure of hormones stored in this tissue that play a role in some forms of breast cancer (Wynder et al., 1997). This also may play a role in decreasing circulating insulin and related growth factors (Bianchini, Kaaks, & Vainio, 2002). Physical activity also assists with peristalsis, which shortens the time exposure of mutagens to the bowel epithelial tissues (Duyff, 1998). Evidence suggests that simply not being sedentary decreases colon cancer risk. Increased activity has been associated with approximately a 40% risk reduction in colon cancer (Vainio & Bianchini). Breast cancer risk evidenced a reduction of as much as 20%–40% for the most physically active group in one study (Vainio & Bianchini).

Diet as Promoter of Carcinogenesis

Fats and Obesity

Cancer risk-reduction research findings are in conflict regarding the association between fat intake and weight or obesity. Questions to be answered include the interactions and connections of fat in diet to

- Total energy intake
- Type of fat
- Obesity
- Energy expenditure
- Fiber
- Vitamins
- Minerals
- Phytochemicals.

Scientific evidence suggests some relationship between fat intake and lung, colorectal, breast, endometrium, and prostate cancers (WCRF & AICR, 1997). Current research on the effects of the type of fat look promising (Byers et al., 2002). Saturated fats should be limited, with more emphasis on mono-unsaturated fats (WCRF & AICR). The evidence is still insufficient regarding the role of polyunsaturated fatty acids in cancer development to draw conclusions on intakes for humans (Willett, 2002). Results from intervention trials are needed.

Fat in the diet can play a significant role in excess calories leading to obesity, but there is speculation that fat itself might not be as much of a culprit as originally suggested (Willett, 2002). Obesity from excess calories (fats, proteins, carbohydrates, alcohol) may be more significant than just fat in the diet. Overweightedness and obesity are associated with an increased risk of cancer at these sites: breast, colon and rectum, endometrium, esophagus, gallbladder, liver, pancreas, and kidney (Byers et al., 2002). Gender-specific research indicates an increased risk in stomach and prostate cancers for men and in breast, uterine, cervical, and ovarian cancers for women (Calle, Rodriguez, Walker-Thurmond, & Thun, 2003).

Additives, Contaminants, and Cooking Methods

Powerful carcinogens can be created or formed in the preservation and preparation of foods. For decades, the public has been concerned about the possibility of cancer risk from additives or contaminants. However, this has not proved to be as great a factor as has been touted. Additives help to make foods safer and improve their stability. Some of the synthetic chemicals used for sweetening, such as saccharin, once were listed as carcinogenic but since have been proved harmful only in laboratory mice (Kiple & Ornelas, 2000). Nitrate (saltpeter) concentrations can lead to the formation of carcinogenic compounds. Salt used in pickling solutions is associated with a high cancer risk, but these additives increase cancer risk from the carcinogens only when consumed in large quantities. Food safety versus the danger of overuse becomes a question. Moderation of all things is the key element in food consumption (Kiple & Ornelas).

It is interesting to note that not all chemicals in foods are disease protective. Some phytochemicals are naturally occurring carcinogens produced possibly to ward off insects, disease, and/or a harsh environment (Shils, Olson, Moshe, & Ross, 1994). In rodent studies, the doses required to cause cancer in humans exceeded dietary intake (Shils et al.). Other chemicals in foods that are not naturally occurring include pesticides and additives, such as artificial sweeteners. Carcinogenic or mutagenic compounds in plants are formed during cooking, such as polycyclic aromatic hydrocarbons, heterocyclic amines (HCAs), and possibly acrylamide (Tareke, Rydberg, Karlsson, Eriksson, & Tornqvist, 2000). The best method for cooking muscle meat is under 400°F (212°C) to reduce these compound formations (Mayo Clinic, UCLA, & Dole Food Company, 2002). Other effective methods are baking, boiling, braising, steaming, and poaching. The effect on cancer rates from these cooking methods is extremely difficult to determine.

AICR (2002) stated that no convincing evidence shows that eating foods containing trace amounts of chemicals such as fertilizers, pesticides, herbicides, and drugs used on farm animals changes cancer risk. AICR (2002) reported environmental pollutants cause less than 1% of all cancers. Byers et al. (2002) stated that pesticides and herbicides can have a health risk if not used properly, but at low doses, pesticides and herbicides do not increase cancer risk. The benefits of a plant-based diet far outweigh any harm from exposure to trace amounts of chemicals that may be found in these foods.

Pesticides are regulated by the following government organizations: Environmental Protection Agency, the U.S. Food and Drug Administration, and the U.S. Department of Agriculture (USDA). These agencies are responsible for approving pesticide levels in food, setting the tolerance levels, and inspecting domestic and imported foods for compliance. They work together to regulate substances and determine the status of "Generally Recognized as Safe." If a concern is raised, the substance must go through a food additive premarket review and approval process (Thompson, 2000).

Genetically modified foods also must satisfy safety requirements. The pros and cons of these foods currently are being researched (Thompson, 2000). A number of valid concerns arise with altering genetic makeup by gene splicing, such as violating dietary restrictions and/or religious beliefs or introducing altered genes to the human food supply. Genetic changes can alter the plant to make it more frost resistant, for example (Beringer, 1999). A plant may be modified so that it is less susceptible to insects with the possible benefit of requiring fewer pesticides (Thompson). Research regarding the safety of consuming genetically modified foods will continue well into the future.

Organic Versus Conventionally Grown Produce

A review by Williams (2002) indicated few compositional differences comparing organically grown vegetables and fruits to conventionally grown produce. Another study stated there is not strong evidence that organic and conventional foods differ in nutritional quality (Bourn & Prescott, 2002). However, some differences in these comparisons include variation in the groups studied as well as differences in growing conditions: organic versus conventional. Organic does not necessarily mean pesticide-free (Baker, Benbrook, Groth, & Benbrook, 2002). A Consumer Union report on unwashed produce indicated 25% of the organic produce contained residues, compared with 77% of the conventional produce (Neville, 1999). The organic foods may be exposed to chemicals carried in the wind or water. The USDA (2002) developed new criteria to receive the stamp of "Certified Organic" in 2002. Farmers must use only government-preapproved, plant-based chemicals; pesticides and herbicides are prohibited. Farmers also must use land that has been free of pesticides or herbicides for several years and be open to inspections, including samples of soil, water, and plant tissue. Individual steps to reduce pesticide residue would include scrubbing fruits and vegetables under running water, removing outer leaves, choosing produce free of holes, eating a variety of foods to lower exposure to any one pesticide, and, if affordable, choosing organic (AICR, 2002). Variety is key, and this will ensure exposure to a number of protective chemicals present in various plant-based foods while decreasing exposure to chemicals that may be used on any one specific crop.

Alcohol

Alcohol's proposed mechanisms in the cancer process include source of free radicals, solvent to carcinogens, and, if abused, depleted nutrient intake (Physician Oncology Education Program, 2001). Molecules in alcohol are being researched for their beneficial effects with reducing the risk of heart disease, but this research has not yet been shown to carry over to cancer risk reduction. Alcohol has been associated with an increased risk of head and neck cancers and gastrointestinal cancers, especially if combined with tobacco (Bal, Woolam, & Seffrin, 1999). Alcohol also has been associated with an increased risk of cancers of the lung, liver, and breast (WCRF & AICR, 1997). Currently, both ACS and AICR suggest moderate consumption of no more than two drinks per day for men and no more than one drink per day for women (Byers et al., 2002; WCRF & AICR). Typically, a serving size for one drink is the equivalent to 12 oz. of beer, 5 oz. of wine, or 1.5 oz. of liquor (Byers et al.).

Food Preparation

American culture includes meat preparation in the form of barbecuing, grilling, and frying, which involve cooking foods at a high temperature. Heat greater than 374°F (212°C) in contact with muscle meat produces HCAs (AICR, 2002; Lan & Chen, 2002). HCAs are associated with gastrointestinal (stomach, pancreatic, colon), breast, and prostate cancers (Lan & Chen; Sugimura, Wakabayashi, Nakagama, & Nagao, 2004). Other sources of protein, such as dairy products, eggs, or organ meats, do not have significant HCA amounts naturally or when cooked (NCI, 1996). Microwaving briefly (one to two minutes) or marinating the meat before placing it in contact with a high heat source reduces the formation of HCAs (Kiple & Ornelas, 2000; Mayo Clinic et al., 2002; Salmon, Knize, & Felton, 1997).

The Promotion of Prevention

Public Campaign

Education of the public about the need for cancer prevention as a priority is paramount. NCI recognizes the key role of prevention in the War on Cancer, and prevention has been one of ACS's primary concerns. Funding for prevention trials must be lobbied.

Knowledge of the prevention and protection benefits of foods must be brought to the public. The 2002 revised ACS guidelines included recommendations for community action for the first time (Byers et al., 2002). Current lifestyle trends related to adverse effects on the long-term health of children include sedentary lifestyle, increased use of electronic entertainment, increased reliance on automobiles, reduced leisure time, consumption of high-calorie convenience foods, and declining levels of physical activity. Recommendations include a challenge to healthcare professionals to be active in their communities to promote lifestyle changes. A unique challenge for communities includes implementation of community and work-site health promotion programs and policies for planning to ensure that all groups have access to healthful food choices and opportunities for physical activity (Byers et al.).

Counseling

With respect to reducing cancer risk, the role of the healthcare professional is that of a counselor in assessing baseline and guiding clients in making healthy behavior changes. The thinking is that "the combined effects of nutrients as contained in the mixtures commonly known as whole foods seem to be more effective in reducing cancer risk than are nutrients contained in supplements. This simple conclusion can be a sound basis for broad nutritional advice to the population, as well as for clinical counseling of individual patients" (Bal, Woolam, & Seffrin, 1999, p. 328).

Common Foods and Their Cancer-Fighting Activity

Research continues to identify numerous anticancer activities from the established essential nutrients as well as from phytochemicals (non-nutrient chemicals that help to ward off disease). The mechanisms of protection still are being studied, but experts have grouped these foods and herbs according to their level of cancer-fighting activity. The following foods and ingredients are thought to decrease cancer risk (Craig, 1997).

Highest anticancer activity
- Garlic
- Soybeans
- Cabbage
- Ginger
- Licorice
- Umbelliferous vegetables (carrots, celery, cilantro, parsley, and parsnips)

Modest anticancer activity
- Onions, flax, citrus, and turmeric
- Cruciferous vegetables (broccoli, brussels sprouts, and cauliflower)
- Solanaceous vegetables (tomatoes and peppers)
- Brown rice and whole wheat

A lesser but still measurable amount of protection
- Oats and barley
- Mint, rosemary, thyme, oregano, sage, and basil
- Cucumber, cantaloupe, and berries

Summary

The full connection between diet and cancer still is incomplete. Results from ongoing control trials are needed. Unfortunately, these trials are time consuming and costly. Patients desire nutritional direction at the time of their sessions. Findings will need to be blended with the complexities of genetic predisposition risk, environmental risk factors, infection, pollution, occupational risk factors, and other lifestyle risk factors for individualized diet plans to reduce cancer risk. Research estimates that two-thirds of cancer deaths in the United States can be linked to poor diet, obesity, lack of exercise, and tobacco use, all of which can be changed at an individual level.

References

Alpha-Tocopherol, Beta Carotene Cancer Prevention Study Group. (1994). The effect of vitamin E and beta-carotene on the incidence of lung cancer and other cancers in male smokers. *New England Journal of Medicine, 330,* 1029–1035.

American Cancer Society. (1996). Guidelines on diet, nutrition, and cancer prevention: Reducing the risk of cancer with healthy food choices and physical activity. *CA: A Cancer Journal for Clinicians, 46,* 325–341.

American Institute for Cancer Research. (1999a). *Taking a closer look at antioxidants* (AICR Publication No. E9B-TLA/E62). Washington, DC: Author.

American Institute for Cancer Research. (1999b). *Taking a closer look at phytochemicals* (AICR Publication No. E9B-TLP/E79). Washington, DC: Author.

American Institute for Cancer Research. (2002). *Pesticides: Facts on preventing cancer* (AICR Publication No. E8H-FSP/F45). Washington, DC: Author.

Baker, B., Benbrook, C., Groth, E., & Benbrook, K. (2002). Pesticide residues in conventional, integrated pest management (IPM)-grown and organic foods: Insights from three U.S. data sets. *Food Additives and Contaminants, 19,* 427–446.

Bal, D., Woolam, G., & Seffrin, J. (1999). Dietary change and cancer prevention: What don't we know and when didn't we know it? *CA: A Cancer Journal for Clinicians, 49,* 327–330.

Beringer, J. (1999). Keeping watch over genetically modified crops and foods. *Lancet, 353,* 605–606.

Beyond vitamins: The new nutrition revolution. (1999, April). *University of California Berkeley Wellness Letter.*

Bianchini, F., Kaaks, R., & Vainio, H. (2002). Weight control and physical activity in cancer prevention. *Obesity Reviews, 3*(1), 5–8.

Block, G., Patterson, B., & Subar, A. (1992). Fruit, vegetables and cancer prevention: A review of the epidemiological evidence. *Nutrition and Cancer, 18*(1), 1–29.

Boik, J. (2001). *Natural compounds in cancer therapy.* Princeton, MN: Oregon Medical Press.

Bourn, D., & Prescott, J. (2002). A comparison of the nutritional value, sensory qualities, and food safety of organically and conventionally produced foods. *Critical Reviews in Food Science and Nutrition, 42*(1), 1–34.

Byers, T., Nestle, M., McTieman, A., Doyle, C., Currie-Williams, A., Gransler, T., et al. (2002). American Cancer Society guidelines on nutrition and physical activity for cancer prevention: Reducing the risk of cancer with healthy food choices and physical activity. *CA: A Cancer Journal for Clinicians, 52,* 92–119.

Calle, E., Rodriguez, D., Walker-Thurmond, K., & Thun, M. (2003). Overweight, obesity, and mortality from cancer in a prospectively studied cohort of U.S. adults. *New England Journal of Medicine, 348,* 1625–1638.

Caragay, A. (1992). Cancer-preventative foods and ingredients. *Food Technology, 46*(4), 65–68.

Cataldo, C.B., DeBruyne, L.K., & Whitney, E.N. (2003). *Nutrition and diet therapy: Principles and practice* (6th ed.). Belmont, CA: Wadsworth/Thomson Learning.

Clifford, C.K., & McDonald, S.S. (2001). Proper nutritional habits for reducing the risk of cancer. In T. Wilson & N.J. Temple (Eds.), *Nutritional health strategies for disease prevention* (pp. 494–496). Minneapolis, MN: Chronimed Publishing.

Commission on Life Sciences. (1982). *Diet, nutrition, and cancer.* Washington, DC: National Academies Press.

Courneya, K. (2002, March 4). *Physical activity and the cancer survivor.* Lecture presented at the conference on Nutrition After Cancer, sponsored by the American Institute for Cancer Research, Houston, TX.

Craig, W. (1997). Phytochemicals: Guardians of our health. *Journal of the American Dietetic Association, 97*(10 Suppl. 2), S199–S204.

Doll, R., & Peto, R. (1981). The causes of cancer: Quantitative estimates of avoidable risks of cancer in the United States today. *Journal of the National Cancer Institute, 66,* 1191–1308.

Duyff, R.L. (1998). *The American Dietetic Association's complete food and nutrition guide.* Minneapolis, MN: Chronimed Publishing.

Gollman, B., & Pierce, K. (1998). *The phytopia cookbook. A world of plant-centered cuisine.* Dallas, TX: Phytopia Inc.

Goodman, G., Omenn, G., Thornquist, M., Lund, B., Metch, B., & Gylys-Colwell, I. (1993). The carotene and retinol efficacy trial (CARET) to prevent lung cancer in high-risk populations: Pilot study with cigarette smokers. *Cancer Epidemiology, Biomarkers and Prevention, 2*, 389–396.

Health Science Institute. (1997a). *An introduction to diet, nutrition and cancer* (vol. 1). McLean, VA: Author.

Health Science Institute. (1997b). *Phytochemicals: Teacher's guide* (vol. 2). McLean, VA: Author.

Hermann, J. (2002). *Dietary reference intakes for energy, carbohydrates, fiber, fat, fatty acids, cholesterol, protein, and amino acids (macronutrients).* Washington, DC: Food and Nutrition Board, Institute of Medicine, and National Academy of Sciences.

Kiple, K.F., & Ornelas, K.C. (Eds.). (2000). *The Cambridge world history of food* (vol. 1). New York: Cambridge University Press.

Lan, C., & Chen, B. (2002). Effect of soy sauce and sugar on the formation of heterocyclic amines in marinated foods. *Food and Chemical Toxicology, 40*, 989–1000.

Leaf, C. (2004, March 22). Why we're losing the war on cancer (and how to win it). *Fortune, 149*(6), 77–92.

Mayo Clinic, UCLA, & Dole Food Company. (2002). *Encyclopedia of foods: A guide to healthy nutrition.* San Diego, CA: Academic Press.

Moss, R. (2000). *Antioxidants against cancer.* Brooklyn, NY: Equinox Press.

National Cancer Institute. (1996, July 22). *Heterocyclic amines in cooked meats.* Retrieved June 30, 2004, from http://cis.nci.nih.gov/fact/3_25.htm

Neville, K. (1999, August). Worried about pesticides on produce? EN offers advice on minimizing risk. *Environmental Nutrition, 22*, 8.

Patterson, B., Block, G., Rosenberger, W., Pee, D., & Kahle, L. (1990). Fruit and vegetables in the American diet: Data from the NHANES II survey. *American Journal of Public Health, 80*, 1443–1447.

Physician Oncology Education Program. (2001). *Nutrition and reduction of cancer risk.* Austin, TX: Texas Medical Association.

Polunin, M. (1999). *Healing foods.* New York: DK Publishing.

Ruoslahti, E. (1996). How cancer spreads. *Scientific American, 275*(3), 72–77.

Salmon, C., Knize, M., & Felton, J. (1997). Effects of marinating on heterocyclic amine carcinogen formation in grilled chicken. *Food and Chemical Toxicology, 35*, 433–441.

Shils, M., Olson, J., Moshe, S., & Ross, A. (1994). *Modern nutrition in health and disease* (8th ed.). Philadelphia: Lippincott Williams & Wilkins.

Sugimura, T., Wakabayashi, K., Nakagama, H., & Nagao, M. (2004). Heterocyclic amines: Mutagens/carcinogens produced during cooking of meat and fish. *Cancer Science, 95*, 290–299.

Tareke, E., Rydberg, P., Karlsson, P., Eriksson, S., & Tornqvist, M. (2000). Acrylamide: A cooking carcinogen? *Chemical Research in Toxicology, 13*, 517–522.

Thompson, L. (2000, January–February). *Are bioengineered foods safe?* Retrieved December 1, 2004, from http://vm.cfsan.fda.gov/~dms/

U.S. Department of Agriculture. (2002). *National Organic Program standards and guidelines.* Retrieved December 20, 2004, from http://www.ams.usda.gov/nop/NOP/NOPhome.html

Vainio, H., & Bianchini, F. (Eds.). (2002). *IARC handbooks of cancer prevention. Vol. 6: Weight control and physical activity.* Lyon, France: IARC Press World.

Wang, Y., Corr, J., Thaler, H., Tao, Y., Fair, W., & Heston, W. (1995). Decreased growth of established human prostate LNCaP tumors in nude mice fed a low-fat diet. *Journal of the National Cancer Institute, 87*, 1456–1457.

Weil, A. (2000). *Eating well for optimum health.* New York: Knopf.

Willett, W. (1999). Goals for nutrition in the year 2000. *CA: A Cancer Journal for Clinicians, 49*, 331–352.

Willett, W. (2002). Harvesting the fruits of research: New guidelines on nutrition and physical activity. *CA: A Cancer Journal for Clinicians, 52*, 66–67.

Willett, W., & Trichopoulos, D. (1996). Summary of the evidence: Nutrition and cancer. *Cancer Causes and Control, 7*(1), 178–180.

Williams, C. (2002). Nutritional quality of organic food: Shades of grey or shades of green? *Proceedings of the Nutrition Society, 61*(1), 19–24.

World Cancer Research Fund & American Institute for Cancer Research. (1997). *Food, nutrition and the prevention of cancer: A global perspective.* Washington, DC: American Institute of Cancer Research.

Wynder, E., Cohne, L., Muscat, J., Winters, B., Dwyer, J., & Blackburn, G. (1997). Breast cancer: Weighing the evidence for a promoting role of dietary fat. *Journal of the National Cancer Institute, 89,* 766–775.

CHAPTER 2

Breast Cancer

Diane M. Fletcher, RN, MA, BSN, OCN®
Michele C. Hayward, RD, LDN

Overview

Few things are more feared in this world than cancer, and breast cancer tops most women's lists. An American woman has a one in eight chance of developing breast cancer in her lifetime (National Cancer Institute, 2004). Most women know someone who has or has had breast cancer, and because of early detection, close surveillance, and increasingly successful treatment options, most people know at least one survivor. This chapter explores the nature of breast cancer, nutrition-based risk reduction, nutritional concerns during and after treatment, and diet in long-term survivorship.

Staging for cancer of the breast follows the American Joint Committee on Cancer's staging system to categorize patients for prognostic purposes. The TNM (tumor, regional lymph node, distant metastasis) classification system is used to gauge tumor size, the number of lymph nodes in the area of the tumor that contain cancer cells, and microscopic spread or metastases to distant body sites. Generally, five stages are identified in breast cancer. The first, stage 0, is ductal carcinoma in situ (DCIS). The cancer has not developed the ability to spread to surrounding tissue and is highly treatable. Lobular carcinoma in situ (LCIS), in which abnormal cells are found in the glands that produce milk, is a marker for increased risk of disease later in life. Once LCIS is confirmed by biopsy, the patient will be examined routinely for disease progression and may be treated with one of a number of agents, such as tamoxifen, to decrease risk of breast malignancy in the future. A more detailed discussion of these agents and their effect on the nutritional status of the patient can be found later in this chapter. Stages I–IV are delineated by increasing tumor sizes, number of positive lymph nodes in the areas surrounding the breast, and/or metastases to distant locations, such as bone, liver, lungs, or brain. With treatment, relative survival rates for breast cancer at five years for each stage are stage 0, in situ, 100%; stage I, 98%; stage IIA, 88%; stage IIB, 76%; stage IIIA, 56%; stage IIIB, 49%; stage IV, 16% (American Cancer Society, 2004).

Incidence

Approximately 212,930 women and men will be newly diagnosed with breast cancer in 2005 in the United States. In 2005, 40,870 deaths from all breast cancers are expected (Jemal et al., 2005). Men account for approximately 1% of diagnoses and deaths. Breast cancer is the number-one cancer for women of all races. White, Hawaiian, and African American women have the highest incidence of breast cancer, and African American women have a disproportionately higher mortality rate (National Cancer Institute, n.d.). Research currently is being conducted to investigate this disparity (Jatoi, Becher, & Leake, 2003).

Risk Factors and Prevention

Many of the theories regarding the etiology of breast cancer are associated with hormone levels, particularly levels of estrogens and insulin-like growth factors, throughout life and during periods of growth. Research has shown that reproductive factors such as early onset of menarche, late onset of menopause, nulliparity or late parity (Russo, Lareef, Balogh, Guo, & Russo, 2003), and short duration of or no breastfeeding (Collaborative Group on Hormonal Factors in Breast Cancer, 2002) increase a woman's risk for breast cancer. All of these factors depend on extended exposure to estrogens. Estrogens in the blood and in tissue have many functions, one being the ability to promote cell division and growth. During puberty, there is a surge of estrogen and other hormones, which brings about a cascade of changes from physical changes in the sex organs to the onset of the menstrual cycle. In pregnancy and lactation, cells within the breast undergo differentiation, the timing of which may be important when related to cancer diagnosis (Okasha, McCarron, Gunnell, & Smith, 2003). Causative factors may differ among patients with breast cancer pre- and postmenopause (Clavel-Chapelon & Gerber, 2002). Substantial evidence has suggested a link between increased plasma estrogen levels throughout life and postmenopausal breast cancer. Adipose tissue synthesizes estrogen and becomes the strongest contributor to body estrogen levels following menopause (Dai et al., 2003). The drug tamoxifen (Nolvadex®, AstraZeneca Pharmaceuticals LP, Wilmington, DE) has been developed to compete with estrogen at the receptor level and therefore decrease the amount of estrogen that feeds the cancer cells. Tamoxifen is a selective estrogen receptor modulator (SERM) and reduces the risk of recurrence and new primary tumors in early-stage breast cancer. It also is used in women at high risk for breast cancer. In breast tissue, tamoxifen competes with estrogen, but in other tissues, it may mimic estrogen's effects, with benefits such as a decrease in bone loss that often accompanies older age. Tamoxifen may increase the risk for endometrial cancer, deep vein thrombosis, pulmonary emboli, and benign ovarian cysts. Raloxifene (Evista®, Eli Lilly & Co., Indianapolis, IN), a newer SERM, currently is under study to evaluate whether it is as effective as tamoxifen but with fewer side effects.

Another hormone, insulin-like growth factor I (IGF-I), works in the breast to promote healthy development. IGF-I also may contribute to the etiology of breast cancer in premenopausal women. There may be a synergistic effect between estradiol and IGF-I (Agurs-Collins, 2002). In addition to examining plasma IGF-I levels, research also has included certain IGF-binding protein (IGFBP-3) levels and the ratio of the two. A positive association with breast cancer incidence in premenopausal women was found with each factor, IGF-I and IGFBP-3 (Bruning et al., 1995; Hankinson et al., 1998). With this mounting evidence, IGF-I and IGFBP-3 may be used as biomarkers, both in future research and in clinical practice, to assess premenopausal breast cancer risk. IGF-I, like estrogen, is produced in adipose tissue. The evidence with regard to IGF-I levels and obesity has been inconsistent, with some studies showing increased levels and others showing decreased levels (Colletti, Copeland, Devlin, Roberts, & McAuliffe, 1991; Copeland, Colletti, Devlin, & McAuliffe, 1990; Voskuil et al., 2001; Waibitsch, Heinze, Debatin, & Blum, 2000). It may be that central obesity is a stronger predictor of increased IGF-I levels (Schapira, Kumar, Lyman, & Cox, 1990; Stoll, 1996). Together, estrogens and IGF-I provide hormone-modulated mechanisms related to breast cancer incidence, and suppressors of these and other hormones hold promise for effective prevention and treatment strategies.

In 1994, the tumor suppressor gene BRCA1 was identified (Miki et al., 1994). Mutations in this gene and in BRCA2, identified in 1995, confer a substantially higher risk for development of invasive breast cancer (Wooster et al., 1995). Inherited cancers account for only 5%–10% of all breast cancer cases. Recent research has suggested that women with these genetic mutations may have a lifetime risk for breast cancer as high as 82% (King, Marks, & Mandell, 2003). King et al. found that increased activity as a teenager and normal weight at menarche and at age 21 were associated with later onset of breast cancer in these women. Diet and exercise become increasingly important prevention techniques for these and other high-risk women.

High fruit and vegetable intake has been shown to have a protective effect against cancer diagnosis in general, but the breast cancer literature has been inconsistent (Malin et al., 2003; Mattisson et al., 2004; Olsen et al., 2003). It is possible that there is a negative side to vegetarianism with regard to breast cancer. Several studies have found either an increase in breast cancer risk or a negative change in biomarkers in vegetarians (Hargreaves et al., 1999; Mills, Beeson, Phillips, & Fraser, 1989). Dietary interventions have been created that aim to decrease the problem of being overweight or obese as a way to decrease circulating estrogen levels. Total fat intake has been studied extensively, in part, because of the positive correlation between total fat intake and breast cancer rates (Willett, 2003). The most recent meta-analysis of studies regarding this issue concluded that total dietary fat has a positive association with breast cancer risk (Boyd et al., 2003). High saturated fat intake, often typified by high red meat intake, also conferred an increased relative risk of cancer diagnosis. Possible mechanisms suggested by Boyd et al. for elevated relative risk estimates include mutagens, free radical and eicosanoid (fatty acids such as prostaglandins and leukotrienes that mediate inflammation) generation, and changes in gene expression.

Recommending a diet for the prevention of breast cancer is not as straightforward as for other cancers (e.g., cancers of the gastrointestinal tract or oral cavity). Because the initiation and progression of breast cancer are intimately linked to estrogen metabolism, much of the research has been conducted with plant sources of chemicals that may influence the carcinogenicity of estrogens. Current research initiatives in phytoestrogens, such as lignans found in flaxseed and soy isoflavones, are under way to better illustrate the effect of weak phytoestrogens in the diet (Dai et al., 2003; Messina, 2003; Teede, Dalais, & McGrath, 2004). The theory (Dai et al.) suggested that phytoestrogens compete with endogenous estrogens for binding to estrogen receptors (ERs). Studies have shown that this may not be the only explanation for phytoestrogens' proposed effect as a protective agent against cancer.

Asian populations have a much lower incidence of breast cancer than the general U.S. population, and one of the reasons often cited is Asians' high intake of soy from the time of birth (Ajiki & Yamamoto, 1999; Lee et al., 1991). This finding has spurred a large amount of research. The main questions include Should women in the United States eat more soy foods to decrease breast cancer risk? At what phase of life are the greatest benefits seen? Are isoflavone supplements safe and effective? The not-so-simple answer to all these questions is "maybe." Soy foods are nutrient-dense. They are a great source of protein, with all the amino acids that are present in animal protein but without the saturated fat. The evidence is scarce when it comes to adding soy foods later in life and the impact of this dietary change on breast cancer risk (Messina, 2003). As a primary prevention strategy, including soy in the diet during adolescence may be beneficial, but it has not been established that initiating or increasing soy intake as an adult can decrease risk (Shu et al., 2001; Wu et al., 2002).

Researchers have targeted the two main isoflavones in soy, genistein and daidzein, over the past decade. Isoflavones bind to ERs and may act as SERMs in a similar way to drugs (e.g., tamoxifen, raloxifene) given to decrease plasma estrogen levels (Messina, 2003). Messina reported that Japanese adults consume approximately 1.5 servings of soy foods daily with a total of 30–45 mg of isoflavones. Studies of isolated isoflavone supplements of limited duration (one year) have not shown effects consistent with breast cancer risk reduction, such as decreased breast density or lengthened menstrual cycles (Maskarinec, Williams, & Carlin, 2003; Maskarinec, Williams, Inouye, Stanczyk, & Franke, 2002). The evidence for soy foods also has not been consistent (Lu, Anderson, Grady, & Nagamani, 1996; Nagata, Takatsuka, Inaba, Kawakami, & Shimizu, 1998). As more research is conducted, the biologic mechanisms of action for soy will be further clarified, and optimal exposure, duration, and timing may be identified. At this point, recommendations for the inclusion of soy in the diets of pre- and postmenopausal healthy women interested in reducing breast cancer risk should be made based on all the available and most current evidence.

An interesting line of research related to soy deals with a bacterial metabolite of daidzein called equol. Not everyone who ingests soy produces a significant amount of equol, but people who produce equol may experience increased estrogenic activity from soy (Setchell, Brown, & Lydeking-Olsen, 2002). Equol acts as a free radical scavenger and has strong antioxidant activity in addition to its ER affinity (Mitchell et al., 1998). Future research may use equol status to group patients for dietary interventions using soy and compare the different groups' outcomes.

Lifelong physical activity appears to reduce breast cancer risk in pre- and postmenopausal women (John, Horn-Ross, & Koo, 2003). It is not clear what amount of exercise and at what age exercise would be most beneficial. There are several plausible explanations for this benefit. Athletes often have disruptions in their menstrual cycles that could affect lifetime estrogen exposure. Additionally, exercise can minimize weight gain as women age. The American Cancer Society has recommended at least 45 minutes of moderate/vigorous activity on five or more days of the week (Byers et al., 2002).

A clear association exists between the consumption of two or more alcoholic drinks per day and an increased risk of breast cancer (Singletary & Gapstur, 2001). In the past decade, there has been speculation that increased dietary folate may decrease breast cancer risk in alcohol drinkers (Rohan, Jain, Howe, & Miller, 2000). Women with a family history of breast cancer who do not drink alcohol and who have adequate amounts of dietary folate have demonstrated rates of breast cancer similar to women with no family history (Sellers et al., 2004).

Treatment Modalities

Treatment options for breast cancer vary among stages. For most patients with DCIS, the recommended treatment is local excision (lumpectomy) followed by radiation therapy. Tumors that do not have ERs (ER-negative tumors) do not need estrogen to grow and typically will not respond to antiestrogen therapy. In women with ER-positive cancers, tamoxifen or other antiestrogen agents may be given. Early-stage (stages I, II, and IIIA) breast cancer treatment has several components.

Primary treatment may include lumpectomy with radiation or mastectomy, with or without reconstruction. At the time of surgery, a single or multiple axillary lymph node(s) also will be removed for evaluation. Adjuvant radiation therapy occasionally is used in patients with an increased risk for localized recurrence following mastectomy. Standard adjuvant systemic therapy for early-stage breast cancer includes chemotherapy and hormone therapy. Chemotherapeutic agents most often are used in various combination regimens that may include cyclophosphamide (Cytoxan®, Bristol-Myers Squibb Oncology, Princeton, NJ), methotrexate (Rheumatrex®, Stada Pharmaceuticals, Cranbury, NJ; Trexall™, Barr Laboratories, Pomona, NY), 5-fluorouracil (5-FU) (Adrucil®, Pfizer, New York, NY), doxorubicin (Adriamycin®, Pfizer), paclitaxel (Taxol®, Bristol-Myers Squibb Oncology), and/or docetaxel (Taxotere®, Aventis Pharmaceuticals, Bridgewater, NJ) (Zangwill, 2003). All of these agents can cause nausea and vomiting and can have an impact on nutritional status. In women with ER-positive tumors, tamoxifen often is given and has significant proven efficacy. Ovarian ablation and aromatase inhibitors, such as anastrozole (Arimidex®, AstraZeneca Pharmaceuticals) and letrozole (Femara®, Novartis, East Hanover, NJ), in postmenopausal women also may be an option for decreasing circulating estrogen levels. Clinical trials are now under way to find out what role ovarian ablation should play in treatment for women who receive chemotherapy and tamoxifen (Arora & Potter, 2004).

Hormone therapy, chemotherapy, and trastuzumab (Herceptin®, Genentech, Inc., South San Francisco, CA) are common treatment options for advanced-stage (stages IIIB, IIIC, IV [metastatic], and recurrent disease) breast cancer treatment. Many of the same agents used for early-stage cancer also are offered as advanced-stage cancer treatments. When a cancer has recurred and the patient has received prior chemotherapy treatment, it may be necessary to use different agents, such as gemcitabine (Gemzar®, Eli Lilly & Co.), carboplatin (Paraplatin®, Bristol-Myers Squibb Oncology), and vinorelbine (Navelbine®, GlaxoSmithKline, Research Triangle Park, NC). Herceptin may be added to the chemotherapy regimen for patients who are *HER2/neu* positive. *HER2/neu* is a protein that has been found to have a great effect on prognosis in advanced-stage cancers. All cells express the *HER2* protein, but tumor cells overexpress this gene. The results of overexpression are faster cell growth and more cell division. Primary and recurrent tumors can be tested for *HER2/neu* status. Tumors that overexpress *HER2/neu* are more aggressive, and patients with these tumors have a poorer prognosis (Sjogren, Inganas, Lindgren, Holmberg, & Bergh, 1998). Herceptin has three proposed mechanisms: (a) it works synergistically with chemotherapy agents, (b) it causes some *HER2* receptors to leave the surface of the cell, decreasing the opportunity for cell growth, and (c) as a monoclonal antibody, it attaches to the cell and attracts natural killer cells, which, over time, consume the cells. The addition of Herceptin to standard treatment protocols has proved to be moderately efficacious and has increased length of survival (Slamon et al., 2001).

Nutritional Implications

Bone loss and decreased bone strength are significant long-term complications of chemotherapy as well as results of the aging process. Adequate intake of calcium and vitamin D is essential to combat the loss of bone mineral density (BMD) in these patients. BMD can be tracked by consecutive dual-energy x-ray absorptiometry scans that will give accurate estimates of current bone density. At this time, there are no recommendations specifically for survivors of breast cancer, but the recommended dietary intake value for women age 30 and older is 1,000–1,200 mg of calcium and 200–600 IU of vitamin D (Food and Nutrition Information Center, 2004). Patients may need to take supplements to reach these levels of intake if they do not consume dairy foods or if they live in a climate where sunlight is not strong enough to initiate endogenous synthesis. The dietitian can evaluate whether needs are being met and can suggest several appropriate ways to increase calcium and vitamin D intake from food and supplements. Weight-bearing exercise may protect against bone loss (Bemben, 1999; Waltman et al., 2003) and should be encouraged if medically appropriate.

Evidence is limited for a connection between alcohol intake following breast cancer diagnosis and impact on survival. One study found a positive association between beer intake and recurrence, but not survival (Hebert, Hurley, & Ma, 1998). Moderate alcohol intake (less than one drink per day) does not appear to increase either risk for recurrence or survival.

Animal research has indicated that soy isoflavones, genistein in particular, may decrease efficacy of the drug tamoxifen (Ju, Doerge, Allred, Allred, & Helferich, 2002). More studies need to be completed, particularly on human subjects, but caution seems necessary. A review of the literature by Messina and Loprinzi (2001) showed positive, synergistic effects in vitro and in some animal studies. A recommendation of no more than one to two servings of soy per week for women taking tamoxifen is prudent until more definitive research is completed.

Assessment Guidelines

It is very important for patients to be evaluated for nutritional status changes during and following treatment. Several tools make this easier for both the patient and the healthcare team. The scored Patient-Generated Subjective Global Assessment (PG-SGA) increasingly is being used in cancer settings (Bauer, Capra, & Ferguson, 2002) (see Appendix A). This tool is completed partially by the patient and partially by the physician, nurse, or dietitian. Not only can the PG-SGA be used to identify malnourished patients, but it also can show the efficacy of nutritional intervention within the clinic setting. Isenring, Bauer, and Capra (2003) found the PG-SGA to be a sensitive tool that was able to show changes in quality of life in patients receiving radiotherapy.

Anthropometric assessment can provide nurses and dietitians with a measure of subtle changes that may occur during and after treatment for breast cancer. Body mass index (BMI) can be calculated and used to assess stages of being overweight or obese (see Appendix B). Another helpful tool, waist-to-hip ratio, can be used to determine abdominal obesity levels. Dietitians can use this measurement to evaluate the effectiveness of their care plans. A recent study found the waist-to-hip ratio to be a marker for increased mortality in ER-positive postmenopausal women but not in premenopausal women (Borugian et al., 2003). Diet should be evaluated by 24-hour usual dietary recall or a short food frequency questionnaire to make sure that basic nutrient levels have been met. If they are motivated, patients can complete a three- or five-day food diary to help to make assessment more individualized. More information on the PG-SGA and other assessment tools can be found in the appendices.

Special Considerations for Nutrition

For the patient with breast cancer, symptoms of fatigue, weight loss or gain, anorexia, depression, nausea, vomiting, diarrhea, and constipation are possible sequelae of sequential or concurrent treatments. As the usual "front line" in cancer care, nurses must recognize the constellation of symptoms that often plague patients with breast cancer. Unlike patients with other cancer diagnoses, a patient with breast cancer may gain, rather than lose, weight during treatment. She also may present with extra weight that made her initially vulnerable to the cancer. Dietitians and nurses then are put in the awkward position of working with a patient who would benefit from weight loss but who will likely be nutritionally compromised during treatment. Also, the patient may be experiencing cancer-related nutritional status changes. As with treatment options, early-stage and advanced-stage patients generally have different nutritional needs and face unique challenges. Thus, for ease of understanding, the discussion will be separated for these two groups of patients.

Patients with early-stage disease often have surgery with radiation and adjuvant chemotherapy. Fiets, van Helvoirt, Nortier, van der Tweel, and Struikmans (2003) compared side effects from concurrent radiation and two chemotherapy regimens (cyclophosphamide, methotrexate, and 5-FU or doxorubicin and cyclophosphamide) or radiotherapy alone. Patients who received chemotherapy (with or without radiation) complained of moderate amounts of nausea, anorexia, malaise, and fever. Fatigue and malaise are key considerations, as they can negatively affect the patient's ability to acquire, prepare, and ingest food.

In recent years, the use of adjuvant chemotherapy in women with node-positive early-stage breast cancer has increased. Significant weight gain during treatment can occur and can have a dramatic effect on body image, self-esteem, and mental status. Between 50%–96% of women who have adjuvant chemotherapy will gain weight, and many of these women will maintain this potentially dangerous new weight (Kutynec, McCargar, Barr, & Hislop, 1999; McInnes & Knobf, 2001). A shift of weight as little as 5%–10% above or below usual body weight would indicate the need for evaluation of clinical and nutritional status.

Weight gain is problematic for many of these women for psychosocial reasons, such as an impaired body image, depression, anxiety, and decreased quality of life. They also may be at increased risk for recurrence, although the evidence is not conclusive (Chlebowski, Aiello, & McTiernan, 2002; Rock & Demark-Wahnefried, 2002). Overweight and obese women (as measured by BMI) also are at increased risk for diabetes, cardiovascular disease, and hypertension (Demark-Wahnefried, Rimer, & Winer, 1997). The cause of this weight gain is still under investigation. It often is difficult to separate the potential factors and to label cause and effect. Nurses and dietitians must work together with these patients to investigate all possible contributing issues and to offer ways to maintain, but not gain, weight. Some likely factors include overeating, depression, low estrogen levels, changes in metabolic rate, decreased physical activity, or a combination of these and other factors (Decker, 2003). The additional weight is predominantly adipose tissue rather than the mix of lean and adipose tissue seen in the healthy population (Demark-Wahnefried et al., 2001). Women reported weight gain while taking tamoxifen, but recent research has found no difference in weight gain between women receiving tamoxifen and those not taking it (Day, 2001; Lankester, Phillips, & Lawton, 2002).

In the patient with advanced-stage breast cancer, cancer cachexia may be an issue. Cancer cachexia is a wasting syndrome characterized by significant weight loss that is not explained by decreased intake. It is metabolically driven and characterized by aberrant carbohydrate and fat metabolism and profound loss of skeletal muscle. Advanced-stage patients who are cachectic often are anemic and have increased C-reactive protein levels (MacDonald, Easson, Mazurak, Dunn, & Baracos, 2003). Caregivers need to understand the process of this wasting so that they can conform to the patient's wishes and meet her comfort level. A dietitian or nurse might be the best person to provide this information to caregivers to ease the burden of trying to persuade the patient to eat. For a more comprehensive look at end-of-life and palliative care issues, see Chapter 19.

Care Planning and Expected Outcomes of Therapy

Patients who experience nutritional side effects from treatment, such as anorexia, nausea, vomiting, diarrhea, constipation, weight gain or loss, or fatigue, would benefit from an evaluation by a dietitian and an individualized nutrition care plan. Cachectic patients can be treated pharmacologically. Oral supplements that contain n-3 fatty acids (with a dose of 2 g per day) also may be useful to increase lean body mass, although research on efficacy for survival has not been consistent (MacDonald et al., 2003). Nurses and dietitians can work with family members to offer foods that appeal to the patient and to ease the burden of food preparation. Once treatment is complete, maintenance of weight or even weight loss may be a major concern for many patients. This is a very vulnerable time in the course of treatment for the patient. The amount of care from the healthcare team will decrease over time, and the patient may become easily attracted to the marketing of diets and supplements, with limited research data to substantiate their efficacy claims. At this time, patients should be introduced to the dietitian to discuss an individualized plan for nutrition. Patients with breast cancer often are interested in using complementary medicine therapies. All patients should be encouraged first to obtain reliable efficacy and safety information from healthcare professionals who have expertise in these therapies. This may include pharmacists, dietitians, nurses, physicians, and naturopaths.

Salminen, Bishop, Poussa, Drummond, and Salminen (2004) reported that 24%–27% of the patients in their study increased their exercise levels following the diagnosis of breast cancer. There is a growing body of literature regarding exercise during and following breast cancer treatment. In a recent review (Courneya, 2003), 12 intervention studies were highlighted that showed multidimensional, significant, positive effects of exercise during treatment. Less research has been done on exercise following treatment; however, the trials measuring psychosocial issues have reported a decrease in anxiety, depression, and fatigue and better mood and self-esteem (Courneya). The American Cancer Society has established exercise recommendations for cancer survivors: (a) Resolve anemia before starting an exercise program, (b) avoid public gyms if immune function is compromised, (c) stretch for 10 minutes when extremely fatigued from treatment, (d) avoid swimming pools when undergoing radiotherapy, (e) avoid water if you have an indwelling catheter, and (f) try to accommodate peripheral neuropathy by decreasing use of the affected limbs (Brown et al., 2003).

Dietitians should counsel patients with an elevated BMI to slowly decrease weight once treatment is complete. A recent study suggested that one-on-one counseling by a dietitian and group counseling by Weight Watchers™ were successful strategies for weight loss (Jen et al., 2004). Breast cancer survivors are particularly interested in dietary change, and this can be used advantageously (Thomson et al., 2002). Saturated fat and red meat intake should be limited, and although the data are equivocal about its direct effects on recurrence and metastasis, a diet that includes less total fat with more of a balance of n-3 and n-6 fatty acids could be beneficial. To take advantage of the various chemicals found in plants that are currently being studied, five to nine daily servings of fruits and vegetables with a wide variety of deep colors (to maximize phytochemical content) should be eaten. In the future, it is likely that diet will be shown to make a significant impact, not only on primary but also on secondary prevention of breast cancer. Nurses and dietitians alike should be aware of this potential impact and should address this important factor.

References

Agurs-Collins, T. (2002). The role of insulin-like growth factors and breast cancer risk. *On-Line: A Publication of the Oncology Nutrition Dietetic Practice Group, 10*(4), 1–8.

Ajiki, J.M., & Yamamoto, S. (1999). Breast cancer incidence in Japan. *Japanese Journal of Clinical Oncology, 4,* 238–241.

American Cancer Society. (2004). *Overview: Breast cancer. After the tests: Staging.* Retrieved February 17, 2004, from http://www.cancer.org/docroot/CRI/content/CRI_2_2_3X_After_the_tests_Staging_5.asp?sitearea=

Arora, A., & Potter, J.F. (2004). Aromatase inhibitors: Current indications and future prospects for treatment of postmenopausal breast cancer. *Journal of the American Geriatrics Society, 52,* 611–616.

Bauer, J., Capra, S., & Ferguson, M. (2002). Use of the scored Patient-Generated Subjective Global Assessment (PG-SGA) as a nutrition assessment tool in patients with cancer. *European Journal of Clinical Nutrition, 56,* 779–785.

Bemben, D.A. (1999). Exercise interventions for osteoporosis prevention in postmenopausal women. *Journal of the Oklahoma State Medical Association, 92,* 66–70.

Borugian, M.J., Sheps, S.B., Kim-Sing, C., Olivoto, I.A., Van Patten, C., Dunn, B.P., et al. (2003). Waist-to-hip ratio and breast cancer mortality. *American Journal of Epidemiology, 158,* 963–968.

Boyd, N.F., Stone, J., Vogt, K.N., Connelly, B.S., Martin, L.J., & Minkin, S. (2003). Dietary fat and breast cancer risk revisited: A meta-analysis of the published literature. *British Journal of Cancer, 89,* 1672–1685.

Brown, J.K., Byers, T., Coyle, C., Courneya, K.S., Demark-Wahnefried, W., Kushi, L.H., et al. (2003). Nutrition and physical activity during and after cancer treatment: An American Cancer Society guide for informed choices. *CA: A Cancer Journal for Clinicians, 53,* 268–291.

Bruning, P.F., Van Doorn, J., Bonfrer, J.M., Van Noord, P.A., Korse, C.M., Linders, T.C., et al. (1995). Insulin-like growth factor–binding protein 3 is decreased in early-stage operable pre-menopausal breast cancer. *International Journal of Cancer, 62,* 266–270.

Byers, T., Nestle, M., McTiernan, A., Doyle, C., Currie-Williams, A., Gansler, T., et al. (2002). American Cancer Society guidelines on nutrition and physical activity for cancer prevention. *CA: A Cancer Journal for Clinicians, 52,* 92–119.

Chlebowski, R.T., Aiello, E., & McTiernan, A. (2002). Weight loss in breast cancer patient management. *Journal of Clinical Oncology, 20,* 1128–1143.

Clavel-Chapelon, F., & Gerber, M. (2002). Reproductive factors and breast cancer risk. Do they differ according to age at diagnosis? *Breast Cancer Research and Treatment, 72,* 107–115.

Collaborative Group on Hormonal Factors in Breast Cancer. (2002). Breast cancer and breastfeeding: Collaborative reanalysis of individual data from 47 epidemiological studies, in 30 countries, including 50,302 women with breast cancer and 96,973 women without the disease. *Lancet, 360,* 187–195.

Colletti, R.B., Copeland, K., Devlin, J.T., Roberts, J.D., & McAuliffe, T.L. (1991). Effect of obesity on plasma insulin-like growth factor-I in cancer patients. *International Journal of Obesity, 39,* 523–587.

Copeland, K.C., Colletti, R.B., Devlin, J.T., & McAuliffe, T.L. (1990). The relationship between insulin-like growth factor-I, adiposity, and aging. *Metabolism, 39,* 584–587.

Courneya, K.S. (2003). Exercise in cancer survivors: An overview of research. *Medicine and Science in Sports and Exercise, 35,* 1846–1852.

Dai, Q., Franke, A.A., Yu, H., Xiao-ou, S., Jin, F., Hebert, J.R., et al. (2003). Urinary phytoestrogen excretion and breast cancer risk: Evaluating potential effect modifiers endogenous estrogens and anthropometrics. *Cancer Epidemiology, Biomarkers and Prevention, 12,* 497–502.

Day, R. (2001). Quality of life and tamoxifen in a breast cancer prevention trial: A summary of findings from the NSABP P-1 study. *Annals of the New York Academy of Sciences, 949,* 143–150.

Decker, G.M. (2003). Weight gain: An inevitable consequence of breast cancer or breast cancer therapy? *Oncology Nutrition Connection, 11*(4), 10–11, 13.

Demark-Wahnefried, W., Peterson, B.L., Winer, E.P., Marks, L., Aziz, N., Marcom, P.K., et al. (2001). Changes in weight, body composition, and factors influencing energy balance among premenopausal breast cancer patients receiving adjuvant chemotherapy. *Journal of Clinical Oncology, 19,* 2381–2389.

Demark-Wahnefried, W., Rimer, B.K., & Winer, E.P. (1997). Weight gain in women diagnosed with breast cancer. *Journal of the American Dietetic Association, 97,* 519–526, 529.

Fiets, W.E., van Helvoirt, R.P., Nortier, J.W.R., van der Tweel, I., & Struikmans, H. (2003). Acute toxicity of concurrent adjuvant radiotherapy and chemotherapy (CMF or AC) in breast cancer patients: A prospective, comparative, non-randomized study. *European Journal of Cancer, 39,* 1081–1088.

Food and Nutrition Information Center. (2004). *Dietary reference intakes (DRI) and recommended dietary allowances (RDA).* Retrieved February 17, 2004, from http://www.nal.usda.gov/fnic/etext/000105.html

Hankinson, S.E., Willett, W.C., Colditz, G.A., Hunter, D.J., Michaud, D.S., Deroo, B., et al. (1998). Circulating concentrations of insulin-like growth factor-I and risk of breast cancer. *Lancet, 351,* 1393–1396.

Hargreaves, D.F., Potten, C.S., Harding, C., Shaw, L.E., Morton, M.S., Roberts, S.A., et al. (1999). Two-week dietary soy supplementation has an estrogenic effect on normal premenopausal breast. *Journal of Clinical Endocrinology and Metabolism, 84,* 4017–4024.

Hebert, J.R., Hurley, T.G., & Ma, Y. (1998). The effect of dietary exposures on recurrence and mortality in early stage breast cancer. *Breast Cancer Research and Treatment, 51,* 17–28.

Isenring, E., Bauer, J., & Capra, S. (2003). The scored Patient-Generated Subjective Global Assessment (PG-SGA) and its association with quality of life in ambulatory patients receiving radiotherapy. *European Journal of Clinical Nutrition, 57,* 305–309.

Jatoi, I., Becher, H., & Leake, C.R. (2003). Widening disparity in survival between white and African-American patients with breast carcinoma treated in the U.S. Department of Defense healthcare system. *Cancer, 98,* 894–899.

Jemal, A., Murray, T., Ward, E., Samuels, A., Tiwari, R.C., Ghafoor, A., et al. (2005). Cancer statistics, 2005. *CA: A Cancer Journal for Clinicians, 55,* 10–30.

Jen, K.L., Djuric, Z., DiLaura, N.M., Buison, A., Redd, J.N., Maranci, V., et al. (2004). Improvement of metabolism among obese breast cancer survivors in differing weight loss regimens. *Obesity Research, 12,* 306–312.

John, E.M., Horn-Ross, P.L., & Koo, J. (2003). Lifetime physical activity and breast cancer risk in a multiethnic population: The San Francisco Bay area breast cancer study. *Cancer Epidemiology, Biomarkers and Prevention, 12,* 1143–1152.

Ju, Y.H., Doerge, D.R., Allred, K.F., Allred, C.D., & Helferich, W.G. (2002). Dietary genistein negates the inhibitory effect of tamoxifen on growth of estrogen-dependent human breast cancer (MCF-7) cells implanted in athymic mice. *Cancer Research, 62,* 2474–2477.

King, M.C., Marks, J.H., & Mandell, J.B. (2003). Breast and ovarian cancer risks due to inherited mutations in BRCA1 and BRCA2. *Science, 302,* 643–646.

Kutynec, C.L., McCargar, L., Barr, S.I., & Hislop, T.G. (1999). Energy balance in women with breast cancer during adjuvant treatment. *Journal of the American Dietetic Association, 99,* 1222–1227.

Lankester, K.J., Phillips, J.E., & Lawton, P.A. (2002). Weight gain during adjuvant and neoadjuvant chemotherapy for breast cancer: An audit of 100 women receiving FEC or CMF chemotherapy. *Clinical Oncology, 14,* 64–67.

Lee, H.P., Gourley, L., Duffy, S.W., Esteve, J., Lee, J., & Day, N.E. (1991). Dietary effects on breast cancer risk in Singapore. *Lancet, 331,* 1197–1200.

Lu, L.J., Anderson, K.E., Grady, J.J., & Nagamani, M. (1996). Effects of soya consumption for one month on steroid hormones in premenopausal women: Implications for breast cancer risk reduction. *Cancer Epidemiology, Biomarkers and Prevention, 5,* 63–70.

MacDonald, N., Easson, A.M., Mazurak, V.C., Dunn, G.P., & Baracos, V.E. (2003). Understanding and managing cancer cachexia. *Journal of the American College of Surgeons, 197,* 143–161.

Malin, A.S., Qi, D., Shu, X.O., Gao, Y.T., Friedmann, J.M., Jin, F., et al. (2003). Intake of fruits, vegetables, and selected micronutrients in relation to the risk of breast cancer. *International Journal of Cancer, 105,* 413–418.

Maskarinec, G., Williams, A.E., & Carlin, L. (2003). Mammographic densities in a one-year isoflavone intervention. *European Journal of Cancer Prevention, 12,* 165–169.

Maskarinec, G., Williams, A.E., Inouye, J.S., Stanczyk, F.Z., & Franke, A.A. (2002). A randomized isoflavone intervention among premenopausal women. *Cancer Epidemiology, Biomarkers and Prevention, 11,* 195–201.

Mattisson, I., Wirfält, E., Johansson, U., Gullberg, B., Olsson, H., & Berglund, G. (2004). Intakes of plant foods, fibre and fat and risk of breast cancer—A prospective study in the Malmö Diet and cancer cohort. *British Journal of Cancer, 90,* 122–127.

McInnes, J.A., & Knobf, M.T. (2001). Weight gain and quality of life in women treated with adjuvant chemotherapy for early-stage breast cancer. *Oncology Nursing Forum, 28,* 675–684.

Messina, M. (2003). Soy intake and breast cancer risk: A review of the animal, epidemiologic and clinical data. *Oncology Nutrition Connection, 11*(4), 1–10.

Messina, M.J., & Loprinzi, C.L. (2001). Soy for breast cancer survivors: A critical review of the literature. *Journal of Nutrition, 131,* 3095S–3108S.

Miki, Y., Swensen, J., Shattuck-Eidens, D., Futreal, P.A., Harshman, K., Tavtigian, S., et al. (1994). A strong candidate for the breast and ovarian cancer susceptibility gene BRCA1. *Science, 266,* 66–71.

Mills, P.K., Beeson, W.L., Phillips, R.L., & Fraser, G.E. (1989). Dietary habits and breast cancer incidence among Seventh-day Adventists. *Cancer, 64,* 582–590.

Mitchell, J.H., Gardner, P.T., McPhail, D.B., Morrice, P.C., Collins, A.R., & Duthie, G.G. (1998). Antioxidant efficacy of phytoestrogens in chemical and biological model systems. *Archives of Biochemistry and Biophysiology, 360,* 142–148.

Nagata, C., Takatsuka, N., Inaba, S., Kawakami, N., & Shimizu, H. (1998). Effect of soymilk consumption on serum estrogen concentrations in premenopausal Japanese women. *Journal of the National Cancer Institute, 90,* 1830–1835.

National Cancer Institute. (2004, October 4). *Lifetime probability of breast cancer in American women.* Retrieved November 23, 2004, from http://cis.nci.nih.gov/fact/5_6.htm

National Cancer Institute. (n.d.). *Breast: U.S. racial/ethnic cancer patterns.* Retrieved January 20, 2004, from http://www.nci.nih.gov/statistics/cancertype/breast-racial-ethnic

Okasha, M., McCarron, P., Gunnell, D., & Smith, G.D. (2003). Exposures in childhood, adolescence and early adulthood and breast cancer risk: A systematic review of the literature. *Breast Cancer Research and Treatment, 78,* 223–276.

Olsen, A., Tjonneland, A., Thomsen, B.L., Loft, S., Stripp, C., Overvad, K., et al. (2003). Fruits and vegetables intake differentially affects estrogen receptor negative and positive breast cancer incidence rates. *Nutritional Epidemiology, 133,* 2342–2347.

Rock, C.L., & Demark-Wahnefried, W. (2002). Nutrition and survival after the diagnosis of breast cancer: A review of the evidence. *Journal of Clinical Oncology, 20,* 3302–3316.

Rohan, T.E., Jain, M.G., Howe, G.R., & Miller, A.B. (2000). Dietary folate consumption and breast cancer risk. *Journal of the National Cancer Institute, 92,* 266–269.

Russo, J., Lareef, M.H., Balogh, G., Guo, S., & Russo, I.H. (2003). Estrogen and its metabolites are carcinogenic agents in human breast epithelial cells. *Journal of Steroid Biochemistry and Molecular Biology, 87,* 1–25.

Salminen, E., Bishop, M., Poussa, T., Drummond, R., & Salminen, S. (2004). Dietary attitudes and changes as well as use of supplements and complementary therapies by Australian and Finnish women following the diagnosis of breast cancer. *European Journal of Clinical Nutrition, 58,* 137–144.

Schapira, D.V., Kumar, N.B., Lyman, G.H., & Cox, C.E. (1990). Abdominal obesity and breast cancer risk. *Annals of Internal Medicine, 112,* 182–186.

Sellers, T.A., Grabrick, D.M., Vierkant, R.A., Harnack, L., Olson, J.E., Vachon, C.M., et al. (2004). Does folate intake decrease risk of postmenopausal breast cancer among women with a family history? *Cancer Causes and Control, 15,* 113–120.

Setchell, K.D.R., Brown, N.M., & Lydeking-Olsen, E. (2002). The clinical importance of the metabolite equol—A clue to the effectiveness of soy and its isoflavones. *Journal of Nutrition, 132,* 3577–3584.

Shu, X.O., Jin, F., Dai, Q., Wen, W., Potter, J.D., Kushi, L.H., et al. (2001). Soyfood intake during adolescence and subsequent risk of breast cancer among Chinese women. *Cancer Epidemiology, Biomarkers and Prevention, 10,* 483–488.

Singletary, K.W., & Gapstur, S.M. (2001). Alcohol and breast cancer: Review of epidemiologic and experimental evidence and potential mechanisms. *JAMA, 286,* 2143–2151.

Sjogren, S., Inganas, M., Lindgren, A., Holmberg, L., & Bergh, J. (1998). Prognostic and predictive value of c-erbB-2 overexpression in primary breast cancer, alone and in combination with other prognostic markers. *Journal of Clinical Oncology, 16,* 462–469.

Slamon, D.J., Leyland-Jones, B., Shak, S., Fuchs, H., Paton, V., Bajamonde, A., et al. (2001). Use of chemotherapy plus a monoclonal antibody against HER2 for metastatic breast cancer that overexpresses HER2. *New England Journal of Medicine, 344,* 783–792.

Stoll, B. (1996). Timing of weight gain and breast cancer risk. *Cancer, 77,* 210.

Teede, H.J., Dalais, F.S., & McGrath, B.P. (2004). Dietary soy containing phytoestrogens does not have detectable estrogenic effects on hepatic protein synthesis in postmenopausal women. *American Journal of Clinical Nutrition, 79,* 396–402.

Thomson, C.A., Flatt, S.W., Rock, C.L., Ritenbaugh, C., Newman, V., & Pierce, J.P. (2002). Increased fruit, vegetable, and fiber intake and lower fat intake reported among women previously treated for invasive breast cancer. *Journal of the American Dietetic Association, 102,* 801–808.

Voskuil, D.W., de Mesquita, H.B., Kaaks, R., van Noord, P.A., Rinaldi, S., Riboli, E., et al. (2001). Determinants of circulating insulin-like growth factor (IGF)-I and IGF binding proteins 1-3 in premenopausal women: Physical activity and anthropology (Netherlands). *Cancer Causes and Control, 12,* 951–958.

Waibitsch, M., Heinze, E., Debatin, K.M., & Blum, W.F. (2000). IGF-I and IGFBP-3 expression in cultured human preadipocytes and adipocytes. *Hormone and Metabolic Research, 32,* 555–559.

Waltman, N.L., Twiss, J.J., Ott, C.D., Gross, G.J., Lindsey, A.M., Moore, T.E., et al. (2003). Testing an intervention for preventing osteoporosis in postmenopausal breast cancer survivors. *Journal of Nursing Scholarship, 35,* 333–338.

Willett, W. (2003). Lessons from dietary studies in Adventists and questions for the future. *American Journal of Clinical Nutrition, 78*(Suppl.), 539S–543S.

Wooster, R., Bignell, G., Lancaster, J., Swift, S., Seal, S., Mangion, J., et al. (1995). Identification of the breast cancer susceptibility gene BRCA2. *Nature, 378,* 789–792.

Wu, A.H., Wan, P., Hankin, J., Tseng, C.C., Yu, M.C., & Pike, M.C. (2002). Adolescent and adult soy intake and risk of breast cancer in Asian-Americans. *Carcinogenesis, 23,* 1491–1496.

Zangwill, M. (2003). Treating early-stage breast cancer. *Cure: Cancer Updates, Research and Education, 2*(3), 21–26.

CHAPTER 3

Colorectal Cancer

Karen Masino, MS, CNP, APRN-BC, OCN®, RD, LDN, CNSD

Overview

Colorectal cancer (CRC) is one of the most commonly occurring cancers in the Western world. Because of the substantial morbidity and mortality associated with CRC and the costs associated with treating it, prevention is a desirable goal. There is increasing evidence that environmental factors, especially dietary factors, are involved in the etiology of CRC. Studies suggest that many of the cancers that surface in later life begin decades before signs and symptoms emerge. Practicing healthy eating habits, performing regular physical activity, and maintaining a healthy weight are considered reasonable guidelines for decreasing the risk of developing cancer (Brown et al., 2003). In the meantime, new therapies to treat CRC provide hope that more people will be cured, even in advanced stages of disease.

Incidence

An estimated 145,290 new cases of CRC and 56,290 deaths will occur in 2005 (Jemal et al., 2005). CRC incidence begins to increase around age 50, with 92% of the cases being diagnosed in people age 50 and older. Although overall mortality has declined, CRC mortality for African Americans remains higher than for other ethnic and racial groups (Jemal et al.). An estimated 65%–85% of cases occur in people with no obvious cause. Another 10%–30% of cases are related to a family history of polyps or CRC. Inherited syndromes such as nonpolyposis CRC, familial adenomatous polyposis, and other rare syndromes contribute to only a small percentage (6%) of all cases of CRC (Jass, Whitehall, Young, & Leggett, 2002).

Risk Factors and Prevention

Several genetic and environmental factors have been identified as increasing the risk of CRC. Nonmodifiable risk factors include a family history of CRC, a personal or family history of colorectal adenomas, familial adenomatous polyposis, inflammatory bowel disease, or ovarian or uterine cancer (Jass et al., 2002). Although a genetic component for CRC is well established, environmental factors are thought to account for most of the variation in rates and incidence in different areas of the world. Lifestyle factors that may increase CRC risk include cigarette smoking (Giovannucci, 2001), physical inactivity, and overweight/obesity (Calle, Rodriguez, Walker-Thurmond, & Thun, 2003), which is associated with an increased risk of death from all cancers. Hyperinsulinism, which is associated with obesity, also is postulated to stimulate the growth of CRC (Kim, 1998). Increased physical activity has been associated with a lower risk of colon cancer (Slattery & Potter, 2002; White, Jacobs, & Daling, 1996). Although a great deal of research has been generated on the role of environmental factors in the contribution to CRC risk, there is significant debate regarding the role of specific nutrients, such as fiber, fat, vegetables, and fruits, among others. A recent comprehensive review identified multiple factors that may modulate risk based on strength of evidence (Levin, 2004). Conclusions were that increased vegetable consumption was the most strongly correlated dietary factor in decreased risk, and red meat and alcohol consumption were probable factors in increasing risk of CRC. This summary also concluded that fiber, fish, calcium, selenium, and carotenoids have only a possible role in decreasing cancer risk. Finally, several substances were identified as possible factors that may have an impact in increasing cancer risk, including sugar, eggs, fat, processed meat, and heavily cooked meat. Many difficulties arise in attempting to identify specific factors in the environment and diet, in particular, that modulate cancer risk. Most of these factors are interrelated, and it is difficult to control the effect of interactions between nutrients versus the effect of individual nutrients. Additional nutrients in the diet that may show promise of decreasing CRC include folate (Rampersaud, Bailey, & Kauwell, 2002) and vitamins E and D. Current consensus appears to reinforce advice consistent with prevention of other chronic diseases, which encourages increased fruit and vegetable consumption and decreased intake of fat.

Treatment Modalities

Determining the appropriate treatment plan for CRC involves setting the appropriate goal and establishing whether treatment is intended to cure the disease, control the disease, or alleviate distressing symptoms. Treatment goals will change necessarily over time as the status of the patient changes. The treatment plan is determined by staging of the disease, effectiveness of available treatment, and the comorbidities and performance status of the patient.

Three different staging systems are used; however, the tumor-node-metastasis (TNM) system is the most common and has been adapted for more precise staging of CRC (American Joint Committee on Cancer, 2002). The most frequent sites for distant metastasis include the liver and lungs, with the bones, brain, kidneys, and adrenal glands being less common (Fong, 2000). Spread to the liver occurs in half of all colon cancers because of its proximity to the capillary network (Fong & Salo, 1999).

Treatment for CRC may consist of any single modality or combination of surgery, radiation therapy, chemotherapy, or biologic therapy. Surgery is the treatment of choice for cure, and the extent of resection frequently determines nutrition impact symptoms. Surgical resection includes removal of the cancer and regional lymph nodes and may include organs invaded locally by tumor (e.g., liver, duodenum, pancreas, ureter, bladder). Selected patients who present with liver- or lung-only disease can undergo potentially curative surgical resection. Resection of isolated liver and lung lesions might be feasible, which can lead to prolonged survival (Scheele, Stang, Altendorf-Hofmann, & Paul, 1995). For patients with advanced disease, surgery may be appropriate for palliative care (e.g., to relieve a bowel obstruction). In general, the more extensive the surgery, the more likely the patient is to experience a negative impact on nutritional status. Because the recovery period typically lasts four to six weeks prior to starting anticancer therapy after surgery, it is important for the healthcare professional to assist in the patient's nutritional recovery from surgery. Residual occult tumor cells can remain after surgery, so chemotherapy may be indicated to reduce the risk of recurrence. Chemotherapy and/or radiation therapy following surgical resection of the primary tumor is standard adjuvant therapy. Approximately 30% of patients have metastatic disease at initial diagnosis, and an additional 25%–30% of patients will subsequently develop metastatic disease (Bengmark & Hafstrom, 1969). This means that many patients will require adjuvant therapy in addition to surgery. Neoadjuvant chemotherapy (given prior to surgery) may be indicated to reduce tumor size so that less extensive resection is necessary. Hepatic intraarterial infusion chemotherapy may be given in selected patients with liver metastasis (Braccia & Heffernan, 2003).

Radiation therapy may be indicated as adjuvant, neoadjuvant, or palliative therapy for CRC with or without chemotherapy. Nutrition impact symptoms produced by radiation are determined by the area of the body being treated, total radiation dose received, comorbid conditions, and performance status of the patient. Additive effects of combining radiation with chemotherapy usually result in more acute and prolonged toxicity.

Generalized side effects from surgery, radiation therapy, and chemotherapy include some degree of fatigue, but fatigue also can be exacerbated by poor performance status, pain, anemia, tumor burden, and combined modality therapies (Ottery, 1996). During the past few decades, knowledge of molecular biology has continued to evolve and has led to the development of therapies targeting tumor cells while sparing normal tissue. Growth factor receptors are important in regulating various cellular processes that are necessary for continued replication of the cell and its survival. The epidermal growth factor receptor (EGFR) normally is expressed on cells of epithelial origin and is overexpressed in several cancers, including CRC. This has been correlated with a more aggressive type of cancer and a worse prognosis (Wood, 2002).

EGFR blockade therapies that inhibit angiogenesis and block the binding of epidermal growth factors to their receptors recently have been approved for treatment of CRC (U.S. Food and Drug Administration, 2004). In general, side effects from these medications are less severe than those associated with chemotherapy, making it possible to administer antiangiogenesis factors in addition to chemotherapy. Therefore, a complete assessment is indicated to evaluate symptoms that may have an impact on nutrition.

Assessment Guidelines

Malnutrition has long been recognized as an important contributor to morbidity, mortality, and decreased quality of life in patients with cancer (Rubin, 2003). Nutrition screening and assessment of patients with cancer should be an ongoing process beginning at the time of diagnosis and continuing throughout treatment. Patients should be screened for nutrition problems with a nutritional management plan developed to correct these problems as quickly as possible. Presenting nutritional symptoms in CRC can include unintentional weight loss, anorexia, anemia, abdominal pain, indigestion, fatigue, and an alteration in bowel habits (Knowles, 2002). Depending on location and size of the lesion, patients may complain of constipation or diarrhea. It is not unusual for patients to initially attempt to control their bowel movements and indigestion by modifying their diet. In some instances, patients will have inadequate diets for an extended period of time because they eliminate foods that they believe are associated with some of their symptoms. Many patients will present with anorexia prior to diagnosis. However, anorexia is a nutrition impact symptom with multiple etiologies, such as pain, stress, psychosocial concerns, physical symptoms (e.g., nausea, vomiting, dysgeusia [altered taste sensation]), and systemic effects of the malignancy caused by increased circulating cytokines (Dinnarello, 2000; Puccio & Nathanson, 1997; Tisdale, 1997). It is important to assess all factors contributing to anorexia and inadequate intake in the patient so that an effective management plan can be implemented. Pharmacologic and nutritional management strategies should be used to correct nutritional deficiencies. For some patients with rectal lesions, an impending bowel obstruction becomes a concern because of a narrowed lumen from the presence of the lesion. These patients need to be counseled to avoid fibrous foods that increase the bulk of the stool as well as bulking agents and medications that slow gut motility to decrease the risk of a bowel obstruction. It is also important to provide education to patients on the signs and symptoms of bowel obstruction and to seek medical attention should these develop.

Nutrition screening and assessment is the responsibility of all healthcare providers involved in management of patients with CRC, with an interdisciplinary process being most efficacious in identifying and managing nutrition impact symptoms. If screening indicates the need for nutritional intervention, a nutrition assessment should be completed with a comprehensive nutrition plan of care developed to address all nutrition impact symptoms.

Special Considerations for Nutrition

After the initial nutrition plan of care has been developed, it is important to maintain ongoing assessment so that the original plan of care can be modified to manage the nutrition impact symptoms that may develop from the different therapies. Most patients with CRC will undergo surgery at some time during their treatment. See Table 3-1 for common surgical procedures for CRC and potential nutrition sequelae. In recent years, the increased use of neoadjuvant chemotherapy and radiation therapy along with newer surgical techniques has permitted the downstaging of cancers with preservation of colon and rectal function. However, although patients may have less morbidity associated with their surgery, the use of multiple therapies increases the likelihood that patients will experience acute nutrition impact symptoms, such as nausea, vomiting, and diarrhea, depending on the therapies provided. An increased risk of infection has been noted in patients receiving preoperative radiation therapy (Ooi, Tjandra, Green, & Church, 1999). Although generalizations can be made regarding the consistency of the stool based on the amount of bowel resected, this will vary depending on a number of factors, including performance status and perioperative nutritional state at the time of surgery, complications related to surgery, age, and comorbid conditions. Adaptation of the large bowel occurs over time, with stool eventually becoming more formed. However, patients have long-term risks for electrolyte and fluid depletion if the entire large colon is resected, resulting in a terminal ileostomy, or if a portion of the small bowel is resected during surgery. If nutritional status and/or performance status is less than optimal, the patient is at increased risk of complications and a protracted recovery (McMahon & Brown, 2000).

Hepatic resection may be indicated for patients with limited hepatic metastasis. The number and location of metastases will determine the extent of resection. Up to six segments of the liver can be safely removed, but enough tissue must be left for regeneration. The liver regenerates within approximately four weeks, with restoration of normal liver function in approximately six weeks (Braccia & Heffernan, 2003; Fong, 2000). Postoperatively, it is important to monitor electrolytes and fluid balance because of the potential for deterioration in liver function. Because of the loss of liver tissue initially, there may not

Table 3-1. Nutrition Sequelae of Surgical Procedures for Colorectal Cancer

Surgery	Nutrition Sequelae	Nutritional Management
Partial colon resection	Loose bowel movements initially	Low-residue diet with patient self-determining foods not well tolerated Progress to regular diet as tolerated.
Total colectomy	Diarrhea, dehydration, electrolyte imbalance	Low-residue diet Adaptation takes place over time, and patient can slowly increase fiber as tolerated. Increased fluid and electrolyte intake
Rectal surgery with colostomy	Psychosocial issues associated with fear of expelling gas, odor-producing foods	Avoidance of potentially gas-producing foods and offending odors
Small bowel resection	Vary depending on length of small bowel resected, potential malabsorption	Determine length and area of bowel resected. If more than 100 cm ileum resected, there is a chance for increased fluid and electrolyte balance problems. Provide total parenteral nutrition—fluid/electrolyte replacement—until patient is able to maintain nutrition orally. Slowly increase diet as tolerated to six small feedings, lactose free, complex carbohydrates included in diet, moderate fat, long-term vitamin use, magnesium, and B_{12} supplementation.
Liver resection	Hypoglycemia	Small, frequent high-protein meals

Note. Based on information from Church et al., 2003; Jeejeebhoy, 2002; Levin, 2004; Lord et al., 2000.

be adequate stored glycogen to buffer the serum glucose when levels decrease between feedings. To avoid hypoglycemia, it is important to provide multiple small, high-protein feedings initially to maintain serum glucose levels.

Adjuvant chemotherapy and radiation therapy continue to be the mainstay of treatment for CRC. Potentially, these regimens can result in significant gastrointestinal toxicity, with diarrhea and mucositis being the most common nutrition-related side effects, depending upon the treatment regimen (Blumberg & Ramanathan, 2002; Marijnen et al., 2002). Table 3-2 lists common chemotherapy regimens for CRC. Many patients may be on multiple chemotherapy medications; however, the side effects encountered may be determined as much by the infusion method as by the dose and number of drugs used, such as 5-fluorouracil, a commonly used chemotherapy medication (Saini et al.,

Table 3-2. Chemotherapy and Biologic Agents Used in Treatment of Colorectal Cancer

Drug	Side Effects
5-fluorouracil (5-FU)	Diarrhea, nausea, vomiting, mucositis, anorexia, pancytopenia, hyperpigmentation with radiation recall, photophobia, integumentary changes including plantar/palmar erythema
Oxaliplatin	Nausea, vomiting, diarrhea, mucositis, pancytopenia, fatigue, anorexia, sensory neuropathy with cold exposure, constipation, increased liver function tests
Cisplatin	Nausea, vomiting, renal and ototoxicity, anorexia, pancytopenia, metallic taste, alopecia, depletion of magnesium, calcium, potassium
Irinotecan	Acute and delayed diarrhea, nausea, vomiting, fatigue, pancytopenia, anorexia, mucositis, skin rash, alopecia
Capecitabine	Pancytopenia, anorexia, mucositis, abdominal pain, fatigue, diarrhea, nausea, vomiting, hand-foot syndrome, integumentary changes
Leucovorin	Mild nausea, vomiting
Floxuridine	Myelosuppression, nausea, vomiting, mucositis or stomatitis of the gastrointestinal tract, alopecia, dermatitis, hepatic dysfunction
Mitomycin-C	Myelosuppression, pulmonary/hepatic/renal toxicity, nausea, vomiting, alopecia, stomatitis
Bevacizumab	Hypertension, fatigue, nausea, vomiting, constipation, anorexia, abdominal pain, leukopenia, asthenia, proteinuria, stomatitis, headache, myalgia, exfoliative dermatitis, gastrointestinal perforation, wound dehiscence
Cetuximab	Acne-like rash, dry skin, fatigue, fever, constipation, abdominal pain

Common protocols
5-FU/leucovorin/oxaliplatin (folfox4)
5-FU/leucovorin
5-FU/leucovorin/irinotecan
5-FU/leucovorin/irinotecan/bevacizumab
Capecitabine
Capecitabine/oxaliplatin
Capecitabine/irinotecan
5-FU/cisplatin
Continuous infusion 5-FU
Hepatic artery infusion—5-FU/leucovorin or floxuridine, continuous 5-FU or floxuridine

2003). The addition of irinotecan can significantly increase toxicity symptoms, including delayed-onset diarrhea, neutropenia, nausea, vomiting, asthenia, alopecia, and an acute cholinergic-like syndrome (sweating, lacrimation, salivation, early diarrhea, abdominal cramps, and bradycardia), which usually is self-limiting but will respond within minutes to subcutaneous administration of atropine. Delayed-onset diarrhea occurs after 24 hours following irinotecan infusion, with peak symptoms at five to six days. If diarrhea is accompanied by neutropenia and dehydration, it can be life threatening. Patients need to be instructed on taking antidiarrheal medications and increasing fluid and electrolyte intake. They should be hospitalized if vomiting or fever develops (Chau & Cunningham, 2002). Oxaliplatin can provoke an oropharyngeal dysesthesia that can be accompanied by muscular and laryngeal spasms when the mucosa comes into contact with cold temperatures or fluids. This is very frightening to patients, and they need to be cautioned about avoiding exposure to a cold environment and fluids (Chau & Cunningham).

Patients typically experience varying degrees of fatigue and anorexia. Intervention strategies for specific nutrition impact symptoms are included in Appendix C. Ongoing trials are evaluating newer surgical techniques to minimize surgery-related morbidity as well as neoadjuvant radiation using more precise techniques to minimize small bowel damage. Trials investigating the use of novel agents with less toxicity are ongoing. Although clinicians anticipate less morbidity with neoadjuvant therapy, long-term complications have not been adequately studied (Church, James, Gibbs, Chao, & Tjandra, 2003). Therefore, it is important to routinely evaluate patients for gastrointestinal toxicity, appetite, and the impact of fatigue on ability to prepare meals and the desire to eat. Acutely, patients can develop diarrhea, skin erythema, or desquamation (Medical Research Council Rectal Cancer Working Party, 1996; Swedish Rectal Cancer Trial, 1997) from radiation therapy to the bowel or rectum. Long-term side effects of radiation therapy can include bowel necrosis and perforation, radiation-induced enteritis, and fistula formation (Allal, Mermillod, Roth, Marti, & Kurtz, 1997; Miller et al., 1999). Clinicians should remember that because radiation therapy has a role in palliative care, patients may be receiving treatment to areas other than the colon or rectum. Radiation therapy is used palliatively to treat symptoms such as pain, obstruction, and bleeding, as well as therapeutically to treat bone metastases and spinal cord compression. Radiation produces local side effects, so toxicity will be determined by the area(s) being treated. Refer to Appendix D for nutritional sequelae of radiation therapy.

Bowel obstruction can occur in this patient population, especially as the disease progresses. Bowel obstruction may result from extrinsic or intrinsic etiologies. Extrinsic compression of the bowel may occur as a result of abdominal carcinomatosis or tumor implantation along the bowel wall and adjacent tissue. Intrinsic compression can occur as a result of progression of the tumor within the bowel lumen (Smothers et al., 2003). Signs and symptoms of bowel obstruction include nausea, vomiting, abdominal pain, and increasing constipation with eventually no bowel movements or bowel sounds over the affected area. Initially, conservative medical management usually is provided along with nasogastric suction and parenteral fluids and electrolytes. Depending on the length of time that the obstruction continues, the patient may need to undergo resection and may even need to have a diverting colostomy created to bypass the area of obstruction as a palliative measure. Although diets for patients with ostomies are not specific and should be individualized, general guidelines are provided in Figure 3-1. Total parenteral nutrition (TPN) may be indicated to provide nutritional support during the perioperative period, but its use in end-stage disease is not supported in the nutrition literature. As a palliative care measure, creation of a gastrostomy may be most appropriate to allow periodic decompression of the stomach when intermittent bowel obstructions occur. With a gastrostomy tube, the patient does not have the discomfort and inconvenience of a large-bore nasogastric tube placed through the nares for extended time periods (Brooksbank, Game, & Ashby, 2002, as cited in Echenique & Correia, 2003).

Fistula formation can be a complication of the disease process, especially in advanced stages. Solid tumors may extend into the bowel from adjacent tissues or burrow from the bowel to the skin, vagina, or other organs to create fistulous communications. The location and presentation of the fistula and the volume of output will determine the nutritional impact. As an example, fistulas originating from the small bowel typically have higher volumes (> 500 ml in 24 hours) of electrolyte-rich output (Jeejeebhoy, 2002). The presence of a fistula is problematic for many reasons, including an increased risk of sepsis, malnutrition, skin breakdown, and fluid and electrolyte imbalance (Rolandelli, & Roslyn, 1996). Patients require constant monitoring to replace fluid and electrolyte losses. TPN with bowel rest may be required to allow spontaneous closure of the fistula or if surgery is necessary to obtain closure. However, if the fistula is caused by malignancy, it is unlikely to close spontaneously (Makhdoom, Komar, & Still, 2000). Case reports have indicated that there may be a role for octreotide in assisting with fistula closure (Martineau, Shwed, &

Figure 3-1. Nutrition Guidelines for Patients With Ostomies

Hydration
Be sure to take adequate fluid to replace losses. The looser the stool, the more fluid that will be needed—at least 8–10 glasses per day.

Odor Control
Odor can be controlled with deodorants and filters. Some foods that may cause odor include asparagus, eggs, cabbage, broccoli, cauliflower, garlic, onions, fish, and coffee. Parsley, cranberry juice, and yogurt may help to decrease odor.

Gas Control
Gas may be a problem for some people. It is important to try small amounts of foods of concern to determine if gas production will be a problem. Some foods that may produce gas include beer, broccoli, cabbage, cauliflower, brussels sprouts, cucumbers, beans, peas, peppers, and highly spiced foods. Avoiding gum chewing and drinking through straws may help to decrease gas, as can limiting pure sugars such as that found in gum, candy, and regular soft drinks.

Denis, 1996). Somatostatin, the naturally occurring peptide hormone, and octreotide, the synthetic hormone, have been shown to exhibit strong inhibitory effects on gastric, pancreatic, biliary, and enteric secretions and thereby decrease gut motility. Adding somatostatin to the TPN regimen may hasten fistula closure because of a reduced volume and decreased enzyme content of digestive secretions (Falconi et al., 1999). For fistulas that are lower in the digestive tract, the patient may be able to continue an oral diet that is low in residue, which should maintain a decreased stool output.

In advanced-stage CRC, malignant ascites can be a complication with significant morbidity. Standard treatment includes diuretics and recurrent large volume paracentesis. The placement of a permanent drainage catheter is a palliative measure that allows the patient and/or caregiver to drain the ascitic fluid routinely, because these patients can experience significant discomfort from the pressure of fluid within the peritoneal cavity (Krouse, 2004). These patients also may experience anorexia and early satiety and may have increased protein losses. Patients need to be monitored for electrolyte and fluid imbalance as well as be encouraged to eat a high-protein diet to replenish losses. Although lymphatic obstruction has been considered the major pathophysiologic mechanism behind its formation, recent evidence suggests that immune modulators, vascular permeability factors, and metalloproteinases contribute significantly to the process. Research now is focused on developing more targeted therapies (Aslam & Marino, 2001).

Chronic radiation enteritis can be a long-term complication of radiation therapy to the pelvic region. Clinical manifestations of chronic radiation enteritis include severe profuse diarrhea, nausea, vomiting, and wave-like abdominal pain and can result in dehydration, weight loss, and malnutrition. Stricture formation and obstruction also can be a complication related to chronic radiation enteritis. Initial signs and symptoms typically occur within 6–18 months of completion of treatment. Findings include submucosal thickening, single or multiple stenoses, adhesions, and sinus or fistula formation. Microscopic findings include villi that are fibrotic or that may be lost altogether. Ulceration is common, varying from simple loss of epithelial layers to ulcers that may penetrate to different depths of the intestinal wall, even to the serosa (National Cancer Institute, 2002). Modifications in radiation treatment techniques to minimize small bowel exposure may be helpful in decreasing incidence, such as three-dimensional conformal radiation therapy (Bismar & Sinicrope, 2002). Limited information is available for nutritional management of chronic radiation enteritis. Older studies have been inconclusive as to the effectiveness of an elemental formula in controlling symptoms (Jain, Scolapio, Wasserman, & Floch, 2002). Medical management of the patient's symptoms, which are similar to those of acute radiation enteritis, is indicated with surgical management reserved for severe damage. TPN also has been evaluated, but its role is unclear. It may be useful mainly as a supportive measure for patients with obstruction (Jain et al.). Other modifications and treatments that are considered anecdotal include low-fat, low-residue, lactose-restricted diets with varying degrees of fiber being tolerated (Sekhon, 2000). An individualized approach is critical, including management by a registered dietitian to help to avoid unnecessary dietary restrictions and increase variety in the diet.

CRC is largely a disease of older adults (Holt, 2003). Therefore, it is important that when determining a nutrition plan of care, the clinician considers nutritional concerns that may be present in the older adult patient with cancer, such as the presence of comorbid disease, physical disability, poor dentition, polypharmacy, limited income, social isolation, decreased sensory acuity, sedentary lifestyle, depression, dementia, and possibly dysphagia (Gary & Fleury, 2002; Persson, Brismar, Katzarski, Nordenstromk, & Cederholm, 2002). Although many older adult patients remain relatively healthy prior to the cancer diagnosis, because of the increased prevalence of nutritional issues, these factors must be considered when completing an assessment.

Nutrition Care Planning

Clinicians caring for patients with cancer recognize the importance of providing nutritional care. Ideally, nutrition care planning should include providing support to the patient before treatment begins to optimize tolerance to cancer therapy, during treatment to prevent nutrition-related complications, and post-treatment to provide for nutrition rehabilitation. To provide optimal nutrition care, an integrated approach is indicated. Patients with CRC will likely receive multimodal treatment in both the inpatient and outpatient settings. Because of the potential for increased nutrition-related toxicity with multiple treatment interventions, there is a risk for developing nutritional compromise throughout the continuum of treatment. Consistent nutrition care planning will depend upon good communication between disciplines. Although numerous screening tools and methods are available for monitoring nutritional status, a validated screening tool for the oncology population is the Patient-Generated Subjective Global Assessment (PG-SGA) (Bauer, Capra, & Ferguson, 2002). This tool is intended to identify and prioritize the nutritional intervention needed. The patient completes a portion of the tool, and the healthcare professional, such as the dietitian, nurse, or physician, completes the remainder (see Appendix A). The PG-SGA then is scored to determine nutritional risk and provide triage guidelines to manage the nutritional needs of the patient. To avoid omission of nutritionally relevant impact symptoms, this tool should be used initially and ongoing to screen for risk factors indicating the need for a comprehensive nutrition assessment. Documentation of nutrition assessments with interventions provided is key to maintaining an interdisciplinary nutrition plan of care because each healthcare professional should be monitoring changes in nutritional status and working within the team to provide intervention. Guidelines for completing a more focused nutrition assessment for patients with CRC are included in Figure 3-2.

Figure 3-2. Nutrition Focus—Colorectal Cancer

Pretreatment
Screen all patients using the PG-SGA (see Appendix A).
  Triage score
  0–1 General nutrition advice; screen each clinic visit for chemotherapy or weekly if
       on radiation
  2–3 General nutrition advice; pharmacologic intervention as indicated
  4 or> Comprehensive assessment by dietetics professional (see Appendix E)

  Focus for assessment
  Bowel pattern (alterations, frequency, diarrhea, constipation)
  Screen for impending bowel obstruction for patients with lesions low in the rectal canal.
  Food intolerance related to bowel movements/abdominal pain

During treatment
  Triage score
  0–3 Continue nutrition screening and triage using PG-SGA.
       Continue general nutrition advice.
  4 or> Comprehensive assessment by dietetics professional (see Appendix E)

  Focus for assessment
  Bowel movement pattern
  Food intolerance
  Treatment-related side effects—nausea, vomiting, diarrhea, mucositis, anorexia,
      fatigue

  Focus for nutritional intervention
  Pharmacologic medications to manage nutrition impact symptoms
  Alteration in food consistency—decrease in soluble fiber for diarrhea
  Alteration in temperature, texture, and irritants for mucositis
  Assess factors contributing to anorexia as appropriate.

Post-treatment
  Triage score
  0–3 Continue nutrition screening and triage using PG-SGA.

  Focus for assessment
  Presence of nutrition impact symptoms and bowel movement pattern

  Focus for nutritional intervention
  Emphasis on correcting nutritional deficits
  Continued intervention for management of nutrition impact symptoms
  Consider long-term nutrition goals.
  Evaluate long-term lifestyle changes to improve risk profile (e.g., increased fruit and
      vegetable intake, exercise, weight reduction).

Expected Outcomes of Therapy

At the present time, stage at diagnosis and potential for resection are the main factors in determining long-term prognosis. However, with new therapies to treat late-stage CRC and distant metastasis, clinicians are more optimistic regarding opportunities for cure or long-term palliation. With therapies becoming more targeted and the availability of newer methods of providing radiation therapy to minimize toxicity, patients will likely experience decreased short-term and long-term toxicity that has, in the past, been so severe it has interfered with ongoing treatment. In the meantime, nutrition researchers will continue to focus on determining optimal lifestyle changes to decrease modifiable risk factors in the hope of decreasing the numbers of new CRC cases. It will be the challenge of healthcare professionals to educate and assist patients on the importance of implementing lifestyle changes with the goal of preventing the development or recurrence of CRC.

References

Allal, A., Mermillod, B., Roth, A., Marti, M., & Kurtz, J. (1997). Impact of clinical and therapeutic factors on major late complications after radiotherapy with or without concomitant chemotherapy for anal carcinoma. *International Journal of Radiation Oncology, Biology, Physics, 39,* 1099–1105.

American Joint Committee on Cancer. (2002). *AJCC cancer staging manual* (6th ed.). New York: Springer.

Aslam, N., & Marino, C. (2001). Malignant ascites: New concepts in pathophysiology, diagnosis and management. *Archives of Internal Medicine, 161,* 2733–2737.

Bauer, J., Capra, S., & Ferguson, M. (2002). Use of the scored Patient-Generated Subjective Global Assessment as a nutrition assessment tool in patients with cancer. *European Journal of Clinical Nutrition, 56,* 779–785.

Bengmark, S., & Hafstrom, L. (1969). The natural history of primary and secondary malignant tumors of the liver: The prognosis for patients with hepatic metastases from colonic and rectal carcinoma diagnosed by laparotomy. *Cancer, 23,* 198–202.

Bismar, M., & Sinicrope, F. (2002). Radiation enteritis. *Current Gastroenterology Reports, 4,* 361–365.

Blumberg, D., & Ramanathan, R.K. (2002). Treatment of colon and rectal cancer. *Journal of Clinical Gastroenterology, 34*(1), 15–26.

Braccia, D., & Heffernan, N. (2003). Surgical and ablative modalities for the treatment of colorectal cancer metastatic to the liver. *Clinical Journal of Oncology Nursing, 7,* 178–184.

Brooksbank, M., Game, P., & Ashby, M. (2002). Palliative venting gastrostomy in malignant intestinal obstruction. *Palliative Medicine, 16,* 520–526.

Brown, J., Byers, T., Doyle, C., Courneya, K.S., Demark-Wahnefried, W., Kushi, L.H., et al. (2003). Nutrition and physical activity during and after cancer treatment: An American Cancer Society guide for informed choices. *CA: A Cancer Journal for Clinicians, 53,* 268–291.

Calle, E., Rodriguez, C., Walker-Thurmond, K., & Thun, M. (2003). Overweight, obesity, and mortality from cancer in a prospectively studied cohort of U.S. adults. *New England Journal of Medicine, 348,* 1625–1638.

Chau, I., & Cunningham, D. (2002). Chemotherapy in colorectal cancer: New options and new challenges. *British Medical Bulletin, 64,* 159–180.

Church, C., James, M., Gibbs, P., Chao, M., & Tjandra, J. (2003). Optimizing the outcome for patients with rectal cancer. *Diseases of the Colon and Rectum, 46,* 389–402.

Dinnarello, C. (2000). Proinflammatory cytokines. *Chest, 118,* 503–508.

Echenique, M., & Correia, M. (2003). Nutrition in advanced digestive cancer. *Current Opinion in Clinical Nutrition and Metabolic Care, 6,* 577–580.

Falconi, M., Sartori, N., Caldiron, E., Salvia, R., Bassi, C., & Pederzoli, P. (1999). Management of digestive tract fistulas: A review. *Digestion, 60*(3), 51–58.

Fong, Y. (2000). Hepatic colorectal metastasis: Current surgical therapy, selection criteria for hepatectomy, and role for adjuvant therapy. *Advances in Surgery, 34,* 351–381.

Fong, Y., & Salo, J. (1999). Surgical therapy of hepatic colorectal metastasis. *Seminars in Oncology, 26,* 514–523.

Gary, R., & Fleury, J. (2002). Nutritional status: Key to preventing functional decline in hospitalized older adults. *Topics in Geriatric Rehabilitation, 17*(3), 40–71.

Giovannucci, E. (2001). An updated review of the epidemiological evidence that cigarette smoking increases risk of colorectal cancer. *Cancer Epidemiology, Biomarkers and Prevention, 10,* 725–731.

Holt, R. (2003). Gastrointestinal diseases in the elderly. *Current Opinion in Clinical Nutrition and Metabolic Care, 6*(1), 41–48.

Jain, G., Scolapio, J., Wasserman, E., & Floch, M. (2002). Chronic radiation enteritis: A ten-year follow-up. *Journal of Clinical Gastroenterology, 35*(3), 214–217.

Jass, J., Whitehall, V., Young, J., & Leggett, B. (2002). Emerging concepts in colorectal neoplasia. *Gastroenterology, 123,* 862–876.

Jeejeebhoy, K. (2002). Short bowel syndrome: A nutritional and medical approach. *Canadian Medical Association Journal, 166,* 1297–1302.

Jemal, A., Murray, T., Ward, E., Samuels, A., Tiwari, R.C., Ghafoor, A., et al. (2005). Cancer statistics, 2005. *CA: A Cancer Journal for Clinicians, 55,* 10–30.

Kim, Y. (1998). Diet, lifestyle, and colorectal cancer: Is hyperinsulinemia the missing link? *Nutrition Reviews, 56,* 275–279.

Knowles, G. (2002). The management of colorectal cancer. *Nursing Standard, 16*(17), 47–52.

Krouse, R. (2004). Advances in palliative surgery for cancer patients. *Journal of Supportive Oncology, 2*(1), 80–87.

Levin, B. (2004). *Colorectal cancer.* Retrieved April 2, 2004, from http://www.medscape.com/viewarticle/472093

Lord, L., Schaffner, R., DeCross, A., Sax., H., Verger, J., & Schears, G. (2000). Management of the patient with short bowel syndrome. *Advanced Practice in Acute and Critical Care, 11,* 604–618.

Makhdoom, Z., Komar, M., & Still, C. (2000). Nutrition and enterocutaneous fistulas. *Journal of Clinical Gastroenterology, 31*(3), 195–204.

Marijnen, C., Kapiteijn, E., Van de Velde, C., Martijnen, H., Steup, W., Wiggers, T., et al. (2002). Acute side effects and complications after short-term preoperative radiotherapy combined with total mesorectal excision in primary rectal cancer: Report of a multicenter randomized trial. *Journal of Clinical Oncology, 20,* 817–825.

Martineau, P., Shwed, J., & Denis, R. (1996). Is octreotide a new hope for enterocutaneous and external pancreatic fistulas closure? *American Journal of Surgery, 172,* 386–395.

McMahon, K., & Brown, J. (2000). Nutritional screening and assessment. *Seminars in Oncology Nursing, 16*(2), 106–112.

Medical Research Council Rectal Cancer Working Party. (1996). Randomized trial of surgery alone versus radiotherapy followed by surgery for potentially operable locally advanced rectal cancer. *Lancet, 348,* 1605–1610.

Miller, A., Martenson, J., Nelson, H., Schleck, C., Ilstrup, D., Gunderson, L., et al. (1999). The incidence and clinical consequences of treatment-related bowel injury. *International Journal of Radiation Oncology, Biology, Physics, 43,* 817–825.

National Cancer Institute. (2002). *Radiation enteritis.* Retrieved June 1, 2004, from http://cancerweb.ncl.ac.uk/cancernet/304093.html

Ooi, B., Tjandra, J., Green, M., & Church, J. (1999). Morbidities of adjuvant chemotherapy and radiotherapy for resectable rectal cancer: An overview. *Diseases of the Colon and Rectum, 42,* 403–418.

Ottery, F. (1996). Supportive nutritional management of the patient with pancreatic cancer. *Oncology, 10*(Suppl. 9), 26–32.

Persson, M., Brismar, K., Katzarski, K., Nordenstromk, J., & Cederholm, T. (2002). Nutritional status using mini nutritional assessment and subjective global assessment to predict mortality in geriatric patients. *Journal of the American Geriatrics Society, 50,* 1996–2002.

Puccio, M., & Nathanson, L. (1997). The cancer cachexia syndrome. *Seminars in Oncology, 24,* 277–287.

Rampersaud, G., Bailey, L., & Kauwell, G. (2002). Relationship of folate to colorectal and cervical cancer: Review and recommendations for practitioners. *Journal of the American Dietetic Association, 2,* 1273–1282.

Rolandelli, R., & Roslyn, J. (1996). Surgical management and treatment of sepsis associated with gastrointestinal fistulas. *Surgical Clinics of North America, 67,* 1111–1122.

Rubin, H. (2003). Cancer cachexia: Its correlations and causes. *Proceedings of the National Academy of Sciences of the United States of America, 100,* 5383–5389.

Saini, A., Norman, A., Cunningham, D., Chau, I., Hill, M., Tait, D., et al. (2003). Twelve weeks of protracted venous infusion of fluorouracil (5-FU) is effective as 6 months of bolus 5-FU and folinic acid as adjuvant treatment in colorectal cancer. *British Journal of Cancer, 88,* 1859–1865.

Scheele, J., Stang, R., Altendorf-Hofmann, A., & Paul, M. (1995). Resection of colorectal liver metastasis. *World Journal of Surgery, 19*(1), 59–71.

Sekhon, S. (2000). Chronic radiation enteritis: Women's food tolerances after radiation treatment for gynecologic cancer. *Journal of the American Dietetic Association, 100,* 941–943.

Slattery, M., & Potter, J. (2002). Physical activity and colon cancer: Confounding or interaction? *Medicine and Science in Sports and Exercise, 34,* 913–919.

Smothers, L., Hynan, L., Fleming, J., Turnage, R., Simmang, C., & Anthony, T. (2003). Emergency surgery for colon carcinoma. *Diseases of the Colon and Rectum, 46*(1), 24–30.

Swedish Rectal Cancer Trial. (1997). Improved survival with preoperative radiotherapy in resectable rectal cancer. *New England Journal of Medicine, 336,* 980–987.

Tisdale, M. (1997). Biology of cachexia. *Journal of the National Cancer Institute, 89,* 1763–1773.

U.S. Food and Drug Administration. (2004, February). *FDA news.* Retrieved April 3, 2004, from http://www.fda.gov/bbs/topics/NEWS/2004/NEW01027.html

White, E., Jacobs, E., & Daling, J. (1996). Physical activity in relation to colon cancer in middle-aged men and women. *American Journal of Epidemiology, 144*(1), 42–50.

Wood, L. (2002). Rationale for EGFR as a target for cancer therapy. *Seminars in Oncology Nursing, 18*(Suppl. 4), 3–10.

CHAPTER 4

Esophageal and Gastric Cancers

Susan Anne Churma, RD, LD
Cindy Jo Horrell, MS, CRNP, AOCN®

Esophageal Cancer

Esophageal cancer is an uncommon malignancy in the United States. The American Cancer Society (ACS) estimates that 14,520 new cases of esophageal cancer will be diagnosed in 2005, and of those, approximately 13,570 will result in death (Jemal et al., 2005). The majority of the cases of esophageal cancer in the United States are categorized into two histologic subtypes: adenocarcinoma and squamous cell carcinoma. During the past few decades, it has become apparent that the epidemiology is changing, with a dramatic increase in adenocarcinomas. Before 1980, adenocarcinomas comprised approximately 15% of esophageal cancers. By 1994, the percentage of cases had risen to 60% (Blot & McLaughlin, 1999). A further analysis of the epidemiology led Thomas Vaughan, MD, of the Fred Hutchinson Cancer Research Center, to report at the 2004 Gastrointestinal Cancers Symposium that the incidence is five times more common in Whites than African Americans, and the male to female incidence is 7:1 (Vaughan, 2004).

Predisposing Conditions

The incidence of esophageal cancer varies among geographic regions, with high rates found in China, central Asia, the Caspian littoral region in north Iran, and the Transkei of South Africa. Esophageal cancers also are more common in Sri Lanka, India, France, and Switzerland. Unlike the United States, in these regions, squamous cell cancer of the esophagus accounts for the majority of the reported cases. This suggests that environmental factors most likely play an important role in the etiology. Several studies suggest that deficiencies of some food and minerals may increase the risk of esophageal cancer (Brown,

1988; Guo et al., 1990; Jaskiewicz, Marasas, Rossouw, Van Niekerk, & Heine Tech, 1988; Yang, 1980). In China, for example, occurrences of esophageal cancer have been attributed to low levels of retinol, riboflavin, alpha-carotene, beta-carotene, alpha-tocopherol, and ascorbate (World Cancer Research Fund & American Institute for Cancer Research, 1997). In addition, low levels of selenium and zinc, as well as a low intake of fruits, particularly citrus, repeatedly are associated with increased risk of esophageal cancer.

Squamous cell carcinoma of the esophagus is associated with a history of heavy tobacco and alcohol use. Alcohol interacts in a multiplicative manner with tobacco, and a near 100-fold increase in the risk of esophageal cancer has been reported (Blot & McLaughlin, 1999). This risk declines with smoking cessation (Siematycki, Krewski, & Franco, 1995). Because of the inverse relationship between caloric intake of alcohol and a healthy diet, it is believed that alcohol may increase the risk of esophageal cancer by decreasing the overall nutrient intake. The histologic type squamous cell carcinoma is seen more often in African Americans and in men and usually is well differentiated and associated with widespread submucosal lymphatic dissemination.

Barrett's esophagus, in which the squamous epithelium is replaced with an intestinal columnar epithelium, is a precursor to adenocarcinoma of the esophagus. Barrett's esophagus has been associated with as high as a 30- to 40-fold increased risk of esophageal cancer (Shaheen & Ransohoff, 2002). Barrett's esophagus tends to be localized in the distal third of the esophagus and presents as fungating masses or stenotic lesions. Many are well differentiated. Swedish researchers conducted a population-based study that evaluated chronic gastroesophageal reflux as a risk factor for esophageal adenocarcinoma. The results confirmed that esophageal reflux independently increased the risk of Barrett's by 5- to 20-fold (Lagergren, Bergstrom, Lindgren, & Nyren, 1999). However, there is insufficient evidence to prove that screening of the general population for gastroesophageal reflux disease can reduce cancer mortality (Gerson & Triadafilopoulos, 2002). Another characteristic of Barrett's esophagus and esophageal adenocarcinoma is the overexpression of Cox-2. Early data suggest that suppression of stomach acid reduces the proliferation seen in Barrett's esophagus (Kaur & Triadafilopoulos, 2002).

Epidemiologic studies have determined that the use of aspirin or nonsteroidal anti-inflammatory drugs is associated with a decreased risk of esophageal cancer, regardless of histology. Diets high in fruits and vegetables also are associated with decreased risk (Siematycki et al., 1995).

Molecular Biology

A number of molecular genetic and cytogenetic abnormalities have been implicated in the development of carcinomas of the esophagus. This information is particularly intriguing when considering drug development and research trials. The oncogenes and tumor suppressor gene mutations disrupt the cell cycle regulation at the G1 restriction point. The overexpression of oncogene cyclin D1 and the inactivation of *p16* (tumor suppressor gene) result in the loss of control of cellular growth and allow continued cell proliferation. There is a significant correlation between overexpression of cyclin D1 and lymph node metastases, advanced tumor stage, and decreased overall survival in patients with esophageal cancer (Roncalli et al., 1998; Takeuchi et al., 1997). More than half of esophageal cancers exhibit *p53* mutations (Koshy, Esiashvili, Landry, Thomas, & Matthews, 2004b). This gene product regulates orderly development of the cell, DNA repair, apoptosis, and neovascularization in tissues. Epidermal growth factor receptor (EGFR) is overexpressed in 70% of squamous cell carcinomas and 30% of adenocarcinomas of the esophagus. Several studies have shown that the overexpression of EGFR significantly increased preference for lymph node metastases and hematogenous recurrence and decreased survival. Many esophageal tumors also overexpress transforming growth factor-α, which binds to EGFR and continues to stimulate the proliferation of cells (Iihara et al., 1993; Itakura et al., 1994; Kitagawa et al., 1996; Shimada et al., 1999). Pharmacologic agents that target these cellular pathways are under development and evaluation in clinical trials.

Screening

At least half of the patients with esophageal cancer are found to have locally advanced or metastatic disease at the time of diagnosis. It has been argued that screening programs could identify cancer at an earlier stage, thereby providing a possibility of cure or increased survival. However, studies have failed to demonstrate the benefit of mass screening. There has been no solid documentation that screening reduces the mortality from adenocarcinomas of the esophagus (Sontag, 2001).

On the other hand, research has suggested that cancer found in Barrett's esophagus during endoscopy has a more favorable prognosis (Sharma, 1999). Recommendations from the American College of Gastroenterology include surveillance endoscopies based on the degree of dysplasia present. With no dysplasia, endoscopies are recommended every three years. If high-grade dysplasia is present, the recommendations include confirmation by a pathologist and the option of esophagectomy versus endoscopy every three months (Spechler, 2002). At this time, it is generally considered that dysplasia is the best pathologic predictor of cancer occurrence.

Clinical Presentation

The most common presenting complaint of patients with esophageal cancer is dysphagia. The patient will describe initial difficulty swallowing solid food. Because of the ability of the esophagus to distend, it can take many months before symptoms finally prompt medical attention. Approximately 75% of the esophageal circumference must be involved before symptoms appear (Schrump, Altorki, Forastiere, & Minsky, 2001). This makes it difficult to discover early-stage esophageal cancer. The majority of patients with limited stage disease are discovered by accident. The second most common complaint is odynophagia, or retrosternal pain associated with swallowing. By the time the patient seeks medical attention, he or she is experiencing progressive weight loss and anorexia. About half of the patients will have locally advanced unresectable disease at the time of diagnosis (Schrump et al.). The physical examination often is negative. A careful examination must be done with attention to checking for evidence of supraclavicular or cervical adenopathy, abdominal mass, or fullness of the liver. A chest x-ray may demonstrate mediastinal widening, evidence of aspiration pneumonia, or presence of pulmonary nodules. Anemia from blood loss, abnormal liver functions, serum lactate dehydrogenase, or alkaline phosphatase levels may indicate visceral or bony metastasis.

For most cases of esophageal cancer, it is typical to see early lymphatic spread. The pattern of lymphatic drainage is primarily longitudinal, so extensive regional dissemination of cancer may occur regardless of the location of the primary tumor. Through hematogenous spread, dissemination is observed in the liver and lungs as well as bones, kidneys, adrenal gland, stomach, heart, omentum, or peritoneum. The single most important prognostic factor is the extent of disease at the time of diagnoses.

Evaluation

Endoscopic evaluation with biopsy and brushings is necessary to establish tissue diagnosis and define the extent of the lesion. Computed tomography (CT) scanning of the chest and abdomen will detect metastatic spread. If the esophageal lesions are in the upper or mid-esophagus, bronchoscopy is performed to assess involvement of the tracheobronchial tree and to rule out recurrent laryngeal nerve involvement. Endoscopy with ultrasound (EUS) is useful in assessing the depth of tumor penetration into the esophageal wall. The EUS is limited by the experience of the ultrasonographer as well as the presence of high-grade obstructions (Schrump et al., 2001).

For staging purposes, FDG PET (fluorodeoxyglucose positron emission tomography) scans are more accurate than CT scans in detecting distant metastases but are less sensitive for identifying locoregional lesions. A study by Meltzer et al. (2000) suggested that PET scanning complements the information obtained by CT scanning. A PET study in Japan (Kato et al., 2002) demonstrated higher sensitivity, specificity, and accuracy of lymph node staging in squamous cell carcinomas of the esophagus. A Belgian study (Lerut et al., 2000) observed that PET significantly improves the detection of stage IV disease in esophageal cancer compared with the conventional staging modalities (i.e., spiral CT scan, EUS). PET also demonstrated improved diagnostic specificity for lymph node staging. One study reported 93% sensitivity and 100% specificity when regional lymph node staging was performed with EUS–fine needle aspiration (Vasques-Sequeiros, Norton, & Clain, 2001).

Treatment

The optimal treatment for esophageal cancer is still controversial. Esophagectomy is the standard of care. Within the surgical literature, controversy exists regarding the best surgical approach. Regardless of the approach, esophagectomy has been associated with considerable morbidity and mortality. The recent advances in the use of minimally invasive surgery has allowed esophagectomy to be performed by both combined laparoscopic and thorascopic and totally laparoscopic transhiatal approaches. These approaches allow for the evaluation of lymph nodes. An intergroup National Cancer Institute (NCI) trial (CALGB 9380) evaluated the feasibility and accuracy of this staging modality. Results demonstrated that the number of positive lymph nodes identified was doubled when compared to conventional, noninvasive staging (Krasna et al., 2001). Although modern anesthetic and surgical care has reduced the risks of esophagectomy, the incidence of major or minor complications is still approximately 70%–80%, and the hospital mortality rate is 4%–7% at experienced centers (Pierre & Luketich, 2002). The technique commonly performed in North America and Europe has been the transhiatal esophagectomy, with five-year survival rates of 20%–25%. Unfortunately, this procedure has been associated with failure to control or eradicate local disease in nearly 40% of the patients. Transthoracic esophagectomy is the approach used worldwide. Survival rates are similar with both approaches.

Many patients with esophageal cancer present with locally advanced or metastatic disease. Attempts have been made to use radiotherapy, chemotherapy, or a combination of these modalities in treatment. The goal of preoperative radiotherapy is to reduce tumor burden, reduce the risk of dissemination at the time of surgery, and sterilize nodal areas. Randomized trials have failed to demonstrate those results (Koshy, Esiashvilli, Landry, Thomas, & Matthews, 2004a). Postoperative radiotherapy is indicated for patients with positive margins at the time of resection, but it has not demonstrated survival benefit (Koshy et al., 2004b). David Kelsen, MD, speaking at the 2004 Gastrointestinal Cancers Symposium, pointed out that there is no established neoadjuvant approach for esophageal carcinomas. The current data support either resection or chemotherapy and radiotherapy without resection (Kelsen, 2004). Many institutions currently are using combined modality treatment with or without adjuvant esophagectomy. The RTOG 85-01 study (Cooper et al., 1999) demonstrated a survival advantage with chemotherapy and radiotherapy compared to radiotherapy alone. Intergroup studies (ECOG 1201) currently are under way in an attempt to prove the effectiveness of neoadjuvant regimens using paclitaxel/cisplatin or paclitaxel/irinotecan combinations given with radiotherapy.

Brachytherapy as a single therapy usually is used as a palliative modality. It is useful in managing symptoms such as dysphagia and bleeding. Several endoluminal techniques also are useful in the palliative setting, including expandable stents placed endoscopically, which are cost effective and provide durable palliation (Cantero et al., 1999; Raijman, Siddique, Ajani, & Lynch, 1998). In addition, photodynamic therapy has proved effective in palliating obstructing esophageal carcinoma lesions with less morbidity and mortality when compared with surgical bypass techniques (Maier, Tomaselli, & Gebhard, 2000).

Nutritional Implications and Treatment

An esophageal cancer diagnosis usually is associated with rapidly progressive dysphagia, weight loss, and malnutrition at time of diagnosis. Treatment may increase patient survival, although patients may experience side effects such as weight loss and malnutrition (see Table 4-1). Conversely, weight loss and poor nutritional status may lead to decreased response to therapies (Dewys et al., 1980). Chemotherapy toxicity may be reduced with improved nutritional status (Torosian, Buzby, & Presti, 1982).

Dysphagia or difficulty swallowing is one of the most frustrating problems that the patient with esophageal cancer may experience. The tumor location as well as the treatment may contribute to dysphagia as well as other nutritional side effects, including nausea, vomiting, and weight loss (Langstein & Norton, 1991). Many patients at presentation are able to tolerate soft foods, although some have difficulty swallowing their own saliva (Lightdale et al., 1995).

A nutrition assessment of a patient with esophageal cancer should examine the patient's past medical history, medications, laboratory analysis, weight history, diet history, and degree of dysphagia present. The dietitian plays an important role with the other healthcare team members in the care and treatment of patients with esophageal cancer. Patients will need to be guided throughout their treatment regarding the types of foods and nutritional supplements that will help them to maintain their nutritional status (see Table 4-2).

Patients with esophageal cancer who are receiving palliative care commonly tolerate and maintain quality of life on oral feeds alone (Litle et al., 2003), but patients usually have a jejunostomy feeding tube placed during surgery (Luketich et al., 2003). Patients with surgically placed jejunostomy tubes after an esophagectomy usually do well on polymeric high-protein standard intact tube formulas (Stralovich, 1993). It is suggested that fiber-containing formulas not be used if the patient has a needle catheter jejunostomy. Feedings are cycled and weaned as the patient is able to tolerate adequate oral caloric intake.

Patients who have undergone esophagectomy or palliative surgery can be expected to eventually tolerate a soft to regular diet. General guidelines can be found in Table 4-3.

If the patient is not receiving 100% of the recommended daily allowance in caloric requirements, vitamin supplementation is recommended. Additional supplementation for wound healing also should be recommended. Zinc sulfate 220 mg (50 mg elemental zinc) for short term (three months) and 500 mg vitamin C daily have been suggested to aid in wound healing (Shepherd, 2003). Newer oral liquid supplements containing the amino acid L-arginine

Table 4-1. Common Side Effects of Esophageal Cancer Treatment, Causes, and Management

Side Effect	Possible Causes	Management
Difficulty or painful swallowing	Tumor location Inflammation/pain in esophagus because of endoscopic surgery, radiation, or chemotherapy Anastamotic stricture after esophagectomy Tumor recurrence Tumor ingrowth in stent	Encourage small, frequent, soft, moist meals and snacks. Encourage patient to drink high-calorie liquid nutritional supplements several times per day if patient is unable to eat enough regular foods to meet his or her nutritional needs. Insert feeding tube if patient is unable to drink and eat sufficient calories to maintain his or her weight.
Early satiety, anorexia, and weight loss	Tumor location, surgical treatment, chemotherapy, and radiation	Encourage small, frequent meals. Encourage patient to consume high-calorie foods such as ice cream, puddings, cheeses, milkshakes, cream soups, eggs, and lunchmeats and spreads, such as tuna and chicken. Limit fluids with meals, but encourage patient to sip fluids throughout the day to meet fluid intake needs. Augment meals with liquid supplements. Patients who have had an esophagectomy must drink slowly to decrease chance of dumping syndrome. Provide appetite stimulants. Cycle or decrease tube feeds to help to increase oral intake.
Gas bloating	Altered anatomy	Use antiflatulence medication, such as simethicone. Encourage small, frequent meals.
Reflux, regurgitation, and esophagitis	Removal of distal esophageal sphincter with esophagectomy Stents and lasers placed at the gastroesophageal junction Increased incidence of heartburn	Follow antireflux diet (i.e., no citrus, tomato, fatty foods, coffee, or chocolate). Encourage small, frequent meals. Encourage patients to stand up or walk after eating. Elevate head of bed 30°–45° during times of rest or bedtime, especially if patient is receiving tube feedings. Use antireflux medications if needed. Try aloe vera liquid before meals.

(Continued on next page)

Table 4-1. Common Side Effects of Esophageal Cancer Treatment, Causes, and Management *(Continued)*

Side Effect	Possible Causes	Management
Dumping syndrome and diarrhea	Occurs in patients who have had an esophagectomy secondary to removal of the distal esophageal sphincter Symptoms that may occur 15–60 minutes after a meal include nausea, vomiting, diarrhea, dizziness, and palpitations. Tube feeding intolerance Infectious diarrhea	Encourage small, frequent meals. Avoid lactose in diet. Avoid large amounts of concentrated sweets. Eat dry meals with fluids consumed 30 minutes after meals. Change tube feeding formula if not tolerated. Begin standard antidiarrheal medications. Use medication if infectious diarrhea is present. Try probiotics, such as Lactinex®, or yogurt. Encourage patients to eat a low-fat and low-roughage diet. Encourage increased fluid intake; patient may need IV hydration.
Constipation	Both pain and anti-nausea medications have a constipating effect. Changes in eating habits or eating a decreased amount Decreased physical activity Decreased fluid intake	Encourage patient to use laxatives and stool softeners as directed. Encourage patient to eat at the same times every day. Encourage patient to drink 8–10 cups of liquid each day, including water, prune juice, and warm liquids. Encourage patient to eat more high-fiber foods. Begin bowel program with stool softeners and laxatives, as needed.
Anastamotic leak	Surgical complication after an esophagectomy (food may be seen leaking out of neck incision)	Nothing by mouth as determined by physician, may be a three- to four-week time period. Begin full nutritional support with jejunal feeds. Retry oral diet as determined by physician.
Chyle leak	Thoracic duct is accidentally nicked during surgery.	Try a very low-fat diet (less than 10 grams) to include flat soft drinks, juices, and broths. Use tube feedings that are semi-elemental and high in MCT oils. Use total parenteral nutrition if drainage persists with the above recommendations. Somatostatin may be of benefit once leak is determined.

Note. Based on information from Bloch, 1990; Kelly & Shumway, 2000; Lerut et al., 2002; National Cancer Institute, 2004; Parrish & McCray, 2004.

Table 4-2. Special Considerations for Nutrition for Endoscopic Palliation

Treatment	Diet Upgrade in Hospital	Diet at Discharge
Stent and photodynamic therapy	After a barium swallow to rule out leak, patient is started on three days of clear liquids, three days of full liquids, and then soft diet as tolerated by postoperative day seven. It may take one to two weeks before swallowing improves secondary to esophageal inflammation secondary to treatment.	Eat small, frequent, soft, moist meals and snacks. Encourage plenty of non-acidic fluids. Encourage high-calorie liquid nutritional supplements several times per day if the patient is unable to eat enough regular foods to meet his or her nutritional needs. Encourage soft foods, such as hot and cold cereals, scrambled and soft-cooked eggs, pasta, casseroles, mashed potatoes and gravy, tender meat and fish, well-cooked vegetables, skinned and canned fruits, crackers, toast, milkshakes, puddings, ice cream, and yogurt. Avoid tough, dry meats; raw vegetables, especially lettuce and cabbage; raw fruits; nuts; seeds; dry foods, such as rice; and most bread products, unless they are toasted.

have shown great enhancement of wound healing and decreased wound infections (Senkal et al., 1999; Snyderman et al., 1999).

Nutrition therapy for the patient with esophageal cancer must start prior to treatment and be an ongoing consideration throughout the patient's lifetime. Because of the patients' altered anatomy, they are especially challenged on amounts and types of foods that can be consumed for an indefinite time frame after surgery.

Gastric Cancer

Gastric cancer is a disease in which malignant cells form in the lining of the stomach. The majority of gastric cancers, approximately 90%, are adenocarcinomas (Karpeh, Kelsen, & Tepper, 2001). The locations of gastric tumors have changed over the past 50 years, with a steady increase in patients diagnosed with proximal gastric and gastroesophageal junction adenocarcinomas (Blot, Devesa, Kneller, & Fraumeni, 1991). During the past half-century, the incidence of gastric cancer has dramatically declined. ACS estimated that approximately 21,860 cases will be diagnosed in the United States in 2005, and that approximately 11,550 people will die from the disease. Incidence of gastric cancer is twice as common in males as in females and occurs one-and-a-half times more frequently in African American males than in white males (Jemal et al., 2005).

Table 4-3. Special Considerations for Nutrition for Patients Who Have Had an Esophagectomy

Treatment	Diet Upgrade in Hospital	Diet Upgrade After Discharge
Esophagectomy	Usually nothing by mouth until postoperative day four On day four, a clear liquid diet, as well as an isotonic feeding, is started. Tube feedings are cycled to night feedings to free the patient through the day and to encourage increased oral intake. The patient may be on tube feedings from two to four weeks. By postoperative day seven or eight, the patient's diet is increased to a full liquid diet. By two to four weeks after surgery, tube feeds will be decreased as soft foods are tolerated.	Suggest two ounces of clear liquids every two hours, and increase until the patient is able to tolerate six ounces every four hours. Continue this schedule as the patient goes to full liquids. Encourage the patient to avoid carbonated soft drinks the first six to eight weeks after surgery. Encourage the patient to drink nutritional supplements several times per day if unable to eat enough regular foods to meet his or her nutritional needs. Avoid dairy products such as milk, cottage cheese, and pudding, as these may cause diarrhea. Encourage small, frequent meals throughout the day. Recommend that the patient sit up straight for one to two hours after each meal. Tell the patient to avoid sweets such as pies, cookies, and pastries that may cause diarrhea or dumping syndrome. Avoid foods that are spicy and gas forming to eliminate gastrointestinal distress.

Note. Based on information from Stralovich, 1993.

Worldwide areas of high incidence include China, South America, and Eastern Europe. Overall survival in the United States and most of the Western world is 5%–15%.

It is generally accepted that gastrointestinal cancers take many years to develop into invasive lesions. The sequential transformation in the gastric mucosa from normal to chronic gastritis progresses to multifocal atrophy, intestinal metaplasia of varying degrees, and finally to invasive carcinoma (Correa, 1992). Several factors have been identified that increase the risk of developing gastric cancer, including nutrition (high salt and nitrate use, low intake of vitamins A and C, and ingestion of salty or cured foods), occupation (workers in the rubber or coal industry), cigarette smoking, genetics (family history, hereditary nonpolyposis colon cancer, Li-Fraumeni syndrome), and the presence of precursor lesions (adenomatous gastric polyps, chronic atrophic gastritis, dysplasia, intestinal metaplasia) (Karpeh et al., 2001; Kurtz & Sherlock, 1985). In addition, infection with *Helicobacter pylori* also is associated with an increased risk of gastric cancer (NCI, 2004).

Clinical Presentation

At the time of presentation, gastric cancer usually is locally advanced or metastatic. The symptoms are vague and nonspecific and typically do not prompt the patient to seek early medical attention. On the other hand, when medical attention is sought, the symptoms do not result in an initial aggressive workup by the healthcare provider. Some of the early symptoms include weight loss, anorexia, and fatigue. As the tumor grows, the patient may complain of upper abdominal or epigastric discomfort. If a tumor is present at the pylorus, there may be vomiting, whereas tumors associated with gastroesophageal junction and cardia lesions typically present with dysphagia.

Physical examination of the patient may detect involvement of regional lymph nodes, such as the supraclavicular or axillary region. Spread along the peritoneal surface may reveal a periumbilical nodule (Sister Mary Joseph node) or malignant ascites. Laboratory results may reveal anemia or abnormal liver function tests.

Initial diagnosing and staging can be accomplished with endoscopy or biopsy. This procedure is useful in staging the depth of invasion of the primary tumor and is more accurate than CT scanning for staging tumor (T) and node (N) status. Pathologic stage remains the most important prognostic factor. There is a strong correlation between depth of invasion and extent and number of involved nodes. CT scanning of the chest and abdomen assists in evaluating the extent of disease. The routine use of PET scanning is not yet standard. One study from Germany described the use of PET scanning in evaluating response to preoperative chemotherapy (Ott et al., 2003). PET scanning, performed 14 days after cisplatin-based chemotherapy, correctly predicted histopathologic responses after three months of therapy in 77% of the responders and 86% of nonresponders. From this study, it was concluded that the use of PET scanning can facilitate the use of preoperative chemotherapy by early identification of those responding to the aggressive chemotherapy, thereby decreasing toxicity and resulting in lessened costs by reducing the number of ineffective therapies.

Another study in Belgium was conducted to assess the value of PET scanning in preoperative lymph node staging in patients with esophageal and gastroesophageal junction cancers (Lerut et al., 2000). This study demonstrated significantly higher accuracy with PET scanning when compared with combined CT and EUS, with a specificity of 90% versus 69%, respectively. Further studies are needed to validate these findings and establish a standard for the use of PET scanning in gastric cancer.

Screening

No prospective, controlled trials have been conducted to evaluate screening populations for gastric cancer. In Japan, where gastric cancer is endemic, screening programs have been successful in detecting early-stage lesions in

40%–60% of newly diagnosed patients. The five-year survival rates in patients with early-stage disease approached 50% (Karpeh et al., 2001).

Treatment

For early-stage gastric cancers, surgical resection with regional lymphadenectomy is standard therapy. The incidence of local failure in the tumor bed and regional lymph nodes as well as distant failure has remained high. Evaluations of clinical trials using adjuvant chemotherapy or radiotherapy as single modalities have not documented a significant impact on overall survival. In a phase III intergroup trial (INT-0166) (Meyerhardt & Fuchs, 2003), patients with completely resected adenocarcinomas of the stomach and gastroesophageal junction were randomized to receive surgery alone or surgery plus postoperative chemotherapy and concurrent radiotherapy. At five-year follow-up, a significant survival benefit was reported for the adjuvant combined modality treatment arm (MacDonald, Smalley, & Benedetti, 2001). Neoadjuvant chemoradiation therapy currently is under evaluation (Ajani, 2004). Patients with stage IV disease should be considered for clinical trials. In patients with distant metastases at the time of diagnosis, clinical trials are an option. Chemotherapy may provide palliation, although it has not been shown to prolong survival (Vanhoefer et al., 2000). Palliative techniques include endoluminal stenting and radiotherapy to stop bleeding or to address the issue of pain.

Nutritional Implications and Treatment

Many patients diagnosed with gastric cancer may have little to no symptoms at presentation. If symptoms occur, they may include unexplained weight loss, pain or discomfort in the stomach, dysphagia, indigestion, blood in stool, and decreased appetite.

Gastric tumors that involve the middle or upper part of the stomach may require a total gastrectomy, whereas tumors located in the antrum may be treated with a partial gastrectomy.

Acute postoperative weight loss is a major nutrition problem of both the partial and total gastrectomies (Bozzetti et al., 1990). Weight loss usually is caused by a combination of malabsorption, decreased oral intake, rapid intestinal transit time, and bacterial overgrowth (Bae, Park, Yang, & Kim, 1998; Liedman, Svedlund, Sullivan, Larson, & Lundell, 2001). Table 4-4 shows the common nutritional consequences from gastrectomy.

Nutrition assessment and intervention play a large role in the care of a patient with gastric cancer secondary to the problems of malabsorption and food intolerances that lead to weight loss (Braga, Zuliani, Foppa, DiCarlo, & Cristallo, 1988) (see Table 4-5). General guidelines for assessing nutrient needs are similar to other oncology diagnoses and can be found in Appendices F, G, H, and I. Early enteral nutrition after gastrectomy is necessary to prevent

Table 4-4. Special Considerations for Nutrition for Patients Who Have Had a Gastrectomy

Treatment	Diet Upgrade in Hospital	Diet Upgrade After Discharge
Gastrectomy	Usually nothing by mouth until postoperative day four On day four, a clear liquid diet, as well as an isotonic feeding, is started. Tube feedings are cycled to night feedings to free the patient throughout the day and to help to encourage increased oral intake. Patients may be on tube feedings from two to four weeks. By postoperative day seven or eight, patient's diet is increased to a full liquid diet.	Dietitian should instruct patient on diet progression prior to patient's discharge. Dietitian and nurse should coordinate and instruct patient on details of tube feeding and administration prior to patient's discharge. Suggest two ounces of clear liquids every two hours, and increase until patient is able to tolerate six ounces every four hours. By two to four weeks after surgery, tube feeds will be decreased as soft foods are tolerated. As diet progresses to soft diet, encourage patient to consume six to eight small meals and limit fluid intake (two to four ounces) with meals. No carbonated soft drinks are allowed the first six to eight weeks after surgery. Encourage patient to drink high-calorie liquid nutritional supplements several times per day if he or she is unable to eat enough regular foods to meet his or her nutritional needs. Dairy products such as milk, cottage cheese, and pudding may cause diarrhea and should be temporarily avoided. As patient starts soft foods, encourage small, frequent meals throughout the day. Recommend that the patient sit up straight for one to two hours after each meal. Tell patient to avoid sweets such as pies, cookies, and pastries that may cause diarrhea or dumping syndrome. Tell patient to avoid foods that are spicy and gas forming to eliminate gastrointestinal distress.

Note. Based on information from Stralovich, 1993.

malnutrition (Persson, Johansson, Sjoden, & Glimelius, 2002). Transition from enteral feeds to eating food alone may be difficult because of the nutrition problems associated with surgery. The registered dietitian plays a major role in the assessment and education of the patient who has had a gastrectomy immediately after surgery and beyond. Diet education of the patient after discharge is very important to help patients to maintain their weight and nutritional status.

Weight loss is a common problem after a gastrectomy. A large uncontrolled weight loss could lead to severe malnutrition with detrimental consequences.

Table 4-5. Common Side Effects of Gastric Cancer Treatment, Causes, and Management

Side Effect	Possible Causes	Management
Anemia	Decreased vitamin B_{12} absorption because of loss of intrinsic factor secondary to a total gastrectomy Decreased iron absorption from either a partial or a total gastrectomy. This can be a late complication of a gastrectomy. A folate deficiency may occur secondary to malabsorption.	Patient will need vitamin B_{12} levels measured at baseline and then every three months afterward. In a mild deficiency, may try oral vitamin B_{12}. In a severe deficiency, patient will require vitamin B_{12} internally. Patient will require iron supplementation for about four to six months if a deficiency is present. Patient will require a multivitamin with folate to prevent a deficiency.
Fat malabsorption	Increased transit time that prevents sufficient mixing of food with digestive enzymes Decreased enzyme production	Encourage patient to try a low-fat diet. Patient may need to use medium-chain triglycerides if steatorrhea is present. Patient may need pancreatic enzymes. Fat-soluble vitamins may need to be added to patient's diet.
Lactose intolerance	May occur despite intact jejunum	Encourage patient to try a low-fat diet. Encourage patient to use lactase enzymes.
Metabolic bone disease	Metabolic bone disease can be seen as a late complication after a gastrectomy. This may be caused by malabsorption of fat-soluble vitamins, including vitamin D, and poor food and lactose intake. Patients also may have decreased calcium metabolism.	Patient will need vitamin D and calcium supplementation in addition to a daily multivitamin.
Delayed gastric emptying	Patients with truncal vagotomy may have a higher incidence. Symptoms include discomfort or bloating that may last a few hours and possibly emesis.	Encourage smaller and more frequent meals. Patient may need a prokinetic agent.

(Continued on next page)

Table 4-5. Common Side Effects of Gastric Cancer Treatment, Causes, and Management (Continued)

Side Effect	Possible Causes	Management
Reactive hypo-glycemia	Can be the result of late dumping syndrome Late dumping is caused by a quick rise and then fall of blood sugars secondary to increased insulin. Can occur one to three hours after a meal and cause symptoms of sweating, palpitations, and fatigue	Encourage smaller and more frequent protein-dense meals. Tell patient to avoid large amounts of concentrated sweets.

Note. Based on information from Radigan & Parrish, 2004.

The clinical dietitian plays a large role in the assessment and planning of the patient's diet to help to prevent these side effects. This includes careful patient education to help the patient to manage the many food intolerances after gastrectomy as well as to help to prevent nutritional deficiencies that may lead to anemia and metabolic bone disease.

Summary

Patients who have had a gastrectomy will be challenged throughout their lifetime to maintain their weight and tolerate a varied diet. Close nutritional monitoring is needed for an indefinite time period after surgery to avoid malnutrition, weight loss, and nutritional deficiencies associated with the gastrectomy.

References

Ajani, J.A. (2004). *Phase II study of preoperative chemotherapy and chemoradiotherapy in patients with potentially resectable adenocarcinoma of the stomach.* Radiation Therapy Oncology Group Clinical Trial RTOG 99-04. Retrieved June 30, 2004, from http://www.rtog.org/members/protocols/99-04/99-04.pdf

Bae, J., Park, J., Yang, H., & Kim, J.D. (1998). Nutritional status of gastric cancer patients after total gastrectomy. *World Journal of Surgery, 22,* 254–261.

Bloch, A.S. (1990). Nutrition implications in esophageal and gastric cancer. In A.S. Bloch (Ed.), *Nutrition management of the cancer patient* (pp. 73–78). Sudbury, MA: Jones and Bartlett.

Blot, W.J., Devesa, S.S., Kneller, R.W., & Fraumeni, J.F., Jr. (1991). Rising incidence of adenocarcinomas of the esophagus and gastric cardia. *JAMA, 265,* 1287–1289.

Blot, W.J., & McLaughlin, J.K. (1999). The changing epidemiology of esophageal cancer. *Seminars in Oncology, 26*(5 Suppl. 15), 2–8.

Bozzetti, F., Ravera, E., Cozzaglio, L., Dossena, G., Agradi, E., Bonfanti, G., et al. (1990). Comparison of nutritional status after total or subtotal gastrectomy. *Nutrition, 6,* 371–375.

Braga, M., Zuliani, W., Foppa, L., DiCarlo, V., & Cristallo, M. (1988). Food intake and nutritional status after total gastrectomy: Results of a nutritional follow-up. *British Journal of Surgery, 75,* 477–480.

Brown, L.M. (1988). Environmental factors and high risk of esophageal cancer among men in coastal South Carolina. *Journal of the National Cancer Institute, 80,* 1620–1625.

Cantero, R., Torres, A.J., Hernando, F., Gallego, J., Lezana, A., Suarez, A., et al. (1999). Palliative treatment of esophageal cancer: Self-expanding metal stents versus post lethwait techniques. *Hepatogastroenterology, 46,* 971–976.

Cooper, J.S., Guo, M.D., Herskovic, A., MacDonald, J.S., Martenson, J.A., Al-Sarraf, M., et al. (1999). Chemoradiotherapy of locally advanced esophageal cancer: Long-term follow-up of a prospective randomized trial. Radiation Therapy Oncology Group. *JAMA, 281,* 1623–1627.

Correa, P. (1992). Human gastric carcinogenesis: A multistep and multifactorial process. First American Cancer Society Award Lecture on Cancer Epidemiology and Prevention. *Cancer Research, 5,* 6735–6740.

Dewys, W.D., Begg, C., Lavin, P.T., Band, P.R., Bennett, J.M., Bertino, J.R., et al. (1980). Prognostic effect of weight loss prior to chemotherapy in cancer patients. Eastern Cooperative Oncology Group. *American Journal of Medicine, 69,* 491–497.

Gerson, L.B., & Triadafilopoulos, G. (2002). Screening for esophageal adenocarcinoma: An evidence-based approach. *American Journal of Medicine, 113,* 499–505.

Guo, W., Li, J.Y., Blot, W.J., Hsing, A.W., Chen, J.S., & Fraumeni, J.F. (1990). Correlations of dietary intake and blood nutrient levels with esophageal cancer mortality in China. *Nutrition in Cancer, 13,* 121–127.

Iihara, K., Shiozaki, H., Tahara, H., Kobayashi, K., Inoue, M., Tamura, S., et al. (1993). Prognostic significance of transforming growth factor-alpha in human esophagus cancer. Implication for the autocrine proliferation. *Cancer, 71,* 2902–2909.

Itakura, Y., Sansano, H., Shiga, C., Furukawa, Y., Shiga, K., Mori, S., et al. (1994). Epidermal growth factor receptor overexpression in esophageal cancer. An immunohistochemical study correlated with clinicopathologic findings and DNA amplification. *Cancer, 74,* 795–804.

Jaskiewicz, K., Marasas, W.F., Rossouw, J.E., Van Niekerk, F.E., & Heine Tech, E.W. (1988). Selenium and other mineral elements in populations at risk for esophageal cancer. *Cancer, 62,* 2635–2639.

Jemal, A., Murray, T., Ward, E., Samuels, A., Tiwari, R.C., Ghafoor, A., et al. (2005). Cancer statistics, 2005. *CA: A Cancer Journal for Clinicians, 55,* 10–30.

Karpeh, M.S., Kelsen, D.P., & Tepper, J.E. (2001). Cancer of the stomach. In V.T. DeVita, Jr., S. Hellman, & S.A. Rosenberg (Eds.), *Cancer: Principles and practice of oncology* (6th ed., pp. 1092–1126). Philadelphia: Lippincott.

Kato, H., Kuwano, H., Nakajima, M., Miyazaki, T., Yoshikawa, M., Ojima, H., et al. (2002). Japan comparison between positron emission tomography and computed tomography in the use of the assessment of esophageal carcinoma. *Cancer, 94,* 921–928.

Kaur, B.S., & Triadafilopoulos, G. (2002). Acid- and bile-induced PGE(2) release and hyperproliferation in Barrett's esophagus are COX-2 and PKC-epsilon dependent. *American Journal of Physiology. Gastrointestinal and Liver Physiology, 283,* G327–G334.

Kelly, R.F., & Shumway, S.J. (2000). Conservative management of postoperative chylothorax using somatostatin. *Annals of Thoracic Surgery, 69,* 1944–1945.

Kelsen, D.P. (2004, January 22–24). *Neoadjuvant and adjuvant treatment of esophageal and gastroesophageal junction cancers.* Abstract presented at the Gastrointestinal Cancers Symposium, San Francisco, CA.

Kitagawa, Y., Ueda, M., Ando, N., Ozawa, S., Shimizu, N., & Kitajima, M. (1996). Further evidence for prognostic significance of epidermal growth factor receptor gene amplification in patients with esophageal squamous cell cancer. *Clinical Cancer Research, 2,* 909–914.

Koshy, M., Esiashvilli, N., Landry, J., Thomas, C.R., & Matthews, R.H. (2004a). Multiple management modalities in esophageal cancer: Combined modality management approaches. *Oncologist, 9,* 147–159.

Koshy, M., Esiashvilli, N., Landry, J., Thomas, C.R., & Matthews, R.H. (2004b). Multiple management modalities in esophageal cancer: Epidemiology, presentation and progression, work-up, and surgical approaches. *Oncologist, 9,* 137–146.

Krasna, M.J., Reed, C.E., Nedzwiecki, D., Hollis, D.R., Luketich, J.D., DeCamp, M., et al. (2001). CALGB 9380: A prospective trial of the feasibility of thoracoscopy/laparoscopy in staging esophageal cancer. *Annals of Thoracic Surgery, 71,* 1073–1079.

Kurtz, R.C., & Sherlock, P. (1985). The diagnosis of gastric cancer. *Seminars in Oncology, 12,* 11–18.

Lagergren, J., Bergstrom, R., Lindgren, A., & Nyren, O. (1999). Symptomatic gastroesophageal reflux as a risk factor for esophageal adenocarcinoma. *New England Journal of Medicine, 340,* 825–831.

Langstein, H.N., & Norton, J.A. (1991). Mechanisms of cancer cachexia. *Hematology/Oncology Clinics of North America, 5,* 103–123.

Lerut, T., Coosemans, W., Decker, G., De Leyn, P., Nafteux, P., & Van Raemdonck, D. (2002). Anastomotic complications after esophagectomy. *Digestive Surgery, 19*(2), 92–98.

Lerut, T., Flamen, P., Ectors, N., Van Cutsem, E., Peeters, M., Hiele, M., et al. (2000). Histopathologic validation of lymph node staging with FDG-PET scan in cancer of the esophagus and gastroesophageal junction: A prospective study based on primary surgery with extensive lymphadenectomy. *Annals of Surgery, 232,* 743–752.

Liedman, B., Svedlund, J., Sullivan, M., Larson, L., & Lundell, L. (2001). Symptom control may improve food intake, body composition, and aspect of quality of life after gastrectomy in cancer patients. *Digestive Diseases and Sciences, 46,* 2673–2680.

Lightdale, C.J., Heier, S.K., Marcon, N.E., McCaughan, J.S., Jr., Gerdes, H., Overholt, B.F., et al. (1995). Photodynamic therapy with porfirmer sodium versus thermal ablation with Nd:YAG laser for palliation of esophageal cancer: A multicenter randomized trial. *Gastrointestinal Endoscopy, 42,* 507–512.

Litle, V.R., Luketich, J.D., Christie, N.A., Buenaventura, P.O., Alvelo-Rivera, M., McCaughan, J.S., et al. (2003). Photodynamic therapy as palliation for esophageal cancer: Experience in 215 patients. *Annals of Thoracic Surgery, 76,* 1687–1692.

Luketich, J.D., Alvelo-Rivera, M., Buenaventura, P.O., Christie, N.A., McCaughan, J.S., Litle, V.R., et al. (2003). Minimally invasive esophagectomy: Outcomes in 222 patients. *Annals of Surgery, 238,* 486–494.

MacDonald, J.S., Smalley, S.R., & Benedetti, J. (2001). Chemoradiotherapy after surgery compared with surgery alone for adenocarcinoma of the stomach or gastroesophageal junction. *New England Journal of Medicine, 345,* 725–730.

Maier, A., Tomaselli, F., & Gebhard, F. (2000). Palliation of advanced esophageal cancer by photodynamic therapy and irradiation. *Annals of Thoracic Surgery, 69,* 1006.

Meltzer, C.C., Luketich, J.D., Friedman, D., Charron, M., Strollo, D., Meehan, M., et al. (2000). Whole-body FDG positron emission tomographic imaging for staging esophageal cancer comparison with computed tomography. *Clinical Nuclear Medicine, 25,* 882–887.

Meyerhardt, J.A., & Fuchs, C.S. (2003). Adjuvant therapy in gastric cancer: Can we prevent recurrences? *Oncology, 17,* 714–729.

National Cancer Institute. (2004, May 28). *Nutrition in cancer care.* Retrieved August 20, 2004, from http://www.cancer.gov/cancertopics/pdq/supportivecare/nutrition

Ott, K., Fink, U., Becker, K., Stahl, A., Dittler, H.J., Busch, R., et al. (2003). Prediction of response to preoperative chemotherapy in gastric carcinoma by metabolic imaging: Results of a prospective trial. *Journal of Clinical Oncology, 21,* 4604–4610.

Parrish, C., & McCray, S. (2004). When chyle leaks: Nutrition management options. *Practical Gastroenterology, 17,* 60–76.

Persson, C.R., Johansson, B.B., Sjoden, P.O., & Glimelius, B.L. (2002). A randomized study of nutritional support in patients with colorectal and gastric cancer. *Nutrition and Cancer, 42*(1), 48–58.

Pierre, A.F., & Luketich, J.D. (2002). Technique and role of minimally invasive esophagectomy for premalignant and malignant diseases of the esophagus. *Surgical Oncology Clinics of North America, 11,* 337–350.

Radigan, A.E., & Parrish, C.R. (2004). Post-gastrectomy: Managing the nutrition fall-out. *Practical Gastroenterology, 18,* 63–75.

Raijman, I., Siddique, I., Ajani, J., & Lynch, P. (1998). Palliation of malignant dysphagia and fistulae with coated expandable metal stents: Experience of 101 patients. *Gastrointestinal Endoscopy, 48,* 172–179.

Roncalli, M., Bosari, S., Marchetti, A., Buttitta, F., Bossi, P., Graziani, D., et al. (1998). Cell cycle related gene abnormalities and product expression in esophageal cancer. *Laboratory Investigations, 78,* 1049–1057.

Schrump, D.S., Altorki, N.K., Forastiere, A.A., & Minsky, B.D. (2001). In V.T. DeVita, S. Hellman, & S.A. Rosenberg (Eds.), *Cancer: Principles and practice of oncology* (6th ed., pp. 1051–1091). Philadelphia: Lippincott.

Senkal, M., Zumtobel, V., Bauer, K.H., Marpe, B., Wolfram, G., Frei, A., et al. (1999). Outcome and cost-effectiveness of perioperative enteral immunonutrition in patients undergoing elective upper gastrointestinal tract surgery: A prospective randomized trial. *Archives of Surgery, 134,* 1309–1316.

Shaheen, N., & Ransohoff, D.F. (2002). Gastroesophageal reflux, Barrett's esophagus, and esophageal cancer: Scientific review. *JAMA, 287,* 1972–1981.

Sharma, P. (1999). Barrett's esophagus: Put guidelines into practice. Patient care for the nurse. *Practitioner, 2*(9), 23–26.

Shepherd, A.A. (2003). Nutrition for optimum wound healing. *Nursing Standard, 18*(6), 55–58.

Shimada, Y., Imamura, M., Watanabe, G., Uchida, S., Harada, H., Makino, T., et al. (1999). Prognostic factors of oesophageal squamous cell carcinoma from the perspective of molecular biology. *British Journal of Cancer, 80,* 1281–1288.

Siemiatycki, J., Krewski, D., & Franco, E. (1995). Associations between cigarette smoking and each of 21 types of cancer: A multi-site case-control study. *International Journal of Epidemiology, 24,* 504–514.

Snyderman, C.H., Kachman, K., Molseed, L., Wagner, R., D'Amico, F., Bumpous, J., et al. (1999). Reduced postoperative infections with an immune-enhancing nutritional supplement. *Laryngoscope, 109,* 915–921.

Sontag, S.J. (2001). Preventing death of Barrett's cancer: Does frequent surveillance endoscopy do it? *American Journal of Medicine, 111*(Suppl. 8A), 137S–141S.

Spechler, S.J. (2002). Clinical practice: Barrett's esophagus. *New England Journal of Medicine, 34,* 836–842.

Stralovich, A. (1993). Gastrointestinal and pancreatic disease. In M.M. Gottschlich, L.E. Matarese, & E.P. Shronts (Eds.), *Nutrition support dietetics: Core curriculum* (2nd ed., pp. 275–284). Silver Spring, MD: American Society for Parenteral and Enteral Nutrition.

Takeuchi, H., Ozawa, S., Ando, N., Shih, C.H., Koyanagi, K., Ueda, M., et al. (1997). Altered p16/MTSI/CDKN2 and cyclin D1/PRAD-1 gene expression is associated with the prognosis of squamous cell carcinoma of the esophagus. *Clinical Cancer Research, 3,* 2229–2236.

Torosian, M.H., Buzby, G.P., & Presti, M.E. (1982). Reduction of methotrexate toxicity with improved nutritional status. *Surgical Forum, 33,* 109–112.

Vanhoefer, U., Rougier, P., Wilke, H., Ducreux, M.P., Lacave, A.J., Van Cutsem, E., et al. (2000). Final results of a randomized phase III trial of sequential high-dose methotrexate, fluorouracil, and doxorubicin versus etoposide, leucovorin, and fluorouracil versus infusional fluorouracil and cisplatin in advanced gastric cancer: A trial of the European Organization for Research and Treatment of Cancer Gastrointestinal Tract Cancer Cooperative Group. *Journal of Clinical Oncology, 18,* 2648–2657.

Vasques-Sequeiros, E., Norton, I.D., & Clain, J.E. (2001). Impact of EUS-guided fine-needle aspiration of lymph node staging in patients with esophageal carcinoma. *Gastrointestinal Endoscopy, 53,* 751–757.

Vaughan, T. (2004). *Molecular epidemiology of esophageal adenocarcinoma.* Abstract presented at the Gastrointestinal Cancers Symposium, San Francisco, CA.

World Cancer Research Fund & American Institute for Cancer Research. (1997). *Food, nutrition and the prevention of cancer: A global perspective*. Washington, DC: American Institute for Cancer Research.

Yang, C.S. (1980). Research on esophageal cancer in China: A review. *Cancer Research, 40*, 2633–2644.

CHAPTER 5

Genitourinary Cancers

Erin Dummert, RD, CD
Eileen Milakovic, MA, BSN, RN, OCN®, CHPN

Overview

The malignancies of the genitourinary system are distinctly different from one another and, thus, will be dealt with independently. The only commonalities among them include the absence of specific screening guidelines for any of the three sites (renal, bladder, and testicular) and the role of early detection as the mode of secondary prevention. Incidence, risk factors, prevention, and treatment modalities will be discussed separately for each type of cancer.

Renal Cell Carcinoma

Incidence

Malignancies that originate in the kidney are identified as renal cell carcinoma (RCC), renal adenocarcinoma, hypernephroma, or transitional cell carcinoma of the renal pelvis. New cases in 2005 are expected to be approximately 36,160, with more cases in men than in women. Expected deaths are 12,660, with approximately the same gender proportions as the incidence (American Cancer Society [ACS], 2005).

Risk Factors and Prevention

Occupational exposure to the organic solvent trichloroethylene has been shown to increase the risk of RCC. Exposure to this chemical can occur in a cardboard factory or where workers are greasing or degreasing metals. Asbestos exposure also is being studied with varied results (Golka, Wiese, Assennato, & Bolt, 2004).

Cigarette smoking (Moyad, 2001), obesity (Moyad; Shapiro, Williams, & Weiss, 1999), central adiposity (Nicodemus, Sweeny, & Folsom, 2004), high vitamin C intake (Nicodemus et al.), use of copper supplements in women (Nicodemus et al.), and hypertension (Moyad) are all known to increase the risk of RCC.

Factors known to decrease risk are vitamin E intake (Nicodemus et al., 2004), healthy eating habits (such as high intake of fruits and vegetables), lower caloric intake, and physical activity (Moyad, 2001).

Factors that may have some association but are not well understood or supported in the literature are alcohol and tea consumption. There are indications of effect modification by gender with alcohol consumption (Parker, Cerhan, Lynch, Ershow, & Cantor, 2002) and mixed results on tea consumption and RCC. Patients should be advised to minimize known risk factors and enhance protection against RCC by quitting smoking, avoiding megadose copper and vitamin C supplements, adopting a regular exercise program, eating more plant foods and fewer calories, and ensuring adequate vitamin E intake.

Treatment Modalities

As with most other solid malignancies, kidney cancers are considered curable if detected and treated early and when they are localized in the kidney and surrounding tissues. Primary treatment involves resection, either simple nephrectomy or a more radical procedure up to and including regional lymph node dissection. Surgical intervention (nephrectomy) causes few, if any, nutrition problems. Unilateral nephrectomy can contribute to a chronically decreased glomerular filtration rate without kidney damage; however, it is not certain whether individuals with a chronically decreased glomerular filtration rate (in the range of 60–89 ml/min/1.73 m^2) without kidney damage are at increased risk for adverse outcomes, such as toxicity from drugs excreted by the kidney or acute kidney failure (National Kidney Foundation, 2004). No data are available to support dietary restriction in this situation. Surgery can be considered a curative procedure for stage I or stage II cancers and often for stage III. Curative surgical resection also may be possible for a solitary metastatic lesion, especially in the lung, after a significant period of disease-free survival after initial treatment. Other options, if the patient is not a surgical candidate, involve external beam radiation therapy or arterial embolization.

Chemotherapy regimens generally have little impact on RCCs but can cause a variety of side effects that affect the patient's nutritional status. Some side effects, such as nausea, anorexia, fatigue, and early satiety, are common to many drugs. Knowing the treatment regimen and anticipating related side effects can impact the incidence and severity of side effects, thus decreasing the risk of nutritional deficiency and complications.

Biologic response modifiers are showing a slightly better response, especially in patients with pulmonary metastasis and an excellent performance status, even in stage IV disease. Current regimens involve the use of alpha interferon and interleukin-2 in a variety of dosing and scheduling regimens (National

Cancer Institute, 2003b). Side effects related to these regimens that create nutritional concerns include fever (56%), nausea and vomiting (31%), and diarrhea (25%) (Beveridge et al., 2002), each of which can contribute further to the risk of nutritional deficiency.

Thalidomide (Thalomid®, Celgene Corporation, Warren, NJ) is commonly used in the treatment of RCC. The most common side effects are constipation, drowsiness, somnolence, peripheral neuropathy, and rash (Celgene Corporation, 2003; Eisen, 2000; Motzer et al., 2002; Stebbing et al., 2001). Constipation caused by Thalomid is common but rarely is severe and can be alleviated by increased fluid intake and aggressive laxative therapy (Eisen). Thalomid appears to have some palliative effects on the symptoms of RCC, including enhanced or maintained appetite, improved sleep, and reduced sweating (Eisen). Thalomid also has been shown to help to reduce anorexia caused by immunotherapy treatment (Eisen).

Renal Function

RCC usually does not affect renal function to the extent that it would affect nutritional needs. However, in some cases, it can cause a decrease in renal function warranting dietary restriction. Patients with end-stage renal disease frequently require dialysis, which increases the need for dietary restrictions. The registered dietitian at the dialysis center will follow these patients closely.

Stages of renal disease are difficult to define. The National Kidney Foundation (2004) acknowledges that the proposed definition and classification of chronic kidney disease and stages are arbitrary and can be refined by further research. An elevation of serum creatinine up to more than 2 mg/dl frequently is used to indicate the need for dietary restrictions. Protein and phosphorus may be restricted to protect remaining kidney function; electrolytes may be restricted to avoid toxic serum levels; and fluid needs may be altered to avoid hypervolemia. Frequent monitoring of lab values will be a good guide as to which dietary restrictions are warranted. See Table 5-1 for specific nutrition guidelines.

Special Considerations for Nutrition

Use of herbal supplements may be unsafe for patients with RCC or kidney disease. Because kidney function may be reduced, the body may have a difficult time clearing these substances effectively. Discuss the following points with patients who are using or are considering using herbal supplements.
1. What may be safe for healthy individuals may not be safe for someone with RCC or kidney disease and, in fact, could be dangerous.
2. The government does not regulate herbal supplements, so the exact contents of these products, as well as the purity, safety, and effectiveness, are unknown.
3. Products may contain potassium, a mineral harmful to patients with diminished renal function.

Table 5-1. Energy and Nutritional Requirements in Genitourinary Cancers

Nutritional Factor	Renal Cell Carcinoma	Bladder Carcinoma	Testicular Carcinoma
Calorie needs*			
Weight maintenance	20–25 Kcals/kg dry wt	20–25 Kcals/kg dry wt	20–25 Kcals/kg dry wt
Weight gain	30–35 Kcals/kg dry wt	30–35 Kcals/kg dry wt	30–35 Kcals/kg dry wt
Obese patient	Use adjusted body weight**	Use adjusted body weight**	Use adjusted body weight**
Protein needs***			
Normal kidney function	1.0–1.5 g protein/kg ideal body weight (IBW)	1.0–1.5 g protein/kg IBW	1.0–1.5 g protein/kg IBW
Pre–end-stage renal disease (ESRD)****	0.6–0.8 g protein/kg IBW	–	–
Pre-ESRD with hypoalbuminuria	0.8–1.0 g protein/kg IBW	–	–
Phosphorus	800–1,200 mg/day	–	–
Pre-ESRD	8–12 mg/kg IBW	–	–
Potassium	3.5 g/day	3.5 g/day	–
Urine output < 1,000 ml/day	Specific recommendations depend on size of patient and other factors affecting potassium level.	–	–
Sodium	2,400 mg/day (average intake 4,000–5,000 mg/day)	2,400 mg/day (averge intake 4,000–5,000 mg/day)	–
Pre-ESRD or hypertension	1,000–3,000 mg/day	–	–
Calcium	1,000–1,200 mg/day	–	–
Pre-ESRD	1,200–1,600 mg/day	–	–
Magnesium	300–400 mg/day	–	–

(Continued on next page)

Table 5-1. Energy and Nutritional Requirements in Genitourinary Cancers (Continued)

Nutritional Factor	Renal Cell Carcinoma	Bladder Carcinoma	Testicular Carcinoma
Iron	10–18 mg/day	–	–
Fluids	1 cc/Kcal of estimated calorie needs	1 cc/Kcal of estimated calorie needs	1 cc/Kcal of estimated calorie needs
Pre-ESRD	Typically unrestricted	–	–
Hypertension	Restrict and monitor frequently	–	–
B vitamins			
B$_1$ (thiamine)	1.5 mg/day	–	–
B$_2$ (riboflavin)	1.7 mg/day	–	–
B$_{3/4}$ (niacin/ nicotinamide)	15–20 mg/day	–	–
B$_5$ (pantothenic acid)	10 mg/day	–	–
B$_6$ (pyridoxine)	2–2.5 mg/day	–	–
B$_7$ (biotin)	300 mcg/day	–	–
B$_9$ (folic acid)	400 mcg/day	–	–
B$_{12}$ (cyanocobala-min)	4–6 mg/day	–	–

* These guidelines should be viewed as a starting point for determining energy needs. Actual calorie needs may vary and can be adjusted up or down as needed.
** Adjusted body weight [(actual wt – IBW) x .25] + IBW
*** 2/3 protein should be of high biologic value (meat and dairy products)
**** Pre-ESRD is defined as serum creatinine 2–4 mg/dl (Allen, 1999)

4. Some herbs that may serve as diuretics also may cause kidney irritation or damage. These include bucha leaves and juniper berries. Uva ursi and parsley capsules may have serious side effects (iKidney.com, 2000).
5. Many herbs can interact with prescription drugs, even at low doses. A few examples are St. John's wort, echinacea, ginkgo, garlic, ginseng, ginger, and blue cohosh.
6. Patients should discuss the use of any herbal or nutritional supplement with their oncologist.
7. Remind patients that "natural" does not mean "safe." See Table 5-2 for specific herbs and their safety in kidney disease.

Table 5-2. Unsafe Herbs

Herb Name	Toxic to Kidneys	Harmful in Kidney Disease	Unsafe for All People
Alfalfa		X	
Aloe		X	
Artemisia absinthium (wormwood)	X		
Autumn crocus	X		
Bayberry		X	
Blue cohosh		X	
Broom		X	
Buckthorn		X	
Capsicum		X	
Cascara		X	
Chapparal			X
Chuifong tuokuwan (black pearl)	X		
Coltsfoot		X	
Comfrey			X
Dandelion		X	
Ephedra (ma huang)			X
Epimedium sagittatum		X	
Ginger		X	
Ginseng, panax		X	
Horse chestnut	X		
Horsetail		X	
Licorice		X	
Lobelia			X
Mandrake			X
Mate		X	
Nettle		X	
Noni juice		X	
Pennyroyal			X
Periwinkle	X		
Pokeroot			X
Rhubarb		X	
Sassafras			X
Senna		X	
Tung shueh	X		
Vandelia cordifolia	X		
Vervain		X	
Yohimbe			X

Note. Based on information from iKidney.com, 2000; National Kidney Foundation, 2004.

Bladder Cancer

Bladder cancer is considered to be one of the more curable malignancies, as 70%–80% are diagnosed at an early stage (T1 or less, a superficial presentation) (National Cancer Institute, 2003a). Primary prognostic factors at the time of diagnosis include the depth of invasion and degree of differentiation. Most superficial tumors are well differentiated and, therefore, have a good prognosis. Another positive prognostic indicator includes a complete response to treatment with bacillus Calmette-Guérin (BCG). Adverse prognosis in patients with invasive bladder cancer has been identified with expression of the tumor suppressor gene *p53*. Most bladder cancers are transitional cell carcinomas. Other cell types include squamous cell (6%–8%) and adenocarcinomas (2%) (National Cancer Institute, 2003a).

Incidence

The estimated number of new cases of bladder cancer in 2005 is 63,210, and the estimated number of deaths is 13,180. These statistics have plateaued since 1987–2000. Bladder cancer occurs four times more often in men than in women and one-and-a-half times more often in Whites than in African Americans (ACS, 2005).

Risk Factors and Prevention

Smoking is responsible for approximately 48% of bladder cancer deaths in men and 28% in women. Smokers have twice the risk of bladder cancer as do nonsmokers. Frequency and duration of smoking (number of pack-years) also is an indicator of risk (Zeegers, Kellen, Buntinx, & Van Den Brandt, 2004). Workers who are at risk for bladder cancer because of exposure to chemicals include those involved with processing aromatic amines, rubber industry workers, coke oven workers, dyers in textile and leather industries, and painters and varnishers. The chemical culprits in these industries are benzidine and β-napthylamine. Those who work at dry cleaners also are at an increased risk because of exposure to the known carcinogen perchloroethylene (Golka et al., 2004). People employed in occupations with a high likelihood of exposure to hair dyes over a period of 10 years or more have a fivefold increased risk of bladder cancer. The carcinogenic substance in hair dye is believed to be aromatic amines. Evidence has not supported an increased risk for bladder cancer with personal use of hair dyes (Gago-Domingues, Castelao, Uan, Yu, & Ross, 2001). Patients with bladder cancer should be encouraged to reduce their risk for recurrence by avoiding known risk factors, as noted earlier, and by including foods that have been shown to reduce cancer risk. Dietary factors that have been shown to increase risk are consumption of soft drinks, coffee, and alcohol (Radosavljevic, Jankovic, Marinkovic, & Djokic, 2003). Factors that minimize bladder cancer risk are high doses of vitamins A, B_6, and E and zinc, although no recommendation for amounts has been set (Kamat & Lamm, 2000). Long-term (≥ 10 years) vitamin E supplementation has been associated with a reduced risk of bladder cancer mortality; however, the dosing is not clear (Jacobs et al., 2002). Mineral water, skim milk, yogurt, and frequency of urination all have been identified as protective factors for bladder carcinoma (Radosavljevic et al.). Tea consumption and a high intake of vegetables may be associated with a reduced risk of bladder cancer; however, studies on these subjects have shown mixed results (Bianch et al., 2000; Michaud et al., 2002; Pelucchi, LaVecchia, Negri, Dal Maso, & Franceschis, 2002).

Treatment Modalities

Many bladder cancers are detected at an early stage, with hematuria alarming patients enough to seek care. Prolonged survival for early-stage disease is demonstrated when treated by trans-urethral resection (TUR) with or without intravesicle chemotherapy. Intravesicle chemotherapy treatments for bladder cancer can cause bladder irritation, such as dysuria and frequency. Other unique side effects, such as myelosuppression or contact dermatitis, may be specific to a particular drug (Shipley et al., 2005). Bladder irritation is a distressing side effect for many patients. Irritation may be dramatically decreased by avoiding bladder irritants such as alcohol, caffeine, spicy foods, sugar, milk products, acidic fruit or juice, and carbonated beverages and bladder stimulants such as tea.

More invasive tumors may require segmental cystectomy or radical cystectomy with urinary diversion of some sort. Segmental cystectomy causes a decrease in bladder capacity, which usually is temporary but can be long-lasting. Patients with decreased bladder capacity should avoid drinking large amounts of fluids at any one time and should avoid bladder irritants and stimulants such as tea, alcohol, and caffeine.

Radical cystectomy often is accompanied by a standard ileal conduit in which urine drains directly from the ureters through a segment of ileum to the skin surface, where it is collected. Some patients with this form of diversion develop hypochloremic acidosis, hyperkalemia, hyponatremia, and uremia. Ureteral obstruction and urinary tract infection also are relatively common. More recently, storage reservoirs such as a Koch pouch are being constructed from a section of bowel allowing for a better quality of life.

Patients presenting with multiple or recurring tumors are treated with intravesicle therapy with chemotherapeutic agents such as thiotepa, mitoxantrone, doxorubicin, or BCG after TUR. Standard treatment for stage II cancer and greater usually is radical cystectomy, with or without pelvic lymph node dissection. Other options for these patients with late-stage disease include external beam radiation therapy, possibly with systemic chemotherapy. The chemotherapy regimen used can consist of methotrexate, vinblastine, doxorubicin, and cisplatin and may be used neoadjuvantly (National Cancer Institute, 2003a). Systemic chemotherapy treatments for bladder cancer often cause a reduced appetite, nausea and vomiting, and mouth sores. Systemic chemo-therapy often results in a decreased white blood cell count, thus increasing the risk of infection and resulting in the need for a neutropenic diet, which may decrease the risk of food-borne illness by eliminating potentially unsafe foods. Red blood cell and platelet counts also may be reduced, resulting in decreased energy and easy bruising or bleeding.

Testicular Cancer

Testicular cancer accounts for approximately 1% of cancers in men. Of greatest concern, however, is the age at which it occurs. It is primarily a disease of men younger than 40. The cell types causing testicular cancer are classi-fied as seminoma, nonseminoma, or a combination of the two. Treatment regimens and prognosis differ for each. With prompt, appropriate treatment, even in later stages, it is considered to be potentially curable (National Cancer Institute, 2003c).

Incidence

Testicular cancer is the most common cancer in white men from age 20–34, the third most common in 15–19-year-olds, and the second most common in 35–39-year-olds. It is seen four-and-a-half times more often in Whites than African Americans, with intermediate ranges seen in other ethnic populations (National Cancer Institute, 2003c).

An estimated 8,010 new cases of testicular cancer will be identified in 2005 and approximately 390 deaths (ACS, 2005). Testicular cancer rarely affects nutritional status as other genitourinary cancers can.

Risk Factors

In addition to age and race (and gender), several other distinct risk factors for testicular cancer exist. Males with cryptorchidism have a 3–17 times greater risk of having it. This risk is greatly decreased when correc-tive surgery is performed before age six. Also at risk are those with gonadal dysgenesis, Klinefelter's syndrome, or a family or personal history of tes-ticular cancer.

No prevention measures for testicular cancer currently have been identi-fied. Knowledge of the causes of testicular cancer risk and its association with diet remain limited (Garner et al., 2003) and should be further examined (Sigurdson et al., 1999). Despite this, a few studies have found associations between diet and testicular cancer. Factors that have been shown to increase testicular cancer risk seem to differ by histology, suggesting that seminoma, nonseminoma, and mixed germ cell testicular cancer may have different etiolo-gies (Bonner, McCann, & Moysich, 2002). Diets high in total fat, saturated fat, animal fat, and dairy products (cheese) are associated with an increased risk of seminoma and mixed germ cell testicular cancer (Bonner et al.; Garner et al.; Sigurdson et al.). Vitamin E is suggestive of reduced risk for nonseminoma and mixed germ cell testicular cancer, but it also is suggestive of an increased risk for seminoma testicular cancer (Bonner et al.). Another study found a decreased testicular cancer risk in men who ate more fruits and vegetables (Sigurdson et al.).

Treatment

Treatment choices for testicular cancer are based on cell type. Initial intervention involves radical inguinal orchiectomy, primarily because transscrotal biopsy is not used because of the potential for seeding and local dissemination. This procedure allows for cellular identification of tumor type. Any tumor not able to be conclusively identified as purely seminoma is treated as mixed or nonseminoma.

After surgery, seminomas are treated with radiation therapy, often including radiation therapy to retroperitoneal lymph nodes. Nutritional concerns are related to the impact on other organs in the field of radiation, specifically a risk of diarrhea and nausea. As seminomas are highly sensitive to radiation, cure rates at any stage exceed 90% (National Cancer Institute, 2003c).

In patients with nonseminomas, or a mixture of cell types, treatment plans are aggressive even with widespread metastasis, as they can still be curable. Evaluations of serum tumor markers are a component of care in patients with testicular cancer, in identifying both prognosis and response to treatment. Markers monitored at the time of diagnosis, during treatment, and for the remainder of the patient's life include alpha-fetoprotein, beta human chorionic gonadotropin, and lactate dehydrogenase.

Chemotherapy is the treatment of choice for mixed or nonseminomas after initial surgery. Several chemotherapy regimens currently are in use, and stem cell transplant after high-dose chemotherapy also is being evaluated. Patients receiving the most widely used regimen with bleomycin, etoposide, and cisplatin are at risk for nutritional complications related to nausea and vomiting, as are those receiving a regimen with etoposide, ifosfamide, cisplatin, and mesna. Other regimens include cisplatin, vinblastine, and bleomycin or vinblastine, dactinomycin, bleomycin, cyclophosphamide, and cisplatin.

Patients receiving a preparative regimen for stem cell transplant of carboplatin and etoposide have significant problems (29%) with both diarrhea and mucositis (Beveridge et al., 2002) and may require more aggressive nutritional support throughout the transplant process.

Although studies do not show a strong correlation between testicular cancer and diet, the recommendations to eat less animal fat, total fat, and saturated fat and to eat more fruits and vegetables is consistent with the dietary recommendations for reducing the risk of many chronic diseases, including heart disease, diabetes, and various cancers. Patients should be encouraged to change their eating habits to maximize their quality of life and longevity following treatment.

Assessment Guidelines

The goal of nutrition assessment of the patient with genitourinary cancer is to identify nutritional status with regard to overall nutritional requirements, adequacy of nutrient intake and utilization, as well as any existing nutrient deficiencies or risk of poor nutritional status. The nutrition assessment usually serves as a basis on which a nutrition care plan can be developed. Parameters that should be included in a comprehensive nutrition assessment are patient history, a physical examination, anthropometric measurements, and biochemical data (see Table 5-3).

Useful laboratory tests for evaluation of nutritional status include those pertinent to visceral protein stores, immune competence, nutritional anemias, and vitamin-mineral adequacy (Allen, 1999). Lab values also may identify impaired absorption or utilization of many nutrients. It is important to remember that infection, hepatic and renal disease, dehydration, drugs, treatment, surgery, and stress all may affect the interpretation of lab values (Allen). Table 5-3 lists biochemical measurements that should be considered in renal cell, bladder, and testicular carcinomas.

Care Planning

Care planning is an essential part of health care, but it often is misunderstood or regarded as a waste of time. Without a specific document delineating the plan of care, important issues are likely to be neglected. The nutritional care plan should include proposed nutrient needs, modalities for providing nutrients, and monitoring criteria by which adequacy of nutrient provision and tolerance to therapy are measured. See Table 5-1 for guidelines detailing the nutritional needs of the patient with genitourinary cancer.

Summary

The cancers of the genitourinary system are each distinctly different, with differing incidence rates, risk factors, and treatment modalities. In addition, patients with cancers of the genitourinary system may have distinctly different nutritional needs depending on a variety of factors, including eating habits prior to diagnosis, side effects of the disease, and treatment modality. The nutrition assessment and care plan are essential to ensuring that each patient's nutritional needs are appropriately identified and addressed.

Table 5-3. Biochemical Measurements to Consider in the Treatment of Genitourinary Cancer

Biochemical Measurement	Renal Cell Carcinoma	Bladder Carcinoma	Testicular Carcinoma
Absolute neutrophil count	X	X	X
Albumin (serum)	X	X	X
Alkaline phosphatase	X		
Alanine aminotransferase	X		
Aspartate aminotransferase	X		
Blood glucose	X		
Blood urea nitrogen	X	X	
Calcium (serum)	X		
Chloride	X	X	
Creatinine (serum)	X	X	X
Ferritin (serum)	X		
Hemoglobin and hematocrit	X	X	X
Iron (serum)	X		
Magnesium (serum)	X		
Phosphorus	X		
Potassium	X	X	
Prealbumin (serum)	X	X	X
Sodium	X	X	
Total iron binding capacity	X		
Total protein (serum)	X	X	X
Transferrin (serum)	X		
Platelet count	X	X	X

References

Allen, C. (1999). Protein modifications. In C. Allen (Ed.), *Medical nutrition therapy Cincinnati diet manual* (6th ed., pp. 14–26). Cincinnati, OH: Greater Cincinnati Dietetic Association.

American Cancer Society. (2005). *Cancer facts and figures, 2005*. Atlanta, GA: Author.

Beveridge, R., Reitan, J., Fausel, C., Leather, H., McFarland, H., & Valley, A. (Eds.). (2002).

Guide to selected cancer chemotherapy regimens and associated adverse events (3rd ed.). Thousand Oaks, CA: Amgen.

Bianchi, G.D., Cerhan, J.R., Parker, A.S., Putnam, S.D., See, W.A., Lynch, C.F., et al. (2000). Tea consumption and risk of bladder and kidney cancers in a population-based case-control study. *American Journal of Epidemiology, 151*, 377–383.

Bonner, M.R., McCann, S.E., & Moysich, K.B. (2002). Dietary factors and the risk of testicular cancer. *Nutrition and Cancer, 44*, 35–43.

Celgene Corporation. (2003). Thalomid® [Package insert]. Warren, NJ: Author

Eisen, T.G. (2000). Thalidomide in solid tumors: The London experience. *Oncology, 14*, 17–20.

Gago-Dominguez, M., Castelao, J., Yuan, J., Yu, M., & Ross, R. (2001). Use of permanent hair dyes and bladder cancer risk. *International Journal of Cancer, 91*, 575–579.

Garner, M.J., Birkett, N.J., Johnson, K.C., Shatenstein, B., Ghadirian, P., Krewski, D., et al. (2003). Dietary risk factors for testicular carcinoma. *International Journal of Cancer, 106*, 934–941.

Golka, K., Wiese, A., Assennato, D., & Bolt, H. (2004). Occupational exposure and urological cancer. *World Journal of Urology, 21*, 382–391.

iKidney.com. (2000). *Herbal supplements for renal patients: What do we know?* Retrieved April 9, 2004, from http://www.ikidney.com/nr/ikidney/articles/herbalsupp_herbs1.pdf

Jacobs, E.J., Henion, A.K., Briggs, P.J., Connell, C.J., McCullough, M.L., Jonas, C.R., et al. (2002). Vitamin C and vitamin E supplement use and bladder cancer mortality in a large cohort of U.S. men and women. *American Journal of Epidemiology, 156*, 1002–1010.

Kamat, A.M., & Lamm, D.L. (2000). Diet and nutrition in urologic cancer. *West Virginia Medical Journal, 96*, 449–454.

Michaud, D.S., Pietinen, P., Taylor, P.R., Virtanen, M., Virtamo, J., & Albanes, D. (2002). Intakes of fruits and vegetables, carotenoids and vitamins A, E, in relation to the risk of bladder cancer in the ATBC cohort study. *British Journal of Cancer, 21*, 960–965.

Motzer, R.J., Berg, W., Ginsberg, M., Russo, P., Vuky, J., Yu, R., et al. (2002). Phase II trial of thalidomide for patients with advanced renal cell carcinoma. *Journal of Clinical Oncology, 20*, 302–306.

Moyad, M.A. (2001). Review of potential risk factors for kidney (renal cell) cancer. *Seminars in Urologic Oncology, 19*, 280–293.

National Cancer Institute. (2003a). *Bladder cancer (PDQ®): Treatment.* Retrieved April 16, 2004, from http://www.nci.nih.gov/cancerinfo/pdq/treatment/bladder/healthprofessional

National Cancer Institute. (2003b). *Renal cell cancer (PDQ®): Treatment.* Retrieved April 16, 2004, from http://www.nci.nih.gov/cancerinfo/pdq/treatment/renalcell/healthprofessional

National Cancer Institute. (2003c). *Testicular cancer (PDQ®): Treatment.* Retrieved April 16, 2004, from http://www.nci.nih.gov/cancerinfo/pdq/treatment/testicular/healthprofessional

National Kidney Foundation. (2004). *Use of herbal supplements in chronic kidney disease.* Retrieved April 9, 2004, from http://www.kidney.org/general/news/factsheet.cfm?id=26

Nicodemus, K.K., Sweeny, C., & Folsom, A.R. (2004). Evaluation of dietary, medical and lifestyle risk factors for incident kidney cancer in postmenopausal women. *International Journal of Cancer, 108*, 115–121.

Parker, A.S., Cerhan, J.R., Lynch, C.F., Ershow, A.G., & Cantor, K.P. (2002). Gender, alcohol consumption and renal cell carcinoma. *American Journal of Epidemiology, 155*, 455–462.

Pelucchi, C., La Vecchia, C., Negri, E., Dal Maso, L., & Franceschis, S. (2002). Smoking and other risk factors for bladder cancer in women. *Preventive Medicine, 35*, 114–120.

Radosavljevic, V., Jankovic, S., Marinkovic, J., & Djokic, M. (2003). Fluid intake and bladder cancer. A case control study. *Neoplasma, 50*, 234–238.

Shapiro, J.A., Williams, M.A., & Weiss, N.S. (1999). Body mass index and risk of renal cell carcinoma. *Epidemiology, 10*, 188–191.

Shipley, W.U., Kaufman, D.S., McDougal, W.S., Dahl, D.M., Michaelson, M.D., & Zietman, A.L. (2005). Cancer of the bladder, ureter, and renal pelvis. In V.T. DeVita, S. Hellman, & S.A. Rosenberg (Eds.), *Cancer: Principles and practice of oncology* (7th ed., pp. 1168–1192). Philadelphia: Lippincott Williams & Wilkins.

Sigurdson, A.J., Chang, S., Annegers, J.F., Duphorne, C.M., Pillow, P.C., Amato, R.J., et al. (1999). A case-control study of diet and testicular carcinoma. *Nutrition and Cancer, 34,* 20–26.

Stebbing, J., Benson, C., Eisen, T., Pyle, L., Smalley, K., Bridle, H., et al. (2001). The treatment of advanced renal cell cancer with high-dose oral thalidomide. *British Journal of Cancer, 85,* 953–958.

Zeegers, S., Kellen, M., Buntinx, E., & Van Den Brandt, F. (2004). Associations between smoking, beverage consumption, diet and bladder cancer—A systematic literature review. *World Journal of Urology, 6,* 392–401.

CHAPTER 6

Gynecologic Cancers

Kathryn Hamilton, MA, RD, CDN
Susan M. Roche, CRNP, MSN, OCN®, APRN-BC

Overview

The gynecologic cancers covered in this chapter include ovarian, cervical, and endometrial. Together they account for approximately 12% of the cancers diagnosed in women each year (Jemal et al., 2005).

Ovarian Cancer

Epidemiology

Ovarian cancer has been called the "silent killer" for many decades (Ozols, Schwartz, & Eifel, 2001). The majority of patients present with advanced disease, usually stage III or IV (Barnes, Grizzle, Grubbs, & Partridge, 2002). Ovarian cancer ranks as the number-one cause of death from gynecologic malignancy. In 2005, an estimated 22,220 new cases of ovarian cancer will be diagnosed, and approximately 16,210 women will die from the disease (Jemal et al., 2005). The insidious nature of this disease makes it the fourth leading cause of cancer death in women (Barnes et al.). It is the leading cause of death in industrialized countries with the exception of Japan. However, Japanese women who immigrate to the United States adopt the incidence of U.S. women by the second generation. Women with higher educational and socioeconomic levels tend to delay childbearing, have fewer children, and have a higher incidence of ovarian cancer. Ovarian cancer rarely is seen in developing nations.

Following aggressive surgical resection, chemotherapy can produce clinical responses in 70% of cases, but the majority will relapse. Response to treatment usually is brief (Barnes et al., 2002). Five-year survival rates have modestly increased from 36% in 1970 to 50% in 1994. African American women have a lower incidence than white women, but five-year survival rates are similar (Ozols et al., 2001). Overall, little improvement in long-term survival has been seen over the past 30 years. The disease is still difficult to diagnose, intensive treatment has not been curative, high-risk populations have not been clearly defined, and, essentially, the etiology of this cancer killer of women is unknown (Barnes et al.).

Pathology

The actual carcinogenic process involved in the development of ovarian cancer is quite complex. It involves a multistage process that requires further scientific study (Ozols et al., 2001). In general, epithelial ovarian cancers arise from the ovarian surface epithelium after a malignant transformation. Alterations in DNA quantities and anatomic structure have been demonstrated and linked to alterations in cellular oncogene activity and growth factor signal transformations (Sonoda, 2004). Carcinogenic pathways have been suggested to include uninterrupted ovulation, leading to a growth-stimulating hormonal environment, which increases the probability of genetic lesions and tumor-prone clones (Barnes et al., 2002). Common epithelial tumors account for 60% of all ovarian neoplasms and for 80%–90% of ovarian malignancies; the remaining 10%–20% arise from germ or stromal cells (Ozols et al.).

Epithelial tumors arise from the surface epithelium or serosa of the ovary. During embryogenesis, the lining of the celomic cavity consists of mesothelial cells of mesodermal origin, and the gonadal ridge is covered by serosal epithelium. Mullerian ducts, which give rise to the fallopian tubes, uterus, and vagina, are the result of invagination of the mesothelial lining. When the epithelium becomes malignant, it can express a variety of mullerian-type differentiations. Serous carcinomas can resemble the fallopian tubes, mucinous tumors, and the endocervix, and endometrioid carcinomas can resemble the endometrium. Clear cell malignancies can resemble the endometrial glands occurring in pregnancy, which may be responsible for their worse prognosis (Ozols et al., 2001). Germ cell tumors originate in a primitive streak and can migrate to the gonads. The mesenchyma give rise to the ovarian stromal tumors (Ozols et al.).

Most ovarian malignancies originate from the epithelial surface of the ovary; they invade the stromal tissue and penetrate the capsule of the ovary. The most common mechanisms of disease spread include direct extension, peritoneal seeding, and lymphatic spread. Direct extensions of the malignant cells on the surface of the ovary invade the adjacent structures, including the fallopian tubes, uterus, bladder, rectosigmoid colon, and pelvic peritoneum. Peritoneal seeding occurs when cells exfoliate into the peritoneal cavity, where they are carried in fluid via the posterior paracolic spaces to the subdiaphragmatic surfaces, facilitating widespread dissemination of malignant tumor cells. All of the peritoneal surfaces are at risk, including the omentum, which is a frequent site of tumor involvement (Ozols et al., 2001). Lymphatic spread also is very common. Approximately 10% of women who appear to have localized disease have paraaortic lymphatic metastases. In addition, the retroperitoneal lymph nodes are found to be involved in the majority of advanced ovarian cancer cases (Ozols et al.). Hematogenous spread of ovarian cancer to extra-abdominal sites is uncommon. Dissemination of disease easily can be missed without meticulous histologic examination of visually normal tissues throughout the peritoneal cavity, including the undersurface of the diaphragm (Ozols et al.). Epithelial ovarian cancer usually is diagnosed in postmenopausal women. The median age at diagnosis is 63.

Risk Factors and Prevention

The goal of optimal oncologic intervention for ovarian cancer would be to screen high-risk individuals to identify early-stage disease amenable to curative surgical resection. Early-stage ovarian cancer comprises only approximately one-third of all cases and is associated with a five-year survival rate ranging from 66%–90% (Sonoda, 2004). Unfortunately, the insidious nature of this disease makes early detection an extremely difficult goal. The first obstacle is the low prevalence of ovarian cancer. It is difficult to justify widespread screening when very few cases will be diagnosed. The National Institutes of Health consensus conference held in 1995 concluded that no screening test has proved to be an effective modality to reduce the mortality of ovarian cancer (Sonoda). Prevention strategies provide the only rational approach to reduce overall mortality (Ozols et al., 2001).

Identifying risk factors can be an important tool for assessing an individual's risk of developing ovarian cancer. The strongest risk factor is a history of multiple family members with ovarian cancer. Unfortunately, only about 10% of cases are considered hereditary ovarian cancer. One high-risk population is women of Russian-Jewish descent. These hereditary ovarian cancers may be related to the inherited BRCA1 or BRCA2 gene mutations. Several factors seem to reduce the incidence in this high-risk group of individuals. Use of oral contraceptives or multiparity has been shown to reduce occurrence. Prophylactic oophorectomy at age 35 still leaves the risk for peritoneal carcinomatosis (Barnes et al., 2002). Close surveillance and screening with vaginal ultrasound, pelvic examination, and serial CA-125 levels has been advocated in this population. Another risk factor for ovarian cancer is an uninterrupted ovulation. Incessant ovulation increases the probability of mutational events that lead to promotional factors, contributing to malignant transformation. Women at greater risk include nulliparous women and, to a lesser degree, women who first become pregnant after age 35 (O'Rourke & Mahon, 2003). Higher risk also is associated with high dietary fat intake and low fiber consumption. This link may be related to obesity and the "estrogen storing" properties of adipose tissue, especially in premenopausal women (O'Rourke & Mahon). A personal history of breast or colon cancer, especially before the age of 50, increases the risk three to four times more than the general population for the development of ovarian cancer (O'Rourke & Mahon).

Factors that appear to reduce the incidence of ovarian cancer relate to the reduction of ovulatory events, decreasing the probability of genetically damaged cells (Barnes et al., 2002). Multiparity is associated with decreased risk of ovarian cancer, especially in conjunction with lactation, which also suppresses ovulation (O'Rourke & Mahon). Progestins may influence apoptosis, leading to cellular death of potentially malignant precursor cells (Barnes et al.). Tubal ligation and hysterectomy reduce the risk despite leaving the ovaries intact. It is postulated that these surgeries block direct ovary exposure to the environment (Barnes et al.). Reduced risk has been seen with the use of oral contraceptives, even after they have been used only for a few months. Combination estrogen/progesterone therapy for at least three years reduces the risk by approximately 40%. The greatest benefit in oral contraceptive users occurs in those who have used them longer than four to six years. Reduction in risk diminishes over time after cessation of hormonal influence (Barnes et al.). One chemoprevention trial demonstrated a reduced risk using progesterone alone (Barnes et al.). A reduction in ovarian cancer incidence has been associated with the use of nonsteroidal anti-inflammatory drugs (NSAIDs) (Barnes et al.). Other studies have shown that the regular use of acetaminophen and retinoids can inhibit the processes involved in the transformation of epithelial cells of the ovary (Barnes et al.). Several chemoprevention trials investigating the use of prophylactic oophorectomy followed by oral contraceptives, NSAIDs, and retinoids are under way (Barnes et al.). Further research is needed in this area.

Diagnosis

Diagnosing ovarian cancer is no easy task. Epithelial tumors are the most common type of ovarian cancer. By the time any symptoms develop, 70% of women present with stage III and IV disease outside of the pelvis (Ozols et al., 2001). The most common symptoms of bloating and abdominal discomfort easily can be attributed to many non–life-threatening maladies. Other presenting symptoms include vaginal bleeding, small bowel obstruction, and/or urinary symptoms (Ozols et al.). Epithelial tumors of low malignant potential constitute a separate clinical and pathologic entity and represent approximately 15% of epithelial tumors. These tumors usually occur in women younger than 40 and have a favorable outcome regardless of stage (Sherman et al., 2004). Germ cell tumors, accounting for 4% of ovarian malignancies, are diagnosed 70% of the time in stage I disease. These tumors tend to stretch and twist the infundibulopelvic ligament, causing severe abdominal pain while the disease is still confined to the ovary. The remaining 6% of ovarian malignancies are the sexcord/stromal tumors. They produce symptoms of excessive endogenous estrogen or androgen production (precocious puberty), amenorrhea in premenopausal women, and vaginal bleeding in postmenopausal women (Ozols et al.). Histologic grade is an important predictor of treatment response and survival. It carries greater significance in stage I and II disease, but, overall, more differentiated tumors respond more favorably to treatment (Ozols et al.).

Diagnosis of ovarian cancer begins with a prompt and thorough pelvic exam. The Papanicolaou (Pap) smear is inadequate for detecting ovarian cancer. A palpable ovary in a postmenopausal woman is an indication for an exploratory laparotomy. If an adnexal mass is palpated on routine examination, diagnostic ultrasound and color flow Doppler usually are obtained. Rising serial CA-125 levels need surgical exploration because 80% of advanced cases have an elevated CA-125 level (Ozols et al., 2001). However, elevated CA-125 levels are not specific for ovarian cancer and have been found in nonmalignant gynecologic conditions (i.e., pregnancy, pelvic inflammatory disease, endometriosis, fibroids, menstruation) and other neoplastic diseases of the peritoneum, pleura, pericardium, and bronchus (O'Rourke & Mahon, 2003). If a pelvic mass has been found, a computed tomography (CT) scan can evaluate the extent of disease by assessing the paraaortic and retroperitoneal lymph nodes, mesenteric metastases, and intraperitoneal implants (Ozols et al.). A diagnostic laparotomy is indicated with unexplained pelvic pain and small adnexal masses. Great care must be taken not to rupture the ovarian mass, as peritoneal dissemination can occur if the tumor is not removed en bloc (Ozols et al.). Aspiration of ascetic fluid or saline lavage of all areas of the peritoneal cavity should be sent for peritoneal cytology at the time of surgery. Alpha-fetoprotein and human chorionic gonadotropin can be elevated in endodermal sinus tumors, embryonal carcinomas, choriocarcinomas, or mixed germ cell tumors (Ozols et al.).

Staging

Ovarian cancer is a surgically staged disease. Referral to a gynecologic oncologist has been proved to result in better outcomes, with progression-free and overall survival because of more aggressive cytoreductive techniques and more appropriate surgical staging (Ozols et al., 2001; Sonoda, 2004). Generally, in older women who do not have intraperitoneal carcinomatosis, a total abdominal hysterectomy and bilateral salpingo-oophorectomy are performed, followed by the surgical staging.

Surgical staging involves examination of the entire pelvis and abdominal cavity through an abdominal incision extending from the pelvis to the upper abdomen. First, any fluid present in the abdominal cavity should be aspirated and sent for cytologic studies. Additional cytologic evaluations of peritoneal washings of suspicious areas also are included. Adequate surgical staging involves careful inspection of all abdominal, peritoneal, and subdiaphragmatic surfaces, including intra-abdominal organs such as the liver, spleen, bladder, and large and small intestines (Ozols et al., 2001). If abnormalities are suspected, the surfaces are scraped for histologic evaluation and/or grossly debulked. The omentum is removed and also pathologically evaluated. Retroperitoneal nodes are palpated to determine the extent of disease and are surgically excised if possible (Walczak, Klemm, & Guarnifri, 1997).

Following a comprehensive surgical laparotomy, International Federation of Gynecology and Obstetrics (FIGO) staging is the most important prognostic indicator. A patient with stage I disease who has well or moderately differentiated tumors has a greater than 90% chance of surviving five years (Ozols et al., 2001). Patients with stage II disease (stage I with poor prognostic indicators) have an 80% five-year survival rate, stage III has a 15%–20% five-year survival rate, and stage IV has less than a 5% five-year survival rate. The volume of residual disease after cytoreductive surgery has a significant impact on survival. Stage III disease with optimal debulking (no residual nodule greater than 1 cm in diameter) and adjuvant platinum-based chemotherapy approaches a 35% five-year survival rate (Ozols et al.).

Treatment Modalities

Early-stage disease, stage IA or IB, with well- to moderately well-differentiated tumors has a 90% five-year survival rate with surgery alone (Ozols et al., 2001). Optimal treatment of early-stage disease (stage IC and II) with unfavorable prognostic factors (clear cell histology and grade 3 tumors) still needs to be researched. Some of the modalities that have been studied include external beam radiotherapy, intraperitoneal radioisotopes, or chemotherapy (Ozols et al.; Sherman et al., 2004; Sonoda, 2004). Questions remain whether to treat immediately postoperatively or wait until a recurrence has occurred; these patients are candidates for clinical trials. According to the National Cancer Institute (NCI, 2004a), the standard adjuvant treatment options for stage II disease can be divided into two general categories based upon surgical residuals. If remaining postoperative disease is minimal (less than 1 cm in size), systemic chemotherapy regimens include paclitaxel/cisplatin or carboplatin (TP), cyclophosphamide/cisplatin (CP), or cyclophosphamide/carboplatin (CC). Total abdominal and pelvic radiation therapy may be used (only if no macroscopic upper abdominal disease and minimal residual pelvic disease less than 0.5 cm); intraperitoneal chromic phosphate (P-32) radiation therapy is less frequently used (only if residual disease is less than 1 mm) as it can result in a significant number of late bowel complications, especially small bowel obstruction. If macroscopic pelvic disease remains postoperatively (greater than 2 cm), combination chemotherapy—TP, CP, or CC—should be used.

Treatment of advanced-stage disease, stages III and IV, generally includes cytoreductive surgery, if possible, followed by chemotherapy. Surgical debulking must be aggressive enough to remove virtually all palpable and visible tumors. Adequate debulking increases the remaining tumors' sensitivity to chemotherapy. Patients who are poor surgical candidates include those with liver metastasis, enlarged retrocrural or supraclavicular lymph nodes, mediastinal metastases, parenchymal lung metastases, porta hepatis or suprarenal lymphadenopathy, or omental involvement that extends into the hilum of the spleen. Chemotherapy that follows surgical resection includes several active agents. The "gold standard" therapy is a regimen that includes a combination of platinum and taxane. Carboplatin and paclitaxel used for six cycles is the most widely used regimen. Other active agents include topotecan, oral etoposide, gemcitabine, liposomal doxorubicin, and vinorelbine (Kim, Omura, & Avarez, 2002; Ozols et al., 2001). Palliative radiotherapy can be very helpful in controlling a growing pelvic mass causing pain, bleeding, or rectal narrowing. Radiation can provide rapid relief of symptoms and may prevent or delay the need for a diversional colostomy (Ozols et al.).

Cervical Cancer

Mortality rates from cervical cancer in the United States have declined by 70% over the past 50 years. Cervical cancer now ranks 13th in cancer death of women when it once ranked as the number-one cancer killer (Saslow et al., 2002). Multiple studies have proved that the Pap test has reduced mortality of cervical cancer by identifying premalignant changes of the cervix (Benard et al., 2004). Despite all of the progress to date, cervical cancer remains the second leading cause of cancer death in women age 20–39. It accounts for 18% of deaths from gynecologic cancers and 1.8% of all cancer deaths in women (Eifel, Berek, & Thigpen, 2001). In 2003, approximately 4,100 women died of cervical cancer, and many of the deaths could have been prevented (Likes & Itano, 2003). In the United States, the greatest incidence occurs in American Indians, African Americans, Vietnamese (five times the rate of Caucasians), and Hispanic women (three times the incidence) (Eifel et al.).

Pathophysiology

Human papilloma virus (HPV) is the cause of 90%–100% of cervical cancers (Eifel et al., 2001; Kobayashi, Miaskowski, Wallhagen, & Smith-McCune, 2000; Saslow et al., 2002), a significant fact because HPV infection is the most common sexually transmitted disease in the United States and accounts for 24 million infected Americans. Most infected individuals exhibit no symptoms of their disease. Fortunately, only approximately 11% of women infected with HPV progress to cervical dysplasia, and only 1% of mild dysplasia cases progress to invasive cervical cancer (Kobayashi et al.). Cervical cancer develops over many years after the initial infection with high-risk types of HPV (Benard et al., 2004). According to NCI (2003), once cervical cancer in situ is discovered, 30%–70% of untreated patients will develop invasive carcinoma over a 10–12-year period; another 10% can progress to invasive cancer in less than one year. Most cervical cancers arise from the "transitional zone" between the columnar epithelium of the endocervix and the squamous epithelium of the ectocervix. Once it breaks through the basement membrane of the cervix, it usually progresses in an orderly pattern of metastatic spread beginning in the cervix, on through the pelvic lymph nodes, then to the paraaortic nodes toward sites of distant metastasis. The most common sites of distant spread include the lung, extrapelvic nodes, liver, and bone (Eifel et al.). There are two different types of cervical cancer: squamous cell and adenocarcinoma. Squamous cell carcinomas account for 80%–90% of cervical cancers; the remaining 10%–20% are adenocarcinomas. The highest incidence of adenocarcinomas occurs in women in their 20s and 30s (Eifel et al.).

Clinical Manifestations

Preinvasive disease only can be detected during routine cervical screening with a Pap test. The earliest symptom usually is abnormal vaginal bleeding, often following coitus or vaginal douching. The bleeding can be clear or foul smelling. Pelvic pain can occur when the cancer progresses to locoregionally invasive disease or as a result of pelvic inflammatory disease. Flank pain can indicate ureteral obstruction leading to hydronephrosis. When cancer extensively invades into the pelvic wall, a triad of symptoms occurs: sciatic pain, leg edema, and hydronephrosis. Advanced tumors can produce hematuria or incontinence from cancer extending into the bladder, creating a vesicovaginal fistula (Eifel et al., 2001).

Risk Factors

Risk factors for squamous cell carcinomas of the cervix parallel the typical pattern of other sexually transmitted diseases. Prostitution, early-age coitus, first pregnancy at an early age, multiple sexual partners, diagnosis of other sexually transmitted diseases, promiscuous male partner, or the use of oral contraceptives all increase the risk for cervical cancer. Cigarette smoking may advance infected cells toward a neoplastic process once one is infected with HPV (Likes & Itano, 2003). Women with immunodeficiency, as with HIV infection, are four times more likely to be infected with HPV. Another risk factor is vitamin A and C deficiency (Likes & Itano). Adenocarcinomas of the cervix have a different set of risk factors. Long-term use of oral contraceptives correlates with a higher incidence of adenocarcinomas.

Prevention of cervical cancer begins with routine physical examinations complete with a pelvic exam and Pap smear. All abnormal Pap smears should be followed up appropriately, including a diagnostic colposcopy when indicated. Maintaining proper nutrition can reduce the risk. Modifying alcohol and drug use, stopping cigarette smoking, and using condoms all have been linked to a lower incidence of cervical cancer (Eifel et al., 2001; Kobayashi et al., 2000).

Diagnosis

The most important aspect of diagnosing cervical cancer is routine screening. The majority of cervical cancers have a long preinvasive stage of approximately 10 years, with ample opportunity to intervene before cellular abnormalities transform into a malignant invasion. Cervical cancer rates are highest in unscreened populations (Saslow et al., 2002). Specific guidelines exist for treatment of abnormalities found on Pap smears. Further diagnostic studies include colposcopy, endocervical curettage, and cervical cone biopsy. Positron emission tomography scanning can be a sensitive noninvasive way to detect nodal involvement. Staging laparotomy by a gynecologic oncologist is the most accurate way to diagnose and stage cervical cancer (Eifel et al., 2001).

Prognostic factors, which can help to define the disease course, begin with the stage of the disease. More advanced stages have a worse prognosis. Tumor size criteria are tumors less than or greater than 4 cm. Larger primary tumors are associated with decreased survival. Lymph node and uterine body involvement can indicate distant metastatic spread. In general, adenocarcinomas have a worse prognosis than squamous cell malignancies (Eifel et al., 2001).

Treatment

Treatment of cervical cancer is dictated by the stage of the disease. Early intraepithelial lesions can be managed by superficial ablative techniques, such as cryosurgery, laser surgery, or loop electrosurgical excision procedure. Microinvasive tumors (< 3 mm at a stage IA1) can be treated with conservative surgery, such as excisional conization or extrafascial hysterectomy (without removal of the ovaries). Early invasive cancers (stage IA2 and IB1 and some small stage IIA) require radical hysterectomy or radiotherapy (external beam or brachytherapy) if the surgical risk is too high. For locally advanced cancers (stages IB2–IVA), radiotherapy is used. If a patient is at high risk for locoregional recurrence, cisplatin-containing chemotherapy can be added as a radiosensitizer (Eifel et al., 2001).

Complications of radiotherapy include fatigue, mild to moderate diarrhea, and bladder irritation. If an extended radiation field is used, complications can include nausea, gastric irritation, and myelosuppression. The addition of chemotherapy to radiation exacerbates these complications. Three years after therapy, patients can experience rectal complications (e.g., bleeding, stricture, ulceration, fistula), vaginal shortening, and small bowel obstruction (Eifel et al., 2001).

Endometrial Cancer

Endometrial cancer is the most commonly diagnosed gynecologic cancer in the United States (Campagnutta et al., 2003; Grigsby, 2002). An estimated 7,310 women will die of this disease in 2005 (Jemal et al., 2005). Endometrial cancer is primarily a disease of postmenopausal women, with the average age at diagnosis being 60 years (Burke, Berek, & Thigpen, 2001). An estimated

40,880 new cases of endometrial cancer are expected to be diagnosed in 2005 in the United States (Jemal et al.). The highest incidence rates are among white women (26.5 per 100,000) as compared to African American women (17.8 per 100,000). Women with high-risk or advanced disease have a poor prognosis and account for most of the uterine cancer deaths (Burke et al.). Overall survival and outcomes are related to surgical stage and substage characteristics. In *Cancer Facts and Figures, 2005,* the American Cancer Society (ACS) reported a relative survival rate for endometrial cancer at 94%. The five-year relative survival rate includes 96% for local stage disease, 67% for regional stage, and 26% for distant stages. Relative survival rates for whites are at least 10% higher in each stage category compared to African American women (ACS, 2005).

Pathophysiology

The endometrium tissue is hormone sensitive. Estrogen stimulation produces cellular growth and glandular proliferation. Normally, cyclic hormone shifts balance the proliferation by the maturational effects of progesterone. Abnormal proliferation and neoplastic transformation are associated with "unopposed" estrogen stimulation (Burke et al., 2001). All lesions arise in the glandular component of the uterine lining. Initial growth forms as a polypoid mass within the uterine cavity. Usually the tumor mass is friable and often contains areas of superficial necrosis. Postmenopausal bleeding is the hallmark symptom for more than 90% of women diagnosed with endometrial cancer (Burke et al.). The uterus has a rich and complex lymphatic network, and nodal metastases can occur at any level and in any combination (via the paraaortic or superficial inguinal nodes). Tumors can extend through the uterine serosa and invade adjacent tissues, such as the bladder, colon, and adnexa, or exfoliate into the abdominal cavity to form implant metastases (Burke et al.). Hematogenous spread is uncommon. The most common sites of distant metastases include the lung, liver, bone, and brain. Approximately 90% of endometrial cancers are typical adenocarcinomas, and the remaining 10% are papillary endometrioid carcinoma, mucinous carcinoma, or papillary serous carcinoma. The latter group of diseases is associated with older age at onset, greater risk of extrauterine disease, and an overall poorer prognosis (Burke et al.).

Risk Factors

Risk factors that increase the incidence of endometrial cancer usually are associated with prolonged or excessive exposure to estrogen. Oral intake of exogenous estrogen without progesterone appears to have the highest association with development of uterine cancer. Occurrence of an estrogen-secreting tumor, low parity, and extended periods of anovulation also can increase the risk (Burke et al., 2001). Early onset of menarche or late onset of menopause result in prolonged exposure to estrogens. Extreme obesity with adipose retention of estrogen remains a risk factor. An increased incidence also has been found in women with hypertension and concomitant diabetes (Burke et al.). A personal history of breast cancer, colon cancer, or ovarian cancer can increase one's risk for uterine cancer. Breast cancer risk may be associated with the long-term use of tamoxifen for hormonal therapy (Burke et al.). Genetic predisposition only accounts for a small number of cases.

Diagnosis

Endometrial cancer should be included in the differential diagnosis for any woman who presents with postmenopausal vaginal bleeding, perimenopausal women with heavy or prolonged bleeding, and premenopausal women with abnormal bleeding patterns who are obese or oligo-ovulatory (Burke et al., 2001). The diagnostic "gold standard" for abnormal uterine bleeding is the dilation and curettage (D&C) of the uterine lining. However, with the trend toward less invasive surgical interventions, outpatient endometrial biopsy has replaced the D&C because no anesthesia is required (Burke et al.).

Endometrial cancer is staged both clinically and surgically. Clinical staging involves obtaining a fractional biopsy specimen from both the endocervix and the endometrium and determining the extent of uterine involvement through a thorough gynecologic exam (Burke et al., 2001). Surgical staging includes depth of myometrial invasion, tumor extension into the cervix, spread to the adnexal organs, positive peritoneal cytology, involvement of the retroperitoneal lymph nodes, and spread to the abdomen and distant sites (Burke et al.). Surgical staging remains the most accurate form of staging technique and has been the preferred method since 1988 (Kim et al., 2002).

Treatment

Surgical resection of the primary tumor by total abdominal hysterectomy and bilateral salpingo-oophorectomy is the mainstay of therapy (Grigsby, 2002; Kim et al., 2002). Surgical staging, which includes selective pelvic and paraaortic lymphadenectomy and peritoneal cytology, provides an accurate assessment of the disease spread at the time therapy is initiated (Kim et al.). In women with stage I disease, 60%–70% are cured by hysterectomy alone.

The best clinical outcomes for endometrial cancer can be achieved with either surgery alone or a combination of surgery and radiotherapy (Grigsby, 2002). Radiotherapy can be used preoperatively, postoperatively, and palliatively to treat endometrial cancer. In some high-risk surgical cases (e.g., patients who have severe cardiopulmonary disease or extreme obesity), radiation therapy is used as an alternate therapy for surgery (Grigsby). Preoperative brachytherapy involves cesium sources inserted vaginally for 72 hours. Hysterectomy can safely be performed two to three days postimplant, which can preserve the important prognostic information in the pathologic specimen (Burke et al., 2001). More extensive tumors can be treated preoperatively with combined external beam and intracavitary radiotherapy. Postoperative radiation reduces the incidence of vaginal recurrence from 10%–15% to less than 5% for patients with high-risk disease (Burke et al.). Chemotherapy has not been proved to extend survival when used to treat endometrial cancer (Burke et al.). Chemotherapy is used as an adjuvant therapy when the risk of recurrence exceeds 20%. These include any stage II tumor, clear cell or papillary serous histology, absence of hormone receptors, preoperative elevation of CA-125, and stage I disease with deep myometrial invasion (Burke et al.). Active antineoplastic agents used against endometrial cancer include cisplatin, carboplatin, doxorubicin, epirubicin, cyclophosphamide, ifosfamide, paclitaxel, and oral etoposide (Burke et al.).

Nutritional Implications

If the cancer is caught early, the nutritional implications of ovarian, cervical, and endometrial cancers do not have a significant impact on the patient's health and ability to endure treatment. When the cancers are treated, the treatments can cause nutrition impact symptomology, but the very nature of an early-stage gynecologic cancer usually has limited nutritional implications. Unfortunately, these cancers are not always found at an early stage, and because the areas affected are in the abdominal cavity, the potential for nutrition problems is significant.

Ovarian Cancer

Because ovarian cancer usually is asymptomatic at an early stage, by the time it is detected, most patients exhibit widespread disease. Some nutrition impact symptoms commonly seen in this patient population include bloating, indigestion, abdominal gas, changes in bowel habits, early satiety, nausea, anorexia, ascites, fatigue, and weight loss, which can result in malnutrition upon presentation (Health A to Z, 1999–2004; WomensHealthChannel, 1998–2004).

Presentation with or development of bowel obstruction(s) caused by bulky disease is, unfortunately, a possibility with ovarian cancer, and incidence is reported to be as high as 40% in patients with advanced ovarian cancer. It is the major cause of death in these patients (Letizia & Norton, 2003; Ripamonti & Bruera, 2002). Bowel obstructions can result from mechanical ileus (the occlusion of the intestinal lumen caused by tumor extending into the bowel proper or tumor that is encasing or positioned on the bowel), a functional ileus resulting from paralysis of intestinal muscle, or widespread carcinomatosis causing decreased motility (Adu-Rustum, Barakat, Venkatraman, & Spriggs, 1997; Grandon, 2004). In addition, intestinal blockages can result from progressive intraabdominal disease, inflammatory edema of the bowel from the tumor, prior radiation to the abdomen, or fecal impaction potentially associated with constipating medications, particularly narcotics (Grandon; Letizia & Norton).

Treatment for bowel obstructions depends on the type of obstruction, the condition of the patient, and the predicted prognosis (Letzia & Norton, 2003; Ripamonti & Bruera, 2002). Systemic chemotherapy has been ineffective in restoring bowel function in heavily pretreated patients with ovarian cancer, and surgical intervention remains the primary treatment. However, a significant number of patients with malignant bowel obstructions are not eligible for surgical intervention, so other options must be explored.

Nonpharmacologic inpatient management of blockages includes bowel rest, IV fluid replacement, and possibly a nasogastric drainage and decompression tube. A percutaneous gastrostomy tube may be a more effective palliative treatment strategy, however, because it can be used as a drainage and decompression technique as well as feeding route when the obstruction has resolved (Letizia & Norton, 2003). The more conventional treatment approach is to keep the patient at NPO (nothing by mouth) status while the drainage tube is in place. However, some hospice practitioners have experimented with, in select cases, clamping the tube, providing small amounts of clear liquids, and then resuming the tube suction function (Letizia & Norton).

The use of standard analgesics, antiemetics, and antisecretory agents to control pain, nausea, and vomiting is a challenge with a bowel obstruction. Factors influencing the choice of medications and route of administration must be individualized; additional factors to consider include drug treatment plan, drug cost and type, severity of symptoms, and clinical expertise of the administering practitioner (Letizia & Norton, 2003). Compounding pharmacists have developed recipes for topical administration as well as suppositories. The "Gralla suppository" composed of diphenhydramine hydrochloride, metoclopramide, and dexamethasone is one such prescription preparation (Letizia & Norton). Resolution of obstructions, for some, is possible; slow, steady diet advancement, from liquid to soft, low-residue to possibly regular food (stopping where the diet prescription is tolerated) is recommended (Campagnutta et al., 1996). A study using a soft, low-residue diet to manage the blockages in pancreatic cancer demonstrated good results with the additional deletion of raw fruits and vegetables, nuts, foods with skins, and foods with seeds. Finally, the participants were told to chew their food thoroughly. The authors felt that the diet prescription might be appropriate, in select situations, for others experiencing a malignant bowel obstruction (Grandon, 2004; McCallum, Walsh, & Nelson, 2002).

Another equally difficult side effect of advanced disease is ascites. The occurrence of ascites can greatly affect nutritional status, as it can cause pain, early satiety, nausea, and respiratory distress. In addition to pharmacologic management, a reduced sodium diet and possibly a fluid restriction (fluid restriction usually if the serum sodium is less than 128 mmol/liter) can be recommended in the hope of increasing renal sodium excretion, with the anticipated outcome of a net reabsorption of fluid from the ascites back into the circulating volume (Kumar & Clark, 2002).

Cervical Cancer

Cervical cancer diagnosed at an early stage usually does not cause or present with nutrition problems. Advanced stage disease, however, with metastases beyond the cervix, can cause weight loss possibly caused by anorexia, anemia, fatigue, and abdominal, pelvic, back, and/or leg pain (E*Cure*ME, 2002). Malnutrition with multiple nutrient deficiencies may be a concern given as one possible risk factor for cervical cancer. Although not a significant one, a low intake of vitamins A, C, E, and folate all have been associated with increased risk for cervical cancer (NCI, 2004b; Pence & Dunn, 1998). There has been no evidence to date to prove that supplementation with these nutrients will "treat" the cancer; however, it is prudent to ensure adequate intake of the nutrients in an effort to address potential underlying deficiencies.

Endometrial Cancer

Obesity is a risk factor for endometrial cancer (NCI, 2004c). Obesity, depending on the degree, can bring additional risk to medical treatment because of possible cardiovascular, diabetes, and/or cerebrovascular co-morbid conditions (Kumar & Clark, 2002). Extreme obesity (now used instead of "morbid obesity"), defined as a body mass index of more than 40 (American Medical Association, 2003), can influence the feasibility of treatment plans, making it necessary to deviate from standard protocol. This challenge is addressed on an individual basis by practitioners who are taking into account personal safety and efficacy as well as feasibility with available treatment equipment.

Nutritional Support (All Gynecologic Cancers)

Use of total parenteral nutrition (TPN) is controversial in patients with inoperable bowel obstruction or very advanced disease; issues of hydration and nutritional support must be explored with the patient, family, and health-care team before embarking on an involved plan (Adu-Rustum et al., 1997; Ripamonti & Bruera, 2002). Enteral nutrition, on the other hand, is a more common and a more convenient option even in the palliative setting because the patient may already have a tube in place (formally used for drainage). Enteral nutrition is more economical than TPN, and because it is best to use the gut if it is functional, enteral nutrition is the first option that should be explored (Barton, Woolas, Chan, & Lee, 1999).

Treatment-Related Nutritional Implications

Ovarian Cancer

Surgery

Surgical side effects from ovarian cancer treatment can be extensive, depending on the anticipated clinical outcome of the procedure; the more extensive the disease and the lesser the chance of surgical success usually results in less surgical intervention and, consequently, fewer nutritional implications from the procedure. Nutritional implications from unresectable advanced disease can be extensive. On the other hand, extensive surgical resections or debulking, done for cure or palliation, can include a total abdominal hysterectomy, bilateral salpingo-oophorectomy, omentectomy, removal of the fallopian tubes, and nodal sampling (Runowicz, Petrek, & Gansler, 1999). In addition, extensive surgical resections can include bowel resections that may result in short bowel syndrome and/or an ileostomy or colostomy.

Short bowel syndrome is defined as the malabsorptive condition that arises secondary to removal of significant segments of the small intestine. The type and degree of malabsorption depends on the extent of resection, with resections of 40%–50% of the small intestine usually being well tolerated (Tierney, McPhee, & Papadakis, 2002). Important nutritional considerations with short bowel syndrome are outlined in Table 6-1.

Management of an ileostomy or colostomy is best done with multiple medical disciplines involved. Ostomies can promote significant losses of fluid and electrolytes, depending on the location of the ostomy and the medical condition of the ostomate (McCallum & Polisena, 2000). Ileostomies cause greater losses because the colon, the site of fluid absorption, is bypassed (McCallum & Polisena). Colostomies can result in less fluid and stool output, but both ileostomies and colostomies, in a very sick patient, can be a challenge to manage. Several important tips for successful management include

1. Progress post-op from a clear liquid diet to a bland, low-fiber diet.
2. Gradually add more fiber back to the diet, but avoid foods known to cause additional abdominal gas (see Figure 6-1).
3. Eat small, frequent (or at least regular) meals. Skipping meals will increase gas and fluid output.
4. Eat in a pleasant atmosphere (to decrease aggravation and intestinal upset), chew food thoroughly, and avoid excessive talking or swallowing of air throughout the meal.
5. Drink plenty of fluids (8–12 glasses) each day.
6. Know the foods that can create a strong odor to the output of stool; help to reduce potential for odors by incorporating other foods; help to control mild constipation and diarrhea (see Figure 6-1).

Because the patient with ovarian cancer may have just undergone extensive surgery, the potential for nutrition impact symptoms from adjuvant or palliative chemotherapy is great. Known nutrition impact symptoms of commonly used

Table 6-1. Nutritional Considerations With Short Bowel Syndrome

Consideration	Cause	Recommendation
Bile salts	Possible malabsorption caused by resection of distal ileum or remaining ileum measuring less than 100 cm	Medication: Bile salt-binding resins such as cholestyramine
Vitamin B_{12}	Loss of absorption site with resection of terminal ileum	Supplementation with sublingual or injection of B_{12}
Fat-soluble vitamins (A, E, D, and K)	Reduction of bile salt pool from extensive resection of ileum leads to steatorrhea and malabsorption of fat-soluble vitamins	Low-fat diet with medium chain triglyceride supplementation and vitamin supplementation
Calcium and oxalate	Unabsorbed fatty acids decrease the absorption of calcium, enhancing the absorption of oxalates. Oxalate kidney stones can form.	Calcium supplementation
Overall diet therapy		May benefit from low-fat diet with modifications for low lactose and supplementation of medium chain triglycerides, vitamins (B_{12}, A, E, D, K), and minerals (calcium). Because of possible excessive sodium losses, sodium supplementation (in the form of increased oral sodium intake) also may be needed. Enteral and parenteral nutritional support are appropriate in certain situations.

Note. Based on information from Kumar & Clark, 2002; Tierney et al., 2002.

chemotherapy agents include anorexia, nausea, vomiting (leading to dehydration), fatigue, taste changes, diarrhea, constipation (possibly caused by pain medication), mucositis, esophagitis, and heartburn (McCallum & Polisena, 2000). Chemotherapy usually is given after curative or palliative surgical treatment. It is very difficult for these women to maintain their body weight, and weights should be checked on a regular basis to avoid having significant losses (or unexplained gains) go undetected for even short periods of time.

Figure 6-1. Dietary Management With Colostomies/Iliostomies

Potential gas-producing foods
- Dried beans
- Nuts
- Carbonated soft drinks
- Cruciferous vegetables (e.g., broccoli, cauliflower, cabbage, brussels sprouts)
- Sweet potatoes
- Onions*
- Sugary foods and sweets
- Asparagus*
- Eggs*
- Cheese: Roquefort, Brie, and other strong cheeses
- Beer
- Fish
- Milk

Foods that help to reduce odors
- Cranberry juice
- Yogurt
- Buttermilk

Foods that control mild constipation
- Juices and other fluids
- Cooked fruits and vegetables (eat daily)

Foods that may help to control diarrhea
- Bananas
- Tapioca
- Rice
- Applesauce
- Creamy peanut butter

*These foods, in addition to chicken, may produce strong odors.

Note. Based on information from Northwestern Memorial Hospital, 2001; Vanderbilt Children's Hospital, 2000.

Endometrial and Cervical Cancer

Surgery

Women recovering from surgical treatment for endometrial and cervical cancer can experience the common postsurgical side effects of pain and constipation. These can be effectively managed with pain medication, adequate fluids (six to eight 8-ounce glasses), a fiber-containing diet, and possibly one or more of the following: a psyllium fiber-containing preparation, laxative, or stool softener. Physical activity, with prior approval from a physician, also can help to relieve constipation.

Radiation Therapy

Radiation therapy is a common treatment for more advanced endometrial and cervical cancer and can cause more frequent loose stools, abdominal and perineal/anal pain, and cramping. Evidence-based nutrition recommendations include a bland diet that avoids heavy seasoning and acidic foods and, once more frequent elimination occurs, a decrease in high-fiber foods such as raw fruits, vegetables, coarse grains and cereals, nuts, and seeds for the duration of the treatment and until bowel function normalizes. Some women experience an increase in abdominal gas that can be exacerbated by consumption of carbonated beverages and known gas-producing foods, such as cruciferous vegetables. Consequently, gas-producing foods should temporarily be eliminated during radiation treatment. These foods, as well as high-fiber foods, should be gradually added back to the patient's diet following the cessation of treatment.

Radiation Enteritis

Acute and/or chronic radiation enteritis can occur in patients who have received radiation to the abdomen, pelvis, or lumbar/sacral spine regions, and it can result in mild to severe diarrhea. This condition is caused by radiation-induced injury to the intestinal epithelial cells and can lead to sloughing, inflammation, and ulceration, as well as shortening of the gut villi (Eldridge & Hamilton, 2003). Although the incidence is low because of modern treatment techniques and careful treatment plans, this side effect of radiation therapy can have profound nutritional implications.

Malabsorption of nutrients as well as significant fluid losses can occur. With acute enteritis, some patients may benefit from a regimen of bowel rest for 36–72 hours (Eldridge & Hamilton, 2003). As symptoms lessen, clear liquids can be started, and the diet can progress to small, frequent feedings of a low-fat, low-fiber, low-lactose diet for the remainder of treatment and possibly after (Sekhon, 2003). Symptoms generally resolve within a few weeks post-treatment. If, however, the diarrhea does not lessen with diet intervention, nutritional support with enteral feeding of an elemental formula or TPN may need to be considered.

Chronic enteritis can develop months after radiation treatment has ended and can continue for months or years. Enteritis symptomatology starts as an *acute* problem but persists long after treatment ends and also is referred to as *chronic* enteritis. Symptoms that are typical in this classification include abdominal pain, bloody diarrhea, tenesmus, steatorrhea, vitamin/mineral deficiencies, and weight loss; less common problems include bowel obstructions or perforations, fistulas, and rectal bleeding (Eldridge & Hamilton, 2003).

Chemotherapy

Chemotherapy treatment, given concurrently or concomitantly, presents a physical and psychological challenge to women. In addition to fatigue, common nutrition impact symptoms include nausea, vomiting, diarrhea, constipation, early satiety, and mucositis. Any or all of these can result in weight loss and compound fatigue.

Nutrition Assessment Guidelines

A study published by Santoso et al. (2000) demonstrated that malnutrition was common in the gynecologic population with cancer. Malnutrition, determined by suboptimal findings in serum albumin, transferrin, triceps skin fold, and skin sensitivity tests, was found in 36 of the study participants. Although the study number was small (N = 67), it highlighted the existence of a potential problem, making it a prudent move to provide nutrition screening and, if needed, intervention from the start.

Screening

Nutrition screening is defined as "the process of identifying characteristics known to be associated with nutrition problems with the purpose of identifying individuals who are malnourished or at nutritional risk" (Charney & Malone, 2004, p. 1). Questions pertinent to this population include weight history—has the client lost or gained weight in recent time? Over what period of time and what percentage of body weight has been lost or gained? Is this weight at all influenced by fluid accumulation in the abdomen or extremities (e.g., ascites, lymphedema)? Food intake—is it usual, less than usual, or more than usual? Nutrition impact symptoms—is the client currently experiencing any symptoms or side effects from the disease or treatment that impair food intake? Examples include nausea, vomiting (bowel obstruction or chemotherapy), diarrhea or constipation (pain medication or chemotherapy or hydration), and taste changes (chemotherapy). Special diets—is the client following any particular diet restrictions (complementary and alternative diet)? Medications, vitamin, mineral, and other dietary supplement intake—what and how much? Physical activity—how would the patient describe her daily level of activity:active or sedentary? (Charney & Malone).

A "yes" to any of these questions can put someone at nutritional risk depending on the degree of weight change, the degree of change of food and beverage intake with swallowing problems, the number and severity of nutrition impact symptoms, and the extent of restriction and/or modification of the daily diet. Although most medications and dietary supplements do not put someone at nutritional risk, some can contribute to an underlying problem. In addition, decreased physical activity can compound symptoms such as constipation.

Medical History and Physical Examination

A detailed medical history intake will help to reveal pertinent information for the nutrition assessment. Interviews with the client can be subjective and inconclusive, depending on the patient's health condition. Information may need to be gathered from a number of sources to complete the picture.

Information on recent lab values must be obtained and compared with the institution's normal values. Serum albumin, often used as a biomarker for malnutrition, is not a good reference in this population. Albumin can be affected by chemotherapy treatments and comorbid conditions, such as ascites. Many of the chemotherapy treatments affect common reference points like hemoglobin and hematocrit. Mean corpuscular volume (MCV) and mean corpuscular hemoglobin (MCH) can be affected by the treatment medications, rendering them less than reliable markers for malnutrition. A global picture, however, of an abnormal albumin, hemoglobin, hematocrit, and altered MCV and MCH coupled with high-risk body weight changes and nutrition impact symptoms can more than justify nutritional intervention.

Anthropometric Assessment

It is important in this population to attempt to assess body weight and not to credit fluid accumulation in the extremities or the abdomen as actual body weight. It is very difficult to judge how much weight is lean body mass or fat and how much is fluid. With no chart or reference graph to consult, accept that exact weights are difficult to determine at this time, and assume that real weight (lean and fat) is less than the recorded current body weight if fluid accumulation is present.

Special Considerations for Nutrition

Menopausal Changes and Use of Plant-Derived (Botanical/Herbal) Dietary Supplements

Most patients with gynecologic cancer will experience menopausal changes as the result of treatment for their cancer, whether from chemical (chemotherapy) or surgical (total abdominal hysterectomy and/or bilateral salpingo-oophorectomy) interventions. Women who have been through menopause naturally may experience some symptoms during or following treatment. These menopause-related symptoms can include, but are not limited to, hot flashes, mood alterations such as irritability and nervousness, decreased libido, tingly/prickly skin, vertigo, memory changes/forgetfulness, insomnia, achy joints and muscles, weakness and fatigue, heart palpitations, headaches, weight gain, hair thinning, and fragile skin and nails (Dixon, 2004). Although these potential problems can seriously alter a woman's quality of life, conventional hormone replacement strategies to resolve the issue usually are not viable options following the diagnosis of a hormone-sensitive cancer. Use of plant-derived (botanical/herbal) dietary supplements to manage menopausal symptoms is a common practice (see Table 6-2). Seventy-nine percent of individuals in a 2003 study reported using botanical dietary supplements, of which 36.5% reported daily use (Dixon; Mahady, Parrot, Lee, Yun, & Dan, 2003), but safety and efficacy were not clearly defined. Unfortunately, there is no good replacement for estrogen or progesterone in this patient population. Any attempt to relieve symptoms must be individually determined depending on diagnosis and menopausal symptoms experienced. There is no one product or set of recommendations that will relieve all menopausal

Table 6-2. Commonly Used Plant Medicines and Pertinent Information for Menopausal Symptoms

Dietary Supplement	Available Research	Proposed Use	Common Dose	Potential Problems	Conclusions
Black cohosh	Mixed research results—positive, negative, and neutral studies	Hot flashes, anxiety, depression, and sleep disturbances	1–2 tablets per day of a standardized extract manufactured to contain 1 mg of 27-deoxyacteine per tablet	Weak indications of potential interaction with anti-hypertensive medication Potential for mild stomach aches, headaches, dizziness, weight gain, a feeling of heaviness in the legs, and cramping	May not be efficacious for menopausal symptom management Safety data for long-term use are lacking.
Chaste tree berry	Limited research available; information on menopausal symptom management lacking	Most notable for effect on menopausal cycle No real evidence of therapeutic effect for menopausal symptoms	20–40 mg given in one daily dose; more concentrated extracts are given in different intervals.	One case of mild ovarian hyperstimulation possibly caused by herb Potential gastrointestinal disturbances, nausea, itching and rash, transitory headaches, and intramenstrual bleeding	No research basis is available for this application.
Dong quai	Limited research available; one negative study reported	General gynecologic complaints and a variety of menopausal symptoms	Traditional Chinese recipes Individualized doses; Western herbalists use 10–40 drops of tincture preparations up to three times per day or one capsule three times per day. *This herb is not currently standardized.*	In large doses, can be carcinogenic; may increase photosensitivity	Some in vivo and in vitro studies show increased estrogenic activity. Caution to women with hormone-sensitive cancers
Red clover	Limited research available; two negative studies	General menopausal symptoms	Typical extract provides 40–160 mg of isoflavones daily.	Potential interactions with hormone therapies (phytoestrogenic activity) and anti-coagulant therapies (constituents in the herb)	In vivo and in vitro studies demonstrate endogenous estrogenic activity. Caution to women with hormone-sensitive cancers

Note. Based on information from Bratman & Girman, 2003; Dixon, 2004; Fragakis, 2003.

symptoms; consequently, women may find themselves using any number of medically supervised or unsupervised therapies.

Although herbals cannot be recommended to all women, supervising healthcare professionals should know a little about some of the popular complementary and alternative medicine therapies commonly used (see Table 6-2).

Summary

Although the three gynecologic cancers covered in this chapter account for only 12% of the estimated cancer diagnoses for women in 2005, the prevention and treatment of these diseases uses medical resources across the spectrum of care. It is hoped that better nutrition, more vigilant screening, and innovative treatment methods can reduce the occurrence and mortality of ovarian, cervical, and endometrial cancers in the future, and the incidence will steadily decline.

References

Abu-Rustum, N.R., Barakat, R.R., Venkatraman, E., & Spriggs, D. (1997). Chemotherapy and total parenteral nutrition for advanced ovarian cancer with bowel obstruction. *Gynecologic Oncology, 64,* 493–495.

American Cancer Society. (2005). *Cancer facts and figures, 2005.* Atlanta, GA: Author.

American Medical Association. (2003, November). *Assessment and management of adult obesity: A primer for physicians.* Retrieved April 17, 2004, from http://www.ama-assn.org/ama/pub/category/10931.html

Barnes, M.N., Grizzle, W.E., Grubbs, C.J., & Partridge, E.E. (2002). Paradigms for primary prevention of ovarian carcinoma. *CA: A Cancer Journal for Clinicians, 52,* 216–224.

Barton, D., Woolas, R., Chan, F., & Lee, Y. (1999). Enteral feeding following major surgery in gynaecological cancer patients. *International Journal of Gynecologic Cancer, 9*(Suppl. 1), 142.

Benard, V.B., Eheman, C.R., Lawson, H.W., Blackman, D.K., Anderson, C., Helsel, W., et al. (2004). Cervical screening in the National Breast and Cervical Cancer Early Detection Program, 1995–2001. *Obstetrics and Gynecology, 103,* 564–570.

Bratman, S., & Girman, A.M. (2003). *Mosby's handbook of herbs and supplements and their therapeutic uses.* St. Louis, MO: Mosby.

Burke, T.W., Berek, J.S., & Thigpen, J.T. (2001). Cancers of the uterine body. In V.T. DeVita, S. Hellman, & S.A. Rosenberg (Eds.), *Cancer: Principles and practice of oncology* (6th ed., pp. 1573–1585). Philadelphia: Lippincott Williams & Wilkins.

Campagnutta, E., Cannizzaro, R., Gallo, A., Zarrelli, A., Valentini, M., DeCicco, M., et al. (1996). Palliative treatment of upper intestinal obstruction by gynecologic malignancy: The usefulness of percutaneous endoscopic gastrostomy. *Gynecologic Oncology, 62,* 103–105.

Campagnutta, E., Giorda, G., DePiero, G., Sopracordevole, F., Visentin, M.C., Martella, L., et al. (2003). Surgical treatment of recurrent endometrial carcinoma. *Cancer, 100*(1), 89–96.

Charney, P., & Malone, A. (Eds.). (2004). *ADA pocket guide to nutrition assessment.* Chicago: American Dietetic Association.

Dixon, S. (2004). Plant medicines for managing menopause-related hot flashes. *Oncology Nutrition Connection Newsletter, 12*(1), 11–22.

ECureMe. (2002). *Cervical cancer.* Retrieved April 17, 2004, from http://www.ecureme. com/especial/obgyn/Cervical_Cancer.asp

Eifel, P.J., Berek, J.S., & Thigpen, J.T. (2001). Cancer of the cervix, vagina and vulva. In V.T. DeVita, S. Hellman, & S.A. Rosenberg (Eds.), *Cancer: Principles and practice of oncology* (6th ed., pp. 1526–1548). Philadelphia: Lippincott Williams & Wilkins.

Eldridge, B., & Hamilton, K.K. (2003). *Nutrition impact symptom management.* Chicago: American Dietetic Association.

Fragakis, A.S. (2003). *Popular dietary supplements* (2nd ed.). Chicago: American Dietetic Association.

Grandon, M. (2004). Nutrition therapy in ovarian cancer: Applications for clinical practice. *Oncology Nutrition Connection Newsletter, 12*(1), 7–11.

Grigsby, P.W. (2002). Update on radiation therapy for endometrial cancer. *Oncology, 16,* 777–807.

Health A to Z. (1999–2004). *Ovarian cancer.* Retrieved April 17, 2004, from http://www. healthatoz.com/healthatoz/Atoz/dc/caz/can/ovac/ocsym.html

Jemal, A., Murray, T., Ward, E., Samuels, A., Tiwari, R.C., Ghafoor, A., et al. (2005). Cancer statistics, 2005. *CA: A Cancer Journal for Clinicians, 55,* 10–30.

Kim, R.Y., Omura, G.A., & Alvarez, R.D. (2002). Advances in the treatment of gynecologic malignancies. *Oncology, 16,* 1669–1678.

Kobayashi, A., Miaskowski, C., Wallhagen, M., & Smith-McCune, K. (2000). Recent developments in understanding the immune response to human papilloma virus infection and cervical neoplasia. *Oncology Nursing Forum, 27,* 643–653.

Kumar, P., & Clark, M. (2002). *Clinical medicine* (5th ed.). Philadelphia: Saunders.

Letizia, M., & Norton, E. (2003). Successful management of malignant bowel obstruction. *Journal of Hospice and Palliative Nursing, 5*(3), 152–158.

Likes, W.M., & Itano, J. (2003). Human papillomavirus and cervical cancer: Not just a sexually transmitted disease. *Clinical Journal of Oncology Nursing, 7,* 271–276.

Mahady, G.B., Parrot, J., Lee, C., Yun, G.S., & Dan, A. (2003). Botanical dietary supplement use in peri- and postmenopausal women. *Menopause, 10,* 65–72.

McCallum, P.D., & Polisena, C.G. (Eds.). (2000). *The clinical guide to oncology nutrition.* Chicago: American Dietetic Association.

McCallum, P.D., Walsh, D., & Nelson, K.A. (2002). Can a soft diet prevent bowel obstruction in advanced pancreatic cancer? *Supportive Care in Cancer, 10,* 174–175.

National Cancer Institute. (2003). *Cervical cancer (PDQ®): Treatment. Stage information.* Retrieved January 2, 2005, from http://www.cancer.gov/cancertopics/pdq/treatment/ cervical/HealthProfessional/page3

National Cancer Institute. (2004a). *Ovarian epithelial cancer (PDQ®): Treatment. Stage II ovarian epithelial cancer.* Retrieved January 2, 2005, from http://www.cancer.gov/cancertopics/ pdq/treatment/ovarianepithelial/HealthProfessional/page6

National Cancer Institute. (2004b). *Prevention of cervical cancer.* Retrieved April 17, 2004, from http://www.cancer.gov/cancerinfo/pdq/prevention/cervical /healthprofessional/

National Cancer Institute. (2004c). *Prevention of endometrial cancer.* Retrieved April 17, 2004, from http://www.cancer.gov/cancerinfo/pdq/prevention/endometrial /healthprofessional/

Northwestern Memorial Hospital. (2001). *Ostomy diet guidelines: A patient guide to ileostomy care, a patient guide to colostomy care.* Chicago: American Dietetic Association.

O'Rourke, J., & Mahon, S.M. (2003). A comprehensive look at the early detection of ovarian cancer. *Clinical Journal of Oncology Nursing, 7,* 41–47.

Ozols, R.F., Schwartz, P.E., & Eifel, P.J. (2001). Ovarian cancer, fallopian tube carcinoma and peritoneal carcinoma. In V.T. DeVita, S. Hellman, & S.A. Rosenberg (Eds.), *Cancer: Principles and practice of oncology* (6th ed., pp. 1597–1623). Philadelphia: Lippincott Williams & Wilkins.

Pence, B.C., & Dunn, D.M. (1998). *Nutrition and women's cancers.* Boca Raton, FL: CRC Press.

Ripamonti, C., & Bruera, E. (2002). Palliative management of malignant bowel obstruction. *International Journal of Gynecologic Cancer, 12,* 135–143.

Runowicz, C.D., Petrek, J.A., & Gansler, T.S. (1999). *Women and cancer.* Atlanta, GA: American Cancer Society.

Santoso, J.L., Canada, T., Latson, B., Alladi, K., Lucci, J.A., & Coleman, R.L. (2000). Prognostic nutritional index in relation to hospital stay in women with gynecologic cancer. *Obstetrics and Gynecology, 95*(Part 1), 844–846.

Saslow, D., Runowicz, C.D., Solomon, D., Mosieki, A.B., Smith, R.A., Eyre, H.J., et al. (2002). American Cancer Society guideline for the early detection of cervical neoplasia and cancer. *CA: A Cancer Journal for Clinicians, 52,* 342–361.

Sekhon, S.K. (2003). Women's food tolerances after radiation treatment for gynecologic cancer. *Journal of the American Dietetic Association, 97*(Suppl. 1), A26.

Sherman, M.E., Mink, P.J., Curtis, R., Cote, T.R., Brooks, S., Hartge, P., et al. (2004). Survival among women with borderline ovarian tumors and ovarian carcinoma. *Cancer, 100,* 1045–1051.

Sonoda, Y. (2004). Management of early ovarian cancer. *Oncology, 18,* 343–356.

Tierney, L.M., McPhee, S.J., & Papadakis, M.A. (2002). *CURRENT medical diagnosis and treatment.* New York: Lange Medical Books/McGraw-Hill.

Vanderbilt Children's Hospital. (2000). *Ileostomy and colostomy care: Parent teaching guide.* Nashville, TN: Vanderbilt University.

Walczak, J.R., Klemm, P.R., & Guarnifri, C. (1997). Gynecologic cancers. In S.L. Groenwald, M. Goodman, M.H. Frogge, & C.H. Yarbro (Eds.), *Cancer nursing: Principles and practice* (4th ed., pp. 1145–1198). Sudbury, MA: Jones and Bartlett.

WomensHealthChannel. (1998–2004). *Ovarian cancer symptoms.* Retrieved April 17, 2004, from http://www.womenshealthchannel.com/ovariancancer/symptoms.shtml

CHAPTER 7

Head and Neck Cancers

Sarah H. Kagan, PhD, RN, APRN, BC, AOCN®
Ellen Sweeney-Cordes, MS, RD, LDN

Overview

Head and neck cancers account for approximately 7% of all cancers diagnosed in humans (Jemal et al., 2005). Although relatively uncommon in the United States, it creates a disproportionate amount of disease- and treatment-related symptoms and side effects that are functionally disabling (Forastiere, Koch, Trotti, & Sidransky, 2001). These functional effects include changes in speaking and swallowing, xerostomia, chronic pain, and depression. All of these functional concerns may affect nutritional status in direct and complex ways and contribute to other short- and long-term sequelae of the original cancer (Larsson, Hedelin, & Athlin, 2003).

Incidence

Head and neck cancers are a set of cancer diagnoses grouped anatomically, beginning with the oral cavity and moving through the pharynx and larynx (Forastiere et al., 2001). Cancers of the oral cavity and pharynx are estimated to account for approximately 29,370 new cases in men and women in 2005 (Jemal et al., 2005). Cancer of the larynx is the site most commonly identified, has the highest site-specific incidence (just ahead of oral cavity cancers), and is among the highest in mortality rates (Forastiere et al.; Jemal et al.). In 2005, 9,880 new cases of cancer of the larynx in men and women are expected to occur (Jemal et al.). The group generally also includes the sinonasal passages and upper aerodigestive tract and select aspects of the skull base (Forastiere et al.). The sites that encompass head and neck cancers include those listed in Table 7-1 along with anatomic subsites within them. Head and neck cancers most often exclude the thyroid, which is classified separately, and the esophagus, which is grouped with other gastrointestinal malignancies. Skin cancer of the head and neck often is included in the clinical practice of head and neck oncology. This is anatomically and clinically relevant, because of the frequent exposure of this skin to ionizing solar radiation, yet accurate statistics on incidence, morbidity, and mortality are difficult to isolate.

Table 7-1. Head and Neck Cancer Sites and Subsites With New Cases and Deaths in Both Sexes for Selected Sites, 2005

Site	Estimated New Cases	Estimated Deaths
Oral cavity (includes lip, tongue, gum, floor of mouth, other oral cavity, total palate, tonsil)	20,780	5,190
Pharynx (includes, oropharynx, nasopharynx, pyriform sinus, hypopharynx)	8,590	2,130
Larynx	9,880	3,770

Note. Based on information from Forastiere et al., 2001; Jemal et al., 2005.

Risk Factors and Prevention

The genesis of head and neck cancers is complex, especially given the number of discrete sites and variable histology seen in this diagnostic group (Forastiere et al., 2001). Most cancers of the oral cavity, pharynx, and larynx are squamous cell malignancies. Head and neck cancers involve exposure to widely acknowledged carcinogens, such as tobacco and alcohol, as well as the influence of less well-known viral and chemical carcinogens and oncogene and proto-oncogene mutations (Forastiere et al.).

Exposure to tobacco and alcohol as a significant carcinogen and co-carcinogen pair is well established clinically and scientifically (Forastiere et al., 2001). Tobacco and alcohol together seem to create a phenomenon known as "field cancerization" that creates a greater risk for multiple malignancies in the upper aerodigestive tract or "field" (Forastiere et al.). Opportunities to prevent head and neck cancers linked to tobacco use and the co-carcinogenic effect of alcohol consumption are tightly tied to public health and health education initiatives that regulate availability, encourage abstinence, and teach cessation.

Prevention of malignancies for which issues of carcinogenesis are less well understood is more difficult. For example, Epstein-Barr virus (EBV) is strongly associated with certain types of nasopharyngeal cancers (NPCs), appearing in upward of 90% of undifferentiated NPC tumors (Forastiere et al., 2001; Niedobitek, 2000; Niedobitek, Agathanggelou, & Nicholls, 1996). Nonetheless, EBV infection alone, which is extraordinarily common, infecting more than 90% worldwide, does not account for the high incidence of NPCs in some parts of the world, particularly Southeast Asia (Lechowicz, Lin, & Ambinder, 2002). This implies a complex process that likely involves more than one carcinogen and may rely on somatic genetic mutation or other genetic alterations. Similarly, human papilloma virus (HPV) is linked to approximately one-half of oropharyngeal cancers, especially those found in the tonsils and base of the tongue (Forastiere et al.). HPV infection is common, yet it is impossible to define exactly its incidence or prevalence because of the shifting nature of the infection (Sedlacek, 1999), and the mismatch between benign or asymptomatic infection implies a more intricate equation that results in actual disease.

Genetic evidence for the epidemiology of many head and neck site-specific cancers is growing rapidly (Goepfert, 1998). Evidence reveals a high prevalence, on the order of 50%, of $p53$ mutations in squamous cell head and neck cancers (Forastiere et al., 2001; Le & Giaccia, 2003). Other tumor suppressor genes, including $p16$, PTEN, and Rb, also are implicated in squamous cell cancers of the head and neck. Proto-oncogenes, such as Cyclin D1, $p63$, and epidermal growth factor receptor, which may alter the cell cycle or overall cell growth and proliferation, appear to be involved in head and neck cancers (Forastiere et al.; Le & Giaccia). Emerging knowledge of the interplay between these genetic factors and environmental carcinogenic exposure will greatly aid in identifying the risks of site-specific malignancies and targeting public health and nursing efforts to prevent them.

Treatment Modalities

Treatment modalities for head and neck cancers are advancing as treatment technologies develop and knowledge of site-specific carcinogenesis expands (Forastiere et al., 2001). Early detection remains very limited, with no national guidelines or sensitive and specific technologies currently available beyond the annual cancer-related checkup after age 20, as recommended by the American Cancer Society (Smith, Cokkinides, & Eyre, 2003). Growing translational science in chemoprevention and photodynamic therapies holds promise for treatment or reversal of dysplastic lesions or carcinoma in situ (Forastiere et al.; Goepfert, 1998).

Diagnosis and staging have changed little over time, and head and neck cancers are staged using the tumor-node-metastasis system (American Joint Committee on Cancer, 2002; Forastiere et al., 2001; O'Sullivan & Shah, 2003). Diagnosis is made on the basis of a tissue biopsy. Once staged, individuals diagnosed with a head and neck cancer will be offered a treatment plan that may include multiple modalities or single-modality therapy, such as intensity modulated radiation therapy (IMRT). Surgery and radiation continue to be the mainstays of treatment (Goepfert, 1998). Chemotherapy is increasingly offered as part of combined chemoradiation protocols rather than as a single modality, where it is generally ineffective (Forastiere et al.).

Among the most important surgical advances are organ conservation or preservation using partial laryngectomy or chemoradiation for laryngeal cancers (Goepfert, 1998). There has been movement away from radical neck dissection and its concomitant disability. Modified and selective neck dissection are used to control for nodal spread (Goepfert). Selective neck dissection excises only the lymph nodes that are likely to be involved given the primary site of disease. Surgical reconstruction also is increasingly common, and although it does not offer opportunities for better control of cancers, it bolsters quality of life by improving appearance and, often, function (Forastiere et al., 2001). Techniques include more common local or rotation flaps (e.g., deltopectoralis) to repair oral cavity defects. Newer microvascular free flaps are increasingly used to repair complex or large defects. In these procedures, skin, muscle, and bone distant to the operative site are harvested and then implanted to reconstruct lost tissues. For example, a musculocutaneous flap can be raised from the radial forearm and used to reconstruct the pharynx after ablation of pharyngeal cancer. The monitoring of flap perfusion and the secondary surgical incisions made during flap harvest complicate postoperative care.

Radiotherapeutics are advancing rapidly, making radiation therapy a very prominent part of treatment for head and neck cancers (Forastiere et al., 2001). New techniques for delivery of radiation, protocols to better manage acute and chronic side effects, and related technologies, such as photodynamic therapy, all have a place in treatment of head and neck cancers. Altered fractionation protocols, high-dose radiotherapy, IMRT, and brachytherapy allow the radiation oncologist the means to treat head and neck cancers in more targeted ways, making optimal use of treatment time with better sparing of adjacent tissues. Use of radioprotective drugs such as amifostine offers the possibility of preserving salivary gland function, thereby reducing both acute and chronic side effects related to xerostomia (Seikaly, 2003; Shih, Miaskowski, Dodd, Stotts, & MacPhail, 2003).

Chemoradiation protocols are treatments of choice for select oral and most often oropharyngeal cancers (Forastiere et al., 2001; Le & Giaccia, 2003). Chemoradiation protocols employ concurrent administration of the two modalities. The chemotherapeutic agents most commonly administered are carboplatin and cisplatin with or without fluorouracil, which is given with leucovorin (Forastiere et al.). Side effects and symptom clusters are generally acknowledged to be more pronounced in combined protocols (Lee et al., 1998; Shih et al., 2003). For example, radiation mucositis may be more severe with very thick, tenacious secretions, necessitating enhanced self-care protocols that rely on frequent oral care and medications (e.g., guaifenesin) to thin secretions (McLane, Jones, Lydiatt, Lydiatt, & Richards, 2003). Further, this mucositis may be very painful, mandating enteral feeding support during and after therapy and post-treatment evaluation by a speech language pathologist to ensure rehabilitation of swallowing function.

Nutritional Implications

Patients treated for head and neck cancers are at risk for many side effects that limit their functional ability to swallow, taste, and smell and impact their ability to eat foods and drink liquids (Larsson et al., 2003). Premorbid effects of the disease, such as tumor partly obstructing the oral cavity or esophagus, may alter a patient's overall nutritional status before treatment begins. Multimodality therapies involving surgery and adjuvant radiation or chemoradiation result in acute oral and oropharyngeal side effects that create an inability to eat and require enteral support for the patient through the course of treatment (Lee et al., 1998; Scolapio, Spangler, Romano, McLaughlin, & Salassa, 2001). Side effects that interfere most in maintaining adequate nutrition are oropharyngeal mucositis, dysgeusia, nausea and vomiting from chemotherapy, nausea from increased secretions after surgery or during chemoradiation, pain from surgery or mucositis, and fatigue (Larsson et al.; McLane et al., 2003). The long-term side effects of radiation and chemoradiation—xerostomia, poor dentition, dysphagia, dysgeusia, as well as chronic pain—create the potential for poor nutrition and difficulty eating for years following treatment.

The registered dietitian (RD) is an essential member of the head and neck cancer care team (Lees, 1999). The RD will take the lead in assessing, intervening with, and educating patients and their families about nutrition and diet. The physician relies on the RD and the nurse to discuss the patient's pretreatment state of dentition with him or her, making arrangements for dental care as required. Pretreatment nutrition counseling prepares patients for side effects and corresponding nutritional management. Throughout treatment, the RD emphasizes the goals of the individual's nutrition care plan to maintain optimal body weight, maintain protein stores, support immune function, and contribute to overall treatment tolerance. Post-treatment side effects and disability may present obstacles to eating that, in turn, affect resumption of optimal oral intake and are addressed proactively by the RD.

Proactive nutrition counseling must begin early in treatment while the patient is still able to eat (Lees, 1999). Counseling is focused on maintenance of weight with soft-textured, high-calorie foods and liquid nutritional supplements (e.g., Ensure®, Boost®, Carnation Instant Breakfast®). Patients and their family members should be educated about potential nutritional complications and management of common side effects. Information provided in Table 7-2 details common nutrition-related side effects of head and neck cancer treatment and suggestions for management.

Table 7-2. Common Side Effects of Head and Neck Cancer Treatment: Causes and Management

Side Effect	Possible Causes	Management
Sore mouth/ throat	Mucositis (ir- ritated mucous membranes) from radiation and/or chemotherapy	Follow recommended mouth care regimen as instructed by physician or nurse to keep mouth clean. Eat soft, bland foods such as cream soup, pudding, oatmeal, macaroni and cheese, and ice cream. Avoid eating foods that are extremely hot or cold. Drink through a straw to bypass mouth sores. Avoid irritating spices and condiments such as pepper, chili powder, salsa, horseradish, and vinegar. Eat high-protein foods to speed healing. Avoid alcohol, carbonated beverages, and tobacco, which further irritate mucous membranes. Drink high-calorie liquid nutritional supplements to help to maintain adequate calorie intake. Begin use of tube feedings as ordered to supplement oral intake.
Dry mouth	Decreased saliva production from radiation or surgery	Follow mouth care regimen closely to keep mouth clean and reduce risk for oral lesions and infections. Increase intake of noncaffeinated beverages. Carry a water bottle when away from home. Avoid commercial mouthwashes containing alcohol. Eat soft, moist foods that are cool or at room temperature. Try eating fruit purees, soft cooked chicken and fish, cooked cereals, and plain or flavored ice chips. Moisten foods with broth, non–tomato-based sauces, gravy, cream, or butter. Suck on lemon drops, frozen grapes, or ice pops to moisten mouth. Use Biotene™ (Laclede, Rancho Dominguez, CA) mouthwash and gum to add moisture.
Difficulty swallowing	Tumor location Inflammation/pain in throat or mouth because of surgery, radiation, or chemotherapy Nerve damage from surgery or radiation	See a speech and swallowing therapist for a swallowing evaluation and to receive instructions for special eating techniques. Eat small, frequent, soft, moist meals and snacks. Drink high-calorie liquid nutritional supplements several times per day if you are unable to eat enough regular foods to meet your nutritional needs. A feeding tube may be needed if you are unable to drink and eat enough to maintain your weight.

(Continued on next page)

Table 7-2. Common Side Effects of Head and Neck Cancer Treatment: Causes and Management *(Continued)*

Side Effect	Possible Causes	Management
Thick mucus	Decreased saliva production from salivary glands due to radiation or surgery	Drink 48–64 ounces of fluid per day to help thin mucus. Add lemonade or papaya juice to lemon-lime soda to help to dissolve mucus. Drink pineapple juice before meals (enzymes in pineapple help to dissolve mucus) but not if mouth/throat soreness is present. Try Biotene™ gum and mouthwash. They are alcohol-free and made to correct dry mouth. Moisten foods with soups, gravy, broth, sauces, and butter.
Changes in taste and smell	Inflammation and mucous membrane changes from radiation or taste changes from chemotherapy Lack of smell because of cancer of the nasopharynx	Use plastic utensils if you have a metallic taste in your mouth when eating. Season foods with tart flavors, such lemon wedges, citrus fruits, vinegar, and marinades to overpower bad or "off" tastes (if you do not have mouth/throat soreness). Suck on sugar-free lemon candy or mints to get rid of unpleasant tastes. Flavor foods with onion, garlic, basil, and other herbs/seasonings. Rinse your mouth before eating to help to clear taste buds of "off flavors" or bad tastes. Eat foods cold or at room temperature to decrease food flavor and odor.
Constipation	Both pain and antinausea medications have a constipating effect. Changes in eating habits Decreased physical activity	Use laxatives and stool softeners as directed. Try to eat at the same times every day. Drink 8–10 cups of liquid each day. Try drinking water, prune juice, and warm beverages. Eat more high-fiber foods, such as whole-grain breads and cereals, fruits and vegetables, popcorn, and dried beans, if you can tolerate them.

(Continued on next page)

Table 7-2. Common Side Effects of Head and Neck Cancer Treatment: Causes and Management *(Continued)*

Side Effect	Possible Causes	Management
Decreased appetite	Changes in taste and smell, chewing or swallowing difficulty, nausea, constipation, chemotherapy, medications, pain, fatigue, stress, anxiety, and depression all can lead to poor appetite. Cachexia	Try eating small, frequent meals and snacks every one to two hours. Keep high-calorie, high-protein snacks and foods handy to eat when you are hungry. Try eggs, lunchmeats, ice cream, peanut butter, granola bars, cheese, high-calorie liquid supplements, puddings, and yogurt. Avoid drinking liquids with meals to prevent getting full too soon. Eat with someone else and in a pleasant environment. Add more calories and protein to foods by using oils and other fats in cooking, cheese melted on sandwiches or vegetables, and high-calorie condiments on foods, such as mayonnaise, salad dressing, cream cheese, and jam. Consult your doctor about medications to stimulate appetite and reduce nausea, constipation, pain, and other side effects that may contribute to loss of appetite.
Nausea	Chemotherapy drugs Thick secretions in back of throat	Take antinausea medications as recommended by your doctor to control and prevent nausea. Eat six small meals or snacks per day instead of three large meals. Eat bland, dry foods such as bread, cereal, crackers, and pretzels in the morning and often during the day to prevent nausea. Eat foods that do not have a strong odor. Cool foods, such as sandwiches, are less nauseating than hot, aromatic foods. Avoid greasy, spicy, or overly sweet foods when nauseated. Sit up or recline with your head raised for at least one hour after eating if you need to rest. See Thick Mucus section on tips to thin mucus.

(Continued on next page)

Table 7-2. Common Side Effects of Head and Neck Cancer Treatment: Causes and Management (Continued)

Side Effect	Possible Causes	Management
Weight loss	Inadequate oral or enteral support intake Increased metabolism or cachexia from disease Prolonged decreased food intake caused by tumor location or pain prior to diagnosis	Review your nutritional needs with your nutritionist for ideas about how to increase your intake of calories. Begin use of tube feeding if it has been ordered. Consult you doctor about medications to stimulate appetite.
Fatigue	Chemotherapy and radiation treatment	Ask for help with meal preparation and shopping to conserve energy. Eat a balanced diet with snacks. Use liquid nutritional supplements if you are too tired to eat a meal. Purchase frozen meals for quick, easy preparation.

Maintenance of optimal intake during treatment relies on understanding the site of disease, the treatment plan, and expected side effects, in addition to a detailed individual assessment that accounts for premorbid nutritional compromise (Larsson et al., 2003; Lees, 1999). The ability to maintain adequate oral intake during treatment depends on the involved oral anatomy and presence of oropharyngeal mucositis from radiation or chemoradiation. Although many patients receiving radiation alone to the oral cavity, nasopharynx, or neck may be able to tolerate soft foods early in treatment, most patients must transition to liquid diets using liquid nutritional supplements or have an enteral feeding tube placed. Almost all patients receiving chemoradiation become fully dependent on enteral nutritional support after three to four weeks of therapy (Chandu, Smith, & Douglas, 2003; Lee et al., 1998; Scolapio et al., 2001). Mucositis and resulting odynophagia and dysgeusia make eating and secretion management difficult. Gastrostomy tube placement prior to beginning radiation treatment has been shown to prevent weight loss, treatment interruption, and dehydration (Chandu et al.; Lee et al.; Scolapio et al.). Percutaneous endoscopic gastrostomy (PEG) tubes are most commonly used for enteral support in these patients. The PEG tube often is placed at the time of initial surgical resection and then not used until it becomes necessary during treatment (Lee et al.).

Assessment Guidelines

Nutrition assessment of the patient with head and neck cancer should include fundamental elements of comprehensive nutrition assessment, such as medical history, pertinent laboratory values, current medications, functional or performance status, typical dietary intake, fluid status, and physical indications of malnutrition (e.g., skeletal muscle wasting, temporal wasting), and exploration of concerns specific to this patient group. Assessment of weight history and premorbid weight loss, changes in oral intake, symptoms affecting nutrition (e.g., nausea, vomiting, taste changes, dry mouth, pain, diarrhea, constipation), and use of alcohol, tobacco, and recreational drugs is critical to successful care planning. Assessment ideally is implemented preceding initiation of treatment, and regular follow-up with the RD should be integrated into the overall plan of care.

Calorie, protein, and fluid requirements for patients with cancer can be estimated using standard guidelines (Dempsey & Mullen, 1985; Merrick, Long, Grecos, Dennis, & Blakemore, 1998). The Harris-Benedict equation can be used as an alternate method to estimate caloric needs (Dempsey & Mullen; Merrick et al.). Details of these and other nutrition assessment equations can be found in Appendices F, G, H, and I. These guidelines and equations are only a starting point for initial intervention. Estimates should be adjusted periodically as a patient's nutritional status changes. Actual body weight should be used except for obese patients, in which case ideal body weight should be used.

Special Considerations for Nutrition

Most patients with head and neck cancers come to rely on enteral tube feedings at some point during and after their treatment (Lee et al., 1998). Worsening mucositis with odynophagia and, less commonly, late-onset dysphagia after chemoradiation necessitate the use of tube feeding (Lee et al.). When the patient's oral caloric intake begins to decrease in the context of these symptoms, the RD teaches the patient and family members how to transition to use of the feeding tube, usually placed prior to treatment, to maintain adequate nutrition and fluid. The RD calculates individual nutrient and fluid needs and recommends an appropriate tube feeding formula and feeding method for each patient. The team, then led by the RD, should monitor the patient's adherence to recommendations and tolerance to feeding formula, methods, and intake. Patients with head and neck cancers often have difficulty meeting their tube feeding goals because of several common complications, including nausea, delayed gastric emptying, constipation, diarrhea, and dehydration. Further, some patients and families may find tube feeding difficult to perform and experience feeding schedule conflicts. Table 7-3 outlines problems commonly experienced in enteral feeding along with their possible etiologies and management suggestions.

Table 7-3. Common Enteral Feeding Problems, Possible Causes, and Management Strategies

Problem	Possible Cause	Management
Constipation, causing bloating or fullness when administering tube feeding	Pain medications and/or antinausea medications Decreased activity Lack of fiber Inadequate fluid intake	Use laxative/stool softener according to prescribed schedule. Increase water flushes for adequate hydration.
Diarrhea following tube feeding administration	Tube feeding administered too quickly Tube feeding volume too high	If using bolus feeding technique, switch to gravity drip method to slow rate of feed. Decrease volume of feeding to one can or less every three hours until tolerated. Slowly increase volume up to 1.5–2 cans per feeding maximum. Assess for recent medication changes that may be contributing to diarrhea if volume and rate are not issues. Change tube feeding formula to a lower osmolar type for better tolerance if previously mentioned changes do not help.
Bloating, fullness, nausea, or vomiting	Decreased or delayed gastric emptying caused by medications or treatment Constipation	Change to lower volume, more frequent feeding schedule. Consult physician about use of metoclopramide (Reglan™, A.H. Robins Company, Richmond, VA) for increased gastric emptying. Consider changing to continuous feeds via pump if needed. Keep head of bed elevated greater than 30 degrees. Follow prescribed antiemetic regimen if nausea is chronic. Follow management guidelines (previously mentioned) for constipation if no bowel movement has occurred in two days or more.
Aspiration	Altered gag reflex associated with tumor or surgical resection Poor gastric emptying	Keep head of bed elevated greater than 30 degrees, and check residual volumes. Change to continuous pump feedings if on bolus or gravity feeds. Consider jejunostomy versus gastric tube.

(Continued on next page)

Table 7-3. Common Enteral Feeding Problems, Possible Causes, and Management Strategies *(Continued)*

Problem	Possible Cause	Management
Dehydration	Insufficient free water	Give more free water.
	Diarrhea	Consider more dilute formula if appropriate.

When treatment ends and healing to the radiated site occurs, the patient with head and neck cancer should be instructed on how to make a gradual transition back to oral intake from tube feeding or back to solid foods from a liquid diet. The assistance of a speech and swallowing therapist is an integral part of the patient's nutritional care, as he or she can assess for any swallowing dysfunction resulting from surgery or tissue changes during treatment and prescribe exercises to facilitate maintenance of the swallowing function and optimal transition back to solid foods. Often, tube feedings continue indefinitely post-treatment for those patients who have the greatest swallowing deficits. For others, the road back to eating can happen within weeks after treatment ends. Many patients may request nutrition counseling from the dietitian on how to make their diet more "cancer protective" as they focus on reducing their controllable risk factors for recurrence.

Resuming oral intake is a longer road for some. Patients often are not prepared for the long-lasting effects that treatment has on their quality of life, especially where eating is involved. Patients may avoid participation in events that revolve around eating, resulting in decreased social contact. Most patients will have chronic taste changes, xerostomia, and varying levels of dysphagia that will affect the types of foods they will be able to eat and how they eat. Eating can become more of a chore than a source of enjoyment. Patients also need support for their nutrition problems after their treatment, including coping with the long-term effects of the treatment. Many needs, including nutritional monitoring, can go unmet during this time when the patient is not visiting the clinic or hospital for monitoring as often.

Care Planning and Expected Outcomes of Therapy

Care planning for the patient with head and neck cancer is intensively interdisciplinary and emphasizes nutritional outcomes because both the disease and its treatment create a high risk for poor oral intake, weight loss, and decreased protein intake. The RD will collaborate with nurses or nurse practitioners in surgical, radiation, and medical oncology, the speech language pathologist, and the physician teams across treatment modalities. Additionally, the occupational therapist may be a key collaborator for those patients who need additional support in learning tube feeding or in relearning feeding skills. The team members then must create a plan of care centered on the individual patient, incorporating family and other support, to achieve the goals of optimal nutritional intake, weight maintenance, and resumption of optimal oral intake as treatment concludes. Successful use of enteral tube feeding is a secondary goal to be achieved when the patient's clinical condition warrants it.

References

American Joint Committee on Cancer. (2002). *AJCC cancer staging manual* (6th ed.). New York: Springer-Verlag.

Chandu, A., Smith, A.C., & Douglas, M. (2003). Percutaneous endoscopic gastrostomy in patients undergoing resection for oral tumors: A retrospective review of complications and outcomes. *Journal of Oral and Maxillofacial Surgery, 61,* 1279–1284.

Dempsey, D., & Mullen, J. (1985). Macronutrient requirements in the malnourished cancer patient: How much of what and why? *Cancer, 51,* 6138–6141.

Forastiere, A., Koch, W., Trotti, A., & Sidransky, D. (2001). Medical progress: Head and neck cancer. *New England Journal of Medicine, 345,* 1890–1900.

Goepfert, H. (1998). Squamous cell carcinoma of the head and neck: Past progress and future promise. *CA: A Cancer Journal for Clinicians, 48*(4), 195–198.

Jemal, A., Murray, T., Ward, E., Samuels, A., Tiwari, R.C., Ghafoor, A., et al. (2005). Cancer statistics, 2005. *CA: A Cancer Journal for Clinicians, 55,* 10–30.

Larsson, M., Hedelin, B., & Athlin, E. (2003). Lived experiences of eating problems for patients with head and neck cancer during radiotherapy. *Journal of Clinical Nursing, 12,* 562–570.

Le, Q.T., & Giaccia, A.J. (2003). Therapeutic exploitation of the physiological and molecular genetic alterations in head and neck cancer. *Clinical Cancer Research, 9,* 4287–4295.

Lechowicz, M.J., Lin, L., & Ambinder, R.F. (2002). Epstein-Barr virus DNA in body fluids. *Current Opinion in Oncology, 14,* 533–537.

Lee, J.H., Machtay, M., Unger, L.D., Weinstein, G.S., Weber, R.S., Chalian, A.A., et al. (1998). Prophylactic gastrostomy tubes in patients undergoing intensive irradiation for cancer of the head and neck. *Archives of Otolaryngology—Head and Neck Surgery, 124,* 871–875.

Lees, J. (1999). Incidence of weight loss in head and neck cancer patients on commencing radiotherapy treatment at a regional oncology centre. *European Journal of Cancer Care, 8*(3), 133–136.

McLane, L., Jones, K., Lydiatt, W., Lydiatt, D., & Richards, A. (2003). Taking away the fear: A grounded theory study of cooperative care in the treatment of head and neck cancer. *Psycho-Oncology, 12,* 474–490.

Merrick, H., Long, C.L., Grecos, G.P., Dennis, R.S., & Blakemore, W.S. (1998). Energy requirements for cancer patients and the effect of total parenteral nutrition. *Journal of Parenteral and Enteral Nutrition, 12*(1), 8–14.

Niedobitek, G. (2000). Epstein-Barr virus infection in the pathogenesis of nasopharyngeal carcinoma. *Molecular Pathology, 53,* 248–254.

Niedobitek, G., Agathanggelou, A., & Nicholls, J.M. (1996). Epstein-Barr virus infection and the pathogenesis of nasopharyngeal carcinoma: Viral gene expression, tumour cell phenotype, and the role of the lymphoid stroma. *Seminars in Cancer Biology, 7,* 165–174.

O'Sullivan, B., & Shah, J. (2003). New TNM staging criteria for head and neck tumors. *Seminars in Surgical Oncology, 21,* 30–42.

Scolapio, J., Spangler, P.R., Romano, M.M., McLaughlin, M.P., & Salassa, J.R. (2001). Prophylactic placement of gastrostomy feeding tubes before radiotherapy in patients with head and neck cancer: Is it worthwhile? *Journal of Clinical Gastroenterology, 33*(3), 215–217.

Sedlacek, T.V. (1999). Advances in the diagnosis and treatment of human papillomavirus infections. *Clinical Obstetrics and Gynecology, 42,* 206–220.

Seikaly, H. (2003). Xerostomia prevention after head and neck cancer treatment. *Archives of Otolaryngology—Head and Neck Surgery, 129,* 250–251.

Shih, A., Miaskowski, C., Dodd, M.J., Stotts, N.A., & MacPhail, L. (2003). Mechanisms for radiation-induced oral mucositis and the consequences. *Cancer Nursing, 26,* 222–229.

Smith, R.A., Cokkinides, V., & Eyre, H.J. (2003). American Cancer Society's guidelines for the early detection of cancer, 2003. *CA: A Cancer Journal for Clinicians, 53,* 27–43.

CHAPTER 8

Hepatobiliary Cancer

Helen C. James, MS, APRN, BC, OCN®
Karen P. Kulakowski, MA, RD, LDN

Overview

Hepatobiliary cancers are primary or metastatic tumors of the liver, gall-bladder, and biliary system. Primary tumors of the hepatobiliary tree often are diagnosed at an advanced stage of disease because of vague symptoms of dull right upper quadrant pain, early satiety, weight loss, fatigue, and jaundice. The most frequent causes of hepatic malignancies in the United States are metastatic disease from melanoma and primary tumors of the gastrointestinal tract, lung, and breast (Barber & Fabugais-Nazario, 2003). Individuals with a metastatic tumor present with anorexia, weight loss, fatigue, jaundice, and ascites (Rychcik, 2000). The hepatobiliary system is essential in the metabolism of carbohydrates, proteins, and lipids; the synthesis of hormones, energy, and blood proteins; and the degradation and excretion of toxins and waste products from the blood (Dudrick & Kavic, 2002). Hepatic insufficiency and changes in metabolism result in accelerated weight loss leading to malnutrition (Allison, Eldridge, Polisena, Dixon, & Jinnah, 2000).

Incidence

Although hepatobiliary cancer is rare in the United States, it remains one of the most common malignancies diagnosed worldwide. The incidence of hepatobiliary cancer is much higher in areas of China, Japan, and Subsaharan Africa and is primarily associated with chronic hepatitis B, hepatitis C, and mycotoxin contamination of food sources and drinking water (Rychcik, 2000). The 2005 U.S. cancer statistics for both sexes estimate 17,550 new cases of liver and intrahepatic bile duct tumors and 7,480 cases of gallbladder and other biliary tumors (Jemal et al., 2005). Hepatocellular cancer accounts for 90% of primary tumors secondary to chronic hepatitis B, hepatitis C, and cirrhosis of the liver (Rychcik). The incidence of hepatocellular carcinoma is reported in the literature as higher among men 50–60 years of age and increases with age (Desjardins, 2002). The prognosis is poor, and death usually occurs as a result of local tumor invasion and tissue destruction, leading to malnutrition, gastrointestinal bleeding, and liver failure (Stuart, 2003). Cholangiocarcinoma, bile duct cancer, is the most common malignancy of the biliary tract. It is reported to affect women two times more frequently than men (Coleman, 2000). Incidence increases with age and is associated with a poor prognosis at the time of diagnosis (Misra, Chaturvedi, Misra, & Sharma, 2003).

Risk Factors and Prevention

Risk factors for hepatobiliary cancers are multifactorial, and prevention is related to, but not limited to, the etiology of the disease. Medical circumstances associated with primary hepatobiliary cancers include congenital diseases of infants and children, alcohol-induced cirrhosis of the liver, chronic hepatitis B and C viruses, chronic inflammatory disease of the gallbladder and biliary tree, and ulcerative colitis (Stuart, 2003). Mounting data indicate an apparent association between the prevalence of hepatitis B and C and hepatocellular carcinoma incidence (Desjardins, 2002). Cirrhosis of the liver remains the most prevalent predisposing factor for the development of hepatocellular carcinoma (Desjardins).

Prevention of hepatobiliary cancers begins with limiting exposure to environmental and chemical toxins, receiving hepatitis A and B vaccinations, and practicing primary preventive care for early detection and treatment of associated medical conditions. A natural chemical carcinogen, aflatoxin B1, is the product of *Aspergillus* fungus (Desjardins, 2002). Aflatoxin is found in water and stored food grains of countries with hot, humid climates. Improving grain storage and water purification systems in these countries focuses on reducing the amount of aflatoxin contamination and human exposure.

The main method of prevention is aimed at worldwide vaccination against hepatitis B. Chronic hepatitis B results in cirrhosis of the liver, the most common predisposing factor to the development of hepatobiliary cancer. Unfortunately, there is currently no vaccine against hepatitis C, and prevention focuses on education (Desjardins, 2002).

Primary preventive care is essential in early detection of predisposing conditions and risk factors for the development of metastases associated with hepatic insufficiency. This will provide the individual with the greatest chance for long-term survival.

Treatment Modalities

Treatment modalities focus on surgical resection, systemic chemotherapy, hepatic artery infusion chemotherapy, and limited radiation therapy. The treatment options for hepatobiliary carcinoma are restricted by the extent of disease progression at the time of diagnosis. Nutrition issues of anorexia, malnutrition, and hepatic insufficiency complicate treatment, increasing the risk of liver failure (Allison et al., 2000). Nutrition assessment and interventions must begin at diagnosis and be closely monitored during therapy to potentially improve quality of life and manage complications of therapies (Gabbard, Luthringer, & Eldridge, 2002; Sarhill, Mahmoud, Christie, & Tahir, 2003). Communication among the nutrition professional, patient, family, and healthcare team is essential to implement appropriate medical nutrition therapy consistent with the medical care plan.

Potentially, the only curative intervention for hepatobiliary carcinoma is complete surgical resection. Most hepatobiliary cancers are diagnosed at a late stage of disease with metastases to surrounding tissues, which limits surgical options. Alternate treatment options include radiation, chemotherapy, hepatic artery chemotherapy infusion, and bile duct stent placement for treatment of obstructive jaundice. Advanced stages of metastatic disease are associated with poor prognosis and require alternate treatment modalities for control and palliation of symptoms (Stuart, 2003).

Jaundice often is a presenting symptom at the time of diagnosis. The biliary tree or, if present, biliary stents can become obstructed by an invasive tumor growing in surrounding tissue or by a tumor within the bile ducts, causing jaundice. Jaundice is a poor prognostic indicator and requires immediate intervention. An endoscopic retrograde cholangiopancreaticography is useful for assessing the extent of disease to surrounding tissues, planning palliative care, and placing stents to alleviate obstruction of bile ducts to reduce jaundice. The use of stents to relieve jaundice is considered a temporary solution because of the increased risk of infection and occlusion secondary to inflammation, invasion of tumor cells, and stasis of bile salts (Pack, O'Connor, & O'Hagan, 2001).

The role of radiation in hepatobiliary carcinoma is palliative. It often is used to control pain, reduce tumor size, and improve duration of patency of biliary stents. Radiation therapy's usefulness as a treatment is limited because of the damage that occurs to healthy tissue. The patient receiving radiation therapy must be monitored closely for progression of hepatic insufficiency and complications of nausea, vomiting, and dehydration, which further complicate the delicate nutritional balance and quality of life. A nasogastric tube may be placed to relieve nausea or vomiting associated with bowel obstruction. A percutaneous endoscopic gastrostomy-jejunostomy (PEG-J) tube may be used for decompression and to provide nutrition and hydration (Piazza-Barnett & Matarese, 2000; Schattner, 2003). In situations when radiation therapy is not an option, chemotherapy is used as a palliative treatment.

Chemotherapy provides palliative treatment to reduce tumor size and potentially prolongs survival. Often, the individual with hepatobiliary cancer presents at diagnosis with vague symptoms of nausea, anorexia, and fatigue, making it difficult to evaluate side effects associated with chemotherapy treatments. The side effects of chemotherapy, however, need to be aggressively assessed and treated because of toxicities that complicate hepatic function and nutritional homeostasis (Sarhill et al., 2003). Complications of nausea, vomiting, and diarrhea potentiate the loss of calories and nutrients in an already compromised individual (see Table 8-1).

Table 8-1. Commonly Used Medications in Hepatobiliary Cancers

Drug	Route of Administration	Common Side Effects
Cisplatin	IV, hepatic artery infusion	Nausea, vomiting, diarrhea, peripheral neuropathy, severe nephrotoxicity, hypomagnesemia, hyperuricemia, myelosuppression
Doxorubicin	IV	Myelosuppression, nausea, vomiting, alopecia, mucositis, dose-limiting cardiotoxicity, radiation recall, arrhythmia, hyperuricemia, photosensitivity; drug may turn the urine red
Floxuridine	Intra-arterial, IV	Myelosuppression, nausea, vomiting, diarrhea, mucositis, alopecia, photosensitivity, darkening of the veins, abdominal pain, gastritis, enteritis, hepatotoxicity, hand-foot syndrome
Fluorouracil Leucovorin plus calcium	IV, hepatic artery infusion	Nausea, vomiting, diarrhea, mucositis, anorexia, myelosuppression
Irinotecan	IV	Nausea, vomiting, early and late onset diarrhea, myelosuppression
Lomustine	Oral	Myelosuppression (severe), nausea, vomiting, alopecia, renal toxicity, hepatic toxicity, mucositis, anorexia, pulmonary fibrosis
Mitomycin	IV, hepatic artery infusion	Diarrhea, gastritis, nausea, anorexia, myelosuppression, mucositis, renal toxicity

Note. Based on information from Cahill & Braccia, 2004; Polovich et al., 2005.

Chemotherapy given directly to a localized liver tumor through the hepatic artery is used to reduce systemic chemotherapy side effects and toxicities.

The hepatic artery provides 30% of the blood supply to the liver, making it an ideal entry system for administration of chemotherapy to primary tumors of the liver or metastatic tumors limited to the liver (Barber & Fabugais-Nazario, 2003). Hepatic artery infusion chemotherapy has demonstrated an increase in prolonged survival over standard systemic therapy (Stuart, 2003). The use of hepatic artery infusion reduces the systemic exposure and side effects of the chemotherapy agents. Close monitoring of hepatic function is crucial in identifying early signs of hepatic failure resulting from chemotherapy toxicity in normal hepatic cells. Nutritional support, aggressive hydration, and close monitoring of metabolic status following hepatic artery infusion of chemotherapy remain vital to maintaining and preventing irreversible damage to hepatic failure.

During chemotherapy, the nutrition professional needs to monitor the patient's nutritional intake. Although metabolic status may indicate the need for protein, sodium, or fluid restriction, the amount the patient can consume may be less than optimal. Decreasing the restrictions placed on food may improve palatability of the diet, thereby potentially increasing the amount of food the patient will eat (Martin, 2000; McCallum, 2000).

Nutritional Implications

Malnutrition is common in patients who have hepatobiliary cancers and is manifested most commonly as protein-calorie malnutrition and wasting (Dudrick & Kavic, 2002). Protein functions as reserve metabolic fuel and may become seriously depleted during tumor growth. Alterations in protein metabolism include host nitrogen depletion, decreased protein synthesis, increased protein catabolism in the liver and skeletal muscle, and abnormal plasma amino acid levels. This abnormal amino acid metabolism is hallmark in liver disease and can be characterized by low plasma levels of methionine and branch chain amino acids leucine, isoleucine, and valine. This may be attributed to the altered metabolism of carbohydrates and fat in the patient with liver failure, which is characterized as an increase in rapid transition of substrate utilization from the fed to the starved state (ASPEN Board of Directors & the Clinical Guidelines Task Force, 2002). Considering that human tumors are rarely larger than 1% of body mass, the change in the patient's whole body protein metabolism is attributed to the degree of catabolic response and the type and stage of tumor present.

In patients with cancer, the rate of glucose synthesized from amino acids is increased and muscle protein is degraded; the reasons for this are unknown. The tumor also uses glucose at an increased rate. This, along with an increased energy demand by the tumor, results in a depletion of body fat stores (Nebeling, 2000). Primary hepatocellular tumors, as well as liver metastasis, can potentially alter the liver's capacity to regulate metabolism. The most serious side effect of this is hypoglycemia. A low simple sugar diet with small, frequent feedings will help to prevent hypoglycemic reactions. Foods high in sugar are avoided to prevent stimulation of excessive insulin secretion from the pancreas.

The liver controls fat metabolism. During the fed state, excess dietary carbohydrate is converted into fat by the liver. This fat is sent through the circulatory system to the adipose tissue for storage. During periods of starvation, adipose tissue releases stored fat as fatty acids, which are sent back to the liver and converted into energy (Borum, 2001; Matos, Porayko, Francisco-Ziller, & DiCecco, 2002).

Steatorrhea is common in hepatocellular carcinomas if there is underlying cirrhosis. This may be caused by alcohol, altered pancreatic response to a fatty (meal) challenge, and/or bile salt abnormalities. In cases where no cirrhosis is present, tumor growth often results in obstruction of the biliary drainage system, thus preventing the secretion of bile salts into the gastrointestinal tract.

Assessment Guidelines

All patients undergoing treatment for cancer should have a baseline nutrition evaluation documented to determine whether they are at risk for developing nutrition problems. General guidelines for nutrition evaluation may be found in Appendices E and J. The nutrition assessment should focus on existing or potential nutrition problems but also should take into account the stage of illness and the patient's prognosis. The predominant symptom of advanced liver disease is protein malnutrition, characterized by low plasma albumin and transferrin levels, decreased creatinine/height index, and decreased total lymphocyte count. If cirrhosis is present, micronutrient deficiencies of zinc, vitamin A, B vitamins, and vitamin E may be present. Some patients may have cholestasis or failure to excrete bile, resulting in increased plasma levels of direct and total bilirubin and alkaline phosphatase (Dudrick & Kavic, 2002).

All of these patients are catabolic and most are anorexic, so a high-calorie (30–35 kcal/kg/day) and normal protein (1–1.2 g/kg/day) diet should be administered enterally if possible. Supplemental fat-soluble vitamins (A, D, E, and K) are strongly recommended with prolonged or profound cholestasis (Dudrick & Kavic, 2002). The goals of nutrition therapy should be realistic and consistent with the overall plan of care (McCallum, 2000).

Special Considerations for Nutrition

Hepatocellular carcinoma, cholangiocarcinoma, and carcinomas of the biliary tree may result in mechanical dysfunction of the gastrointestinal tract, malabsorption of micronutrients and macronutrients, ascites (including malignant ascites), or hepatic encephalopathy. If ascites caused by cirrhosis is present, consideration of sodium restriction up to 2,000 mg/day and fluid restriction of 1–1.5 l/day is prudent (Bloch & Charuhas, 2001). However, if intake is poor, the patient may not be consuming enough food or fluid to warrant restrictions (Sawhill et al., 2000).

Malignant ascites can result from extensive intrahepatic metastasis, compression of the hepatic vein, or obstruction of the portal vein. Restrictions are not warranted in this situation.

Gastroparesis may result in nausea and vomiting. Medications that promote gastric emptying, such as metoclopramide and erythromycin, may be of benefit. Severe cases may require placement of a nasogastric or PEG tube for gastric decompression. Jejunal tube feedings or parenteral nutrition may be necessary if consistent with the medical treatment plan. Once the patient can tolerate clamping of the decompression tube, an oral diet consisting of clear liquids would begin and would progress to regular diet in six small meals as tolerated. If nasojejunal or percutaneous endoscopic jejunal tubes are being used to provide nutrition and hydration, the patient should be consuming 70%–75% of nutritional needs via an oral diet before the tube feedings are discontinued (Schattner, 2003).

In hepatocellular cancer, an isotonic tube feeding formula may be used. If hepatic encephalopathy is present, a formula high in branched chain amino acid (BCAA) designed for hepatic failure should be considered. Adequate protein is required to facilitate hepatic cell nutrition without excess ammonia being produced from exogenous and endogenous protein catabolism. Protein should be provided as 0.5 g protein/kg dry weight initially and increased as tolerated. If a formula high in BCAA is used, up to 1.5 g/kg dry weight can be provided.

In cholangiocarcinomas, consider an isotonic tube feeding formula low in long-chain triglycerides and high in medium-chain triglycerides (MCTs). Fat malabsorption may require providing pancreatic lipase supplementation for hydrolysis of dietary fats.

Hyperglycemia may require oral medication or insulin, as well as restriction of simple sugars in the diet. However, if the patient is consuming more than adequate nutrition, a calorie-controlled diet may be indicated for blood sugar management.

Presence of a chylous effusion may necessitate that the patient not take oral nutrition. Trial of a minimal- to no-fat diet by mouth or enteral feeding tube may be prescribed. Supplementation with MCTs may be of benefit. Often, parenteral nutrition is necessary to decrease and seal a chylous leak.

Fluid and electrolyte imbalances often are seen in patients who have hepatocellular carcinomas. Increased losses through gastric tubes and/or diarrhea will require additional IV fluids for hydration.

Malabsorption of fat-soluble vitamins as well as thiamine, folic acid, magnesium and zinc, may require supplementation. Care should be taken not to use megadose vitamins or minerals, as they can further tax an already compromised liver. Supplementation should be by prescription only, and blood levels must be monitored. Herbal preparations aimed at alleviating side effects of treatment should be used with caution and in limited doses, as herbal products are metabolized by the liver.

Perioperative nutritional support should be used in patients undergoing liver resection for hepatocellular carcinoma associated with cirrhosis (Dudrick & Kavic, 2002). Parenteral nutrition also is appropriate in patients who are malnourished, are receiving active anticancer treatment, and are anticipated to be unable to ingest or absorb adequate nutrients for a prolonged period of time (DeChico & Steiger, 2000; DiMaria-Ghalili, 2002). Palliative use of parenteral nutrition in the patient who is terminally ill is rarely indicated (ASPEN Board of Directors & the Clinical Guidelines Task Force, 2002).

Determination of the type of nutritional support should be made by the healthcare provider, patient, and family, as appropriate, and take into account the patient's clinical status, aggressiveness of medical care, and prognosis.

According to the American Dietetic Association (Maillet, Potter, & Heller, 2002), "the development of clinical and ethical criteria for the nutrition and hydration of persons through the life span should be established by the members of the health care team. Registered dietitians should work collaboratively to make nutrition, hydration, and feeding recommendations in individual cases" (p. 716). When palliative care becomes the fundamental goal of care, the plan of care should be constantly reassessed and updated (Dahl, 2002; Meares, 2000; Morita, Tei, Shishido, & Inoue, 2003; Small, Carrera, Danford, Logemann, & Cella, 2002).

References

Allison, G., Eldridge, B., Polisena, C., Dixon, T., & Jinnah, R. (2000). Nutrition implications of surgical oncology. In P.D. McCallum & C.G. Polisena (Eds.), *The clinical guide to oncology nutrition* (pp. 79–89). Chicago: American Dietetic Association.

ASPEN Board of Directors & the Clinical Guidelines Task Force. (2002). Guidelines for the use of parenteral and enteral nutrition in adult and pediatric patients. *Journal of Parenteral and Enteral Nutrition, 26*(Suppl. 1), 1SA–138SA, 144SA.

Barber, F., & Fabugais-Nazario, L. (2003). What's old is new again: Patients receiving hepatic artery infusion chemotherapy. *Clinical Journal of Oncology Nursing, 7*, 647–652.

Bloch, A.B., & Charuhas, P.M. (2001). Cancer and cancer therapy. In M.M. Gottschlich (Ed.), *The science and practice of nutrition support. A case-based core curriculum* (pp. 643–659). Dubuque, IA: Kendall/Hunt Publishing.

Borum, P.R. (2001). Nutrient metabolism. In M.M. Gottschlich (Ed.), *The science and practice of nutrition support. A case-based core curriculum* (pp. 17–29). Dubuque, IA: Kendall/Hunt Publishing.

Cahill, B.A., & Braccia, D. (2004). Current treatment for hepatocellular carcinoma. *Clinical Journal of Oncology Nursing, 8*, 393–400.

Coleman, J. (2000). Gallbladder and bile duct cancer. In C.H. Yarbro, M.H. Frogge, M. Goodman, & S.L. Groenwald (Eds.), *Cancer nursing: Principles and practice* (5th ed., pp. 1192–1209). Sudbury, MA: Jones and Bartlett.

Dahl, M. (2002). Nutrition and hospice. *Healthcare Food and Nutrition Focus, 19*, 6–7.

DeChico, R.S., & Steiger, E. (2000). Parenteral nutrition in medical/surgical oncology. In P.D. McCallum & C.G. Polisena (Eds.), *The clinical guide to oncology nutrition* (pp. 119–126). Chicago: American Dietetic Association.

Desjardins, L. (2002). Hepatocellular carcinoma. *Clinical Journal of Oncology Nursing, 6,* 107–118.

DiMaria-Ghalili, R.A. (2002). Parenteral nutrition in hepatic, biliary, and renal disease. *Journal of Infusion Nursing, 25,* 25–28.

Dudrick, S.J., & Kavic, S.M. (2002). Hepatobiliary nutrition: History and future. *Journal of Hepatobiliary and Pancreatic Surgery, 9,* 459–468.

Gabbard, D., Luthringer, S., & Eldridge, B. (2002). Oncology nutrition standards of care: Integrating nutrition into your cancer program. *Oncology Issues Supplement,* pp. 8–10.

Jemal, A., Murray, T., Ward, E., Samuels, A., Tiwari, R.C., Ghafoor, A., et al. (2005). Cancer statistics, 2005. *CA: A Cancer Journal for Clinicians, 55,* 10–30.

Maillet, J.O., Potter, R.L., & Heller, L. (2002). Position of the American Dietetic Association: Ethical and legal issues in malnutrition, hydration and feeding. *Journal of the American Dietetic Association, 102,* 716–726.

Martin, C. (2000). Calorie, protein, fluid & micronutrient requirements. In P.D. McCallum & C.G. Polisena (Eds.), *The clinical guide to oncology nutrition* (pp. 45–52). Chicago: American Dietetic Association.

Matos, C., Porayko, M., Francisco-Ziller, N., & DiCecco, S. (2002). Nutrition and chronic liver disease. *Journal of Clinical Gastroenterology, 35,* 391–397.

McCallum, P.D. (2000). Patient-generated subjective global assessment. In P.D. McCallum & C.G. Polisena (Eds.), *The clinical guide to oncology nutrition* (pp. 11–23). Chicago: American Dietetic Association.

Meares, C.J. (2000). Nutritional issues in palliative care. *Seminars in Oncology Nursing, 16,* 135–145.

Misra, S., Chaturvedi, A., Misra, N., & Sharma, L. (2003). Carcinoma of the gallbladder. *Lancet Oncology, 4,* 167–176.

Morita, T., Tei, Y., Shishido, H., & Inoue, S. (2003). Treatable complications of cancer patients referred to an inpatient hospice. *American Journal of Hospice and Palliative Care, 20,* 389–391.

Nebeling, L. (2000). Changes in carbohydrate, protein, and fat metabolism in cancer. In P.D. McCallum & C.G. Polisena (Eds.), *The clinical guide to oncology nutrition* (pp. 53–60). Chicago: American Dietetic Association.

Pack, D., O'Connor, K., & O'Hagan, K. (2001). Cholangiocarcinoma: A nursing perspective. *Clinical Journal of Oncology Nursing, 5,* 141–146, 155–156.

Piazza-Barnett, R., & Matarese, L. (2000). Enteral nutrition in medical/surgical oncology. In P.D. McCallum & C.G. Polisena (Eds.), *The clinical guide to oncology nutrition* (pp. 106–118). Chicago: American Dietetic Association.

Polovich, M., White, J.M., & Kelleher, L.O. (Eds.). (2005). *Chemotherapy and biotherapy guidelines and recommendations for practice* (2nd ed.). Pittsburgh, PA: Oncology Nursing Society.

Rychcik, J. (2000). Liver cancer: Primary and metastatic disease. In C.H. Yarbro, M.H. Frogge, M. Goodman, & S.L. Groenwald (Eds.), *Cancer nursing: Principles and practice* (5th ed., pp. 1269–1289). Sudbury, MA: Jones and Bartlett.

Sarhill, N., Mahmoud, F.A., Christie, R., & Tahir, A. (2003). Assessment of nutritional status and fluid deficits in advanced cancer. *American Journal of Hospice and Palliative Care, 20,* 465–473.

Schattner, M. (2003). Enteral nutrition support of the patient with cancer: Route and role. *Journal of Clinical Gastroenterology, 36,* 297–302.

Small, W., Carrera, R., Danford, L., Logemann, J.A., & Cella, D. (2002, March/April). Quality of life and nutrition in the patient with cancer. Integrating nutrition into your cancer program. *Oncology Issues Supplement,* pp. 13–14.

Stuart, K. (2003). Chemoembolization in the management of liver tumors. *Oncologist, 8,* 425–437.

CHAPTER 9

Lung Cancer

Anne Z. Kisak, RN, MBA, BSN
Lesley B. Klein, MS, RD, LD

Overview

Lung cancer is a major public health issue (Thomas, Williams, Cobos, & Turrisi, 2001). It is the leading cause of cancer death in both men and women, accounting for approximately 30% of all cancer deaths in 2005, an estimated 163,510 deaths (Jemal et al., 2005). Patients with lung cancer reported multiple distressing symptoms and have a variety of comorbid conditions and treatment options (Gift, Jablonski, Stommel, & Given, 2004). Lung cancer is associated with significant nutritional implications for patients undergoing treatment.

Incidence

Worldwide, the incidence of lung cancer is still on the rise. According to the American Cancer Society (ACS, 2005), lung cancer is the number-two new cancer diagnosis for both men and women, accounting for 13% of new cancer diagnoses in men and 12% of new cancer diagnoses in women. This translates into an estimated 172,570 new cases in 2005.

Lung and bronchial cancers remain the most common cause of cancer-related deaths. They account for 31% of cancer-related deaths in men and 27% of cancer-related deaths in women (see Figures 9-1 and 9-2). These rates, however, are changing. In men, the lung cancer–related mortality rate has been declining since 1991, whereas mortality rates for women continue to rise (ACS, 2005). Even with changes in male and female and age-adjusted death rates, there has been no significant overall change in lung cancer survival rates in 25 years (ACS). The most important prognostic indicator for lung cancer survival is clinical stage

Figure 9-1. Cancer Death Rates for Women in the United States, 1930–2001

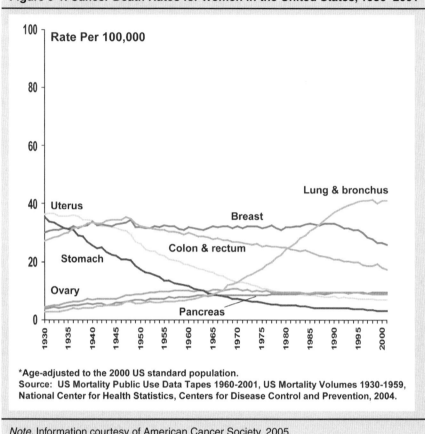

*Age-adjusted to the 2000 US standard population.
Source: US Mortality Public Use Data Tapes 1960-2001, US Mortality Volumes 1930-1959,
National Center for Health Statistics, Centers for Disease Control and Prevention, 2004.

Note. Information courtesy of American Cancer Society, 2005.

(Houlihan, 2004). It is important to note that changes in ICD (International Classification of Diseases) coding practices will play a role in current and future cancer-related mortality statistics. Changes in coding practices using ICD-10 will account for a 0.7% increase in cancer-related deaths (ACS, 2005).

Various pathologic subtypes of lung cancer have been revised and expanded over the years. For practical, but unofficial classification purposes, clinicians often discuss lung cancer as small cell lung cancer or non-small cell lung cancer (Thomas et al., 2001).

Risk and Prevention

Cigarette smoking is the primary risk factor for the development of lung cancer (Thomas et al., 2001). Other risk factors for lung cancer include both occupational and environmental exposures, including exposure to carcinogens such as radon, asbestos, arsenic, and air pollution (ACS, 2005). Patients with some preexisting pulmonary conditions, such as tuberculosis, pulmonary fibrosis, and chronic obstructive pulmonary disease, also are at increased risk for the development of lung cancer (ACS; Thomas et al.).

The primary prevention tool for lung cancer is elimination and reduction of high-risk factors and behaviors. This includes promoting tobacco cessation, changing workplace practices to reduce exposure, and other behavior modification techniques. Tobacco is one of the strongest agents associated with the ability to cause cancer. Based on scientific evidence, cigarette smoking is associated with lung cancer as well as a number of other types of cancers and chronic diseases (National Cancer Institute [NCI], 2004). Tobacco use remains the leading preventable cause of death in the United States, causing more than 440,000 deaths each year and resulting

Figure 9-2. Cancer Death Rates for Men in the United States, 1930–2001

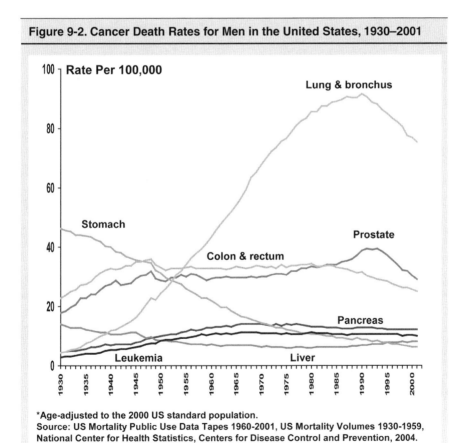

*Age-adjusted to the 2000 US standard population.
Source: US Mortality Public Use Data Tapes 1960-2001, US Mortality Volumes 1930-1959, National Center for Health Statistics, Centers for Disease Control and Prevention, 2004.

Note. Information courtesy of American Cancer Society, 2005.

in an annual cost of more than $75 billion in direct medical costs (Centers for Disease Control and Prevention, 2002). Smoking avoidance and smoking cessation result in decreased incidence and mortality from cancer (NCI, 2004) (see Figures 9-3, 9-4, and 9-5).

Figure 9-3. Tobacco Use in the United States, 1900–2000

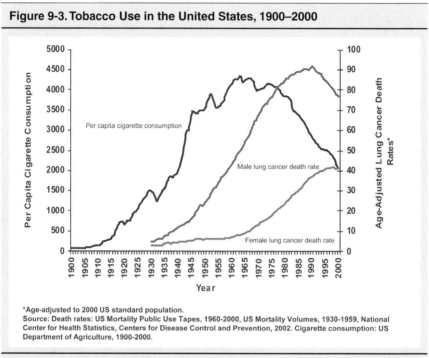

*Age-adjusted to 2000 US standard population.
Source: Death rates: US Mortality Public Use Tapes, 1960-2000, US Mortality Volumes, 1930-1959, National Center for Health Statistics, Centers for Disease Control and Prevention, 2002. Cigarette consumption: US Department of Agriculture, 1900-2000.

Note. Figure courtesy of American Cancer Society, 2005.

Other risk factors for lung cancer include asbestos exposure and various other geographically associated and employment-related exposure issues. These include exposure to radon gas, coal tar derivatives, and other types of irritants. Scientists estimated that approximately 15,000–22,000 lung cancer deaths per year are related to radon. Radon is an odorless, tasteless radioactive gas that seeps up through the soil and is released into the air from the normal decay of uranium in rocks and soil. Radon gas usually exists at very low levels outdoors. However, in areas without adequate ventilation, such as underground mines and basements in some types of homes, radon can accumulate to levels that substantially increase the risk of lung cancer. Although the association between radon exposure and smoking is not well understood, exposure to the combination of radon gas and cigarette smoke creates a greater risk for lung cancer than either factor alone. The majority of radon-related cancer deaths occur among smokers (NCI, 2004).

Figure 9-4. Annual U.S. Deaths Attributable to Cigarette Smoking—1995–1999

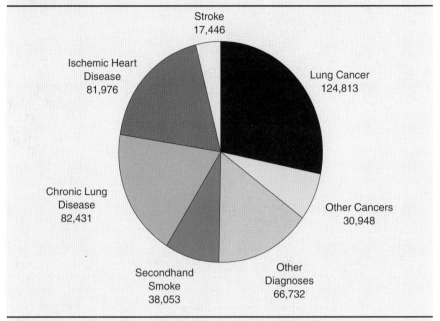

Note. Figure courtesy of the Centers for Disease Control and Prevention, 2002.

Figure 9-5. Trends in Cigarette Smoking Prevalence (%), by Gender, Adults 18 and Older, in the United States, 1965–2002

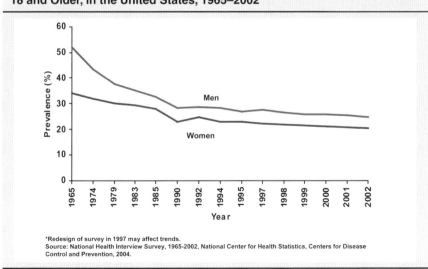

*Redesign of survey in 1997 may affect trends.
Source: National Health Interview Survey, 1965-2002, National Center for Health Statistics, Centers for Disease Control and Prevention, 2004.

Note. Figure courtesy of American Cancer Society, 2005.

Many studies have shown that the combination of smoking and asbestos exposure is particularly hazardous. Smokers who also are exposed to asbestos have an increased risk of lung cancer. Asbestos, the name given to a group of minerals that occurs naturally as bundles of fibers that can be separated into thin threads, was mined and used commercially in North America since the late 1800s as an agent to strengthen cement and plastics, as well as for insulation, fireproofing, and sound absorption. Several different types of asbestos may be associated with different health risks. Starting in the late 1970s, the U.S. Consumer Product Safety Commission banned the use of asbestos in wallboard patching compounds and gas fireplaces because the asbestos fibers in these products could be released into the environment during use. In 1989, the U.S. Environmental Protection Agency banned all new uses of asbestos. Established uses, prior to 1989, are still allowed. Although nearly everyone is exposed to asbestos at some time during his or her life, people who become ill from asbestos usually are those who are exposed to it on a regular basis, most often in a job where they work directly with the material or through substantial environmental contact. As government regulations improve work practices, today's workers (those without previous exposure) are likely to face lower risks than those who were exposed in the past (NCI, 2003).

Lung cancer is primarily diagnosed as a squamous cell histology, which arises from cells that cover organs and form the lining of tissue surfaces. Squamous cells lining the lungs are exposed to external toxins, such as tobacco smoke, but at the same time are exposed to tobacco carcinogens absorbed into the bloodstream. Squamous cell cancers are thought to be cancers of "undernutrition" (Nixon, 1996). In other words, squamous cell cancers appear to be linked to populations that are missing something from their diet. The missing component may be antioxidant vitamins, especially A and E.

Smokers are not necessarily malnourished in the usual sense of the word. They have a much greater need for antioxidants because smoking increases the level of oxidants that damage cells. The body requires more antioxidants to try to reverse the process. However, research shows that taking supplements in megadoses, rather than eating foods containing beta-carotene and other vitamins, may be harmful and increase the risk for lung cancer in people who continue to smoke (WebMD Health, 2004).

Although the role of vitamin supplements in fighting lung cancer is uncertain, studies are beginning to show that eating fruits and vegetables reduces lung cancer risk in smokers and nonsmokers. This protection is probably the result of the ingestion of antioxidants or other phytochemicals.

Treatment Modalities

Lung cancer treatment may involve all aspects of oncology care. Surgery, radiation therapy, and chemotherapy all can be primary components of an individualized, patient-oriented treatment plan. This depends on disease factors, such as the specific subtype of lung cancer and its stage, as well as patient factors, such as the goals of therapy, state of health or comorbid disease states, and course of the disease. In addition, surgery, radiation therapy, and chemotherapy also may have a role in palliation if disease progression continues.

Surgery usually is included as a treatment method for localized and resectable lung cancers (Jemal et al., 2005). Surgery may be done initially or after a course of neoadjuvant chemotherapy. Surgical interventions for patients range from biopsy to vascular access device implantation to lobectomy or wedge resection (Dose & Brueggen, 2001).

Chemotherapy also is a mainstay of lung cancer treatment. Chemotherapy may be used as a neoadjuvant to radiation therapy or surgery, postsurgery concomitantly with radiation therapy, for palliation of symptoms, or for patients with unresectable disease (Thomas et al., 2001). Chemotherapy regimens usually are platinum-based multidrug regimens (Kemper, Haapoja, & Goodman, 2001; Krebs & Russell, 2001).

Radiation therapy has a role in primary treatment and palliative care for patients with lung cancer, especially for inoperable lung cancers (Thomas et al., 2001). Radiation therapy may be used neoadjuvantly to surgery to provide immediate relief of pain or spinal cord compression or to assist with breathing or circulation if superior vena cava syndrome has occurred (Thomas et al.).

Clinical presentation of patients varies widely. Patients may have an underlying lung cancer for several years before the tumor impacts normal function enough to cause symptoms (Houlihan, 2004). Symptoms that may indicate the need to further investigate the possible diagnosis of lung cancer include the following (ACS, 2005).

- Persistent cough that gets worse over time
- Chest pain
- Shortness of breath, wheezing, or hoarseness
- Coughing up blood
- Fever from unknown source
- Frequent pneumonia or bronchitis
- Weight loss and loss of appetite

Nutritional Implications

Lung cancer studies have shown that certain symptoms can occur in clusters. Fatigue, nausea and vomiting, weakness, appetite and weight loss, and altered taste often occur together (Gift et al., 2004). Symptoms can be disease-related or treatment-related. Appendix C provides detailed information regarding these nutrition impact symptoms.

Anorexia

Anorexia is a lack of interest in food or appetite that can lead to substantial weight loss. Suggestions for patients include
- Eat smaller, more frequent meals.
- Concentrate on high-calorie, high-protein foods to make every bite count.
- Consider snacking on cheese on crackers, deviled eggs, peanut butter on an apple, cheesecake with fruit topping, or macaroni and cheese.
- Combine a quart of whole milk with one cup of powdered milk to increase calorie and protein content without increasing portion size. This "double-strength milk" can be used in any food preparation to increase nutrition content.
- Consider pharmacologic therapy, such as megestrol acetate (Megace®, Bristol-Myers Squibb, Princeton, NJ) and dronabinol (Marinol®, Unimed Pharmaceuticals, Marietta, GA), which may increase appetite.

Cachexia

Cachexia is defined as extreme weight loss with severe wasting of muscle and fat. It occurs with malnutrition or a terminal illness. Suggestions for patients include
- Good sources of protein to help to build up and repair tissues that have been damaged by treatment or the cancer itself.
- Good sources of protein include beef, chicken, fish, dairy foods, eggs, beans, legumes, and nuts.

Diarrhea

Often, diarrhea is drug induced. Patients can temporarily become lactose intolerant because of the combination of chemotherapy drugs. Suggestions for patients include
- Follow a low-residue diet.
- Eliminate dairy products and substitute acidophilus milk, Lactaid® milk (McNeil Nutritionals, Fort Washington, PA), or soy products such as soymilk, soy-based ice cream, and "veggie cheese."

Fatigue

Many patients with cancer complain of extreme fatigue during treatment. This symptom has several causes, which can include anemia or a lack of several vitamins and minerals, including iron and vitamins B_2, B_{12}, B_6, E, and C.
- Good sources of iron include calves' livers, chicken livers, eggs, clams, oysters, pork, beef, beans, raisins, spinach, collard greens, apricots, and fortified cereals.

- Food sources of vitamin B_2 include beef, liver, milk, yogurt, cheese, mushrooms, asparagus, and broccoli.
- Sources of vitamin B_{12} include beef liver, clams, oysters, tuna, yogurt, milk, cheese, eggs, and brewer's yeast.
- Foods high in vitamin B_6 include wheat germ, poultry, fish, beef, soybeans, bananas, avocado, whole grain breads, and dried fruit.
- Vitamin E sources include wheat germ, safflower oil, sunflower oil, avocados, broccoli, peaches, and asparagus.
- Vitamin C foods enhance iron absorption and include orange juice and other citrus fruits, brussels sprouts, strawberries, collard greens, tomato juice, potatoes, and lima beans.

Mucositis

Inflammation of the lining of the mouth, or mucositis, can interfere with nutritional intake. Suggestions for patients include
- Modify diet to include more soft foods such as eggs, cooked cereal, pudding, and custard.
- Incorporate commercially prepared or homemade milkshakes to help to meet nutritional needs (Bloch, 1990).

Nausea and Vomiting

Antiemetics are antinausea medications that can reduce nausea/vomiting. In addition, some dietary changes may help to manage these symptoms. These include
- Separate solids from liquids to decrease stomach volume and help to reduce pressure and bloating.
- Avoid sweet foods that may aggravate the nausea and substitute foods that are more tart. Sucking on lemon Italian water ices may be more appealing than sweeter flavored ice pops.
- Marinate meats in a vinegar-based marinade rather than a sweet sauce.
- Reduce odors that can aggravate nausea. Try foods that are cold or room temperature with less offensive odors, such as a turkey sandwich, pudding, or custard. If beverages have an odor, put them in a cup with a lid and drink through a straw.
- Sip on ginger tea or ginger ale, or snack on gingersnap cookies, as ginger has been shown to help to reduce nausea.

Pain

When pain is not controlled, it can greatly reduce appetite. Narcotics can be very useful in managing pain. However, a normal side effect of narcotics is constipation. It is extremely important to encourage activity, fluid replacement, and the use of stool softeners or laxatives on a regular basis. Eating high-fiber foods, such as fruits, vegetables, whole grains (e.g., oats, wheat), and beans, also may aid in easier elimination.

Xerostomia

A decrease in saliva may make eating more difficult. Saliva is important in the first steps of digestion, and lack of saliva can make food stick to teeth or the roof of the mouth and make swallowing difficult. Tart foods may help to stimulate the salivary glands; therefore, sipping on lemonade or sucking on a lemon drop can be helpful.

Special Considerations for Nutrition

Lung cancer is a debilitating disease that can cause involuntary weight loss. Tumor cells produce cytokines, which bind to the cell membrane (Dunlop & Campbell, 2000). Arachidonic acid (AA) is released and metabolized. The AA metabolites stimulate the breakup of the nuclear factor-kappa B/1 kappa B complex (NF-κB/κB complex). These compounds bind to DNA, which signal the production of cytokine mRNA (Lo, Chiu, & Fu, 1999). Cytokines move out of the cell to affect other tissues, such as skeletal muscle, and reactivate NF-κB to continue the cycle. Cytokine production results in decreased appetite, decreased food intake, elevated resting metabolic rate, and eventual weight loss. Some studies show that by incorporating eicosapentaenoic acid, an anti-inflammatory omega-3 fat, into cell membranes, AA production may decrease (Babcock, Helton, & Espat, 2000). With fewer AA metabolites available, there is less breakup of the NF-κB/κB complex. In turn, less NF-κB is available to stimulate production of additional cytokines. Eicosapentaenoic acid is found in fish oils and comes from cold-water fish, such as cod, mackerel, salmon, and shark.

Weight loss can be a primary indicator for outcome. People who have lost < 10% of their body weight in the three to six months prior to diagnosis have a better long-term survival rate. The greater the weight loss before diagnosis, the worse the long-term prognosis (OncoLink, 2001).

The nutrition goals during treatment are maintaining body weight and consuming adequate amounts of protein foods. However, as other side effects occur, adjustments in the diet will become necessary.

Care Planning

Patients with lung cancer can experience multiple symptoms (Gift et al., 2004). Symptoms vary depending on where a patient is in the course of his or her disease. Most patients with lung cancer are diagnosed at an advanced stage. These patients will have more symptoms than newly diagnosed patients at an earlier stage

(Hopwood & Stevens, 1995). Studies have shown that patients with advanced lung cancer experience more severe symptomatic distress when compared to other types of cancers (Gift et al.). Patients require both ongoing disease management as well as treatment-related side effect management, with a focus on quality of life as they move through the disease continuum (Houlihan, 2004).

The most common symptoms patients report are dyspnea, cough, pain, fatigue, nausea, appetite and weight loss, altered taste, and vomiting (Gift et al., 2004). Many of these symptoms are co-occurring, and strategies to manage them must be carefully selected with consideration to how symptoms interact (Gift et al.). Furthermore, additional research is needed with regard to assessment and intervention of clusters of symptoms, which improve the quality of life and function of patients (Gift et al.).

Expected Outcomes of Therapy

Lung cancer requires very aggressive treatment. Surgery, followed by chemotherapy and radiation, can result in the most favorable prognosis (American Society of Clinical Oncology, 2004). However, in small cell lung cancer, surgery is only performed during the biopsy. This type of cancer is so aggressive that surgery usually is not effective. Survival rate is influenced by localization of disease. Patients with metastatic disease at the time of diagnosis have a poorer prognosis than those without metastatic disease (ACS, 2005).

Summary

Although the overall prognosis of lung cancer is poor, medical nutrition therapy can improve the quality of life for patients. The primary nutrition goal for patients should be to maintain body weight and consume adequate protein. Dietitians, nurses, and other healthcare providers should expect to help patients to adjust their diets as side effects occur in order to maintain their weight. Weight loss, including prediagnosis weight loss, should be tracked, as it has been shown to be an indicator for survival.

References

American Cancer Society. (2005). *Cancer facts and figures, 2005*. Atlanta, GA: Author.

American Society of Clinical Oncology. (2004). *People living with cancer*. Retrieved July 12, 2004, from http://www.plwc.org

Babcock, T., Helton, W.S., & Espat, J.J. (2000). Eicosapentaenoic acid (EPA): An anti-inflammatory omega-3 fat with potential clinical applications. *Nutrition, 16*, 1116–1118.

Bloch, A.S. (1990). Nutrition management of the cancer patient. In J.A. Darbinian & A.M. Coulston (Eds.), *Impact of chemotherapy on the nutrition status of the cancer patient* (pp. 161–170). Rockville, MD: Aspen.

Centers for Disease Control and Prevention. (2002). *Deaths attributable to cigarette smoking—United States, 1995–1999.* Retrieved September 1, 2004, from http://www.cdc.gov/tobacco/overview/attrdths.htm

Dose, A.M., & Brueggen, C. (2001). Surgical oncology. In R.A. Gates & R.M. Fink (Eds.), *Oncology nursing secrets* (2nd ed., pp. 27–34). Philadelphia: Hanley and Belfus.

Dunlop, R.J., & Campbell, C.W. (2000). Cytokines and advanced cancer. *Journal of Pain and Symptom Management, 20,* 214–232.

Gift, A.G., Jablonski, A., Stommel, M., & Given, W. (2004). Symptom cluster in elderly patients with lung cancer. *Oncology Nursing Forum, 31,* 203–210.

Hopwood, P., & Stevens, R.J. (1995). Symptom presentation for treatment in patients with lung cancer: Implications for the evaluation of palliative treatment. *British Journal of Cancer, 71,* 633–636.

Houlihan, N.G. (2004). Overview. In N.G. Houlihan (Ed.), *Site-specific cancer series: Lung cancer* (pp. 1–5). Pittsburgh, PA: Oncology Nursing Society.

Jemal, A., Murray, T., Ward, E., Samuels, A., Tiwari, R.C., Ghafoor, A., et al. (2005). Cancer statistics, 2005. *CA: A Cancer Journal for Clinicians, 55,* 10–30.

Kemper, M., Haapoja, I., & Goodman, M. (2001). Principles of chemotherapy. In R.A. Gates & R.M. Fink (Eds.), *Oncology nursing secrets* (2nd ed., pp. 44–52). Philadelphia: Hanley and Belfus.

Krebs, L.U., & Russell, T. (2001). Lung cancer. In R.A. Gates & R.M. Fink (Eds.), *Oncology nursing secrets* (2nd ed., pp. 263–270). Philadelphia: Hanley and Belfus.

Lo, C.J., Chiu, K.C., & Fu, M. (1999). Fish oil decreases macrophage tumor necrosis factor gene transcription by altering the NFkappaB activity. *Journal of Surgical Research, 82,* 216–221.

National Cancer Institute. (2003, August). *Asbestos and cancer: Questions and answers.* Retrieved September 1, 2004, from http://cis.nci.nih.gov/fact/3_21.htm

National Cancer Institute. (2004). *Prevention and cessation of cigarette smoking: Control of tobacco use (PDQ®).* Retrieved September 1, 2004, from http://cancer.gov/cancerinfo/pdq/prevention/control-of-tobacco-use/healthprofessional

Nixon, D.W. (1996). *The Cancer Recovery Eating Plan for people with cancer of the lung, head, neck, esophagus, cervix, bladder, or skin (squamous cancers).* New York: Alison Brown Cerier Book Development.

OncoLink. (2001). *Lung cancer.* Retrieved July 12, 2004, from http://www.oncolink.upenn.edu/resources/article.cfm?

Thomas, C.R., Williams, T., Cobos, E., & Turrisi, A. (2001). Lung cancer. In R.E. Lenhard, R.T. Osteen, & T. Gandsler (Eds.), *Clinical oncology 2001* (pp. 271–295). Atlanta, GA: American Cancer Society.

WebMD Health. (2004). *Lung cancer prevention.* Retrieved May 25, 2004, from http://www.webmd.com

CHAPTER 10

Pancreatic Cancer

Jennifer L. Guy, BS, RN, OCN®
Tracy R. Smith, PhD, RD, LD

Overview

Pancreatic cancer is a deadly disease that is increasing in incidence. Because pancreatic cancer generally develops without symptoms, early detection is rare and survival rates are dismal. For all stages combined, the one-year relative survival rate is 23%, and the five-year rate is 4%. If diagnosed at the localized stage, the five-year relative survival rate is 15% (American Cancer Society [ACS], 2005). Treatment depends on how advanced the disease is at initial diagnosis. Surgery, chemotherapy, and radiation therapy are treatment options that may prolong life and reduce symptoms but rarely cure. Survival rates are greatest for patients who undergo resection of the tumor compared with those who are not surgical candidates (DiMango, Reber, & Tempero, 1999).

People diagnosed with pancreatic cancer may face many nutritional challenges, such as severe cachexia, diabetes, and appetite loss. Proper nutritional management of the patient with pancreatic cancer is a crucial part of the medical care plan that helps to enhance response to treatment, minimize complications, and improve quality of life.

Incidence

In 2005, an estimated 32,180 new cases of pancreatic cancer will be diagnosed in the United States, and nearly as many deaths will occur from this disease (Jemal et al., 2005). Pancreatic cancer is the fourth leading cause of cancer death for men after lung, prostate, and colorectal cancers. It is the fifth leading cause of cancer death for women after lung, breast, colorectal, and ovarian cancers (ACS, 2005). Men have higher incidence and mortality rates than women for all racial and ethnic groups (Miller et al., 1996). Incidence is 50%–90% higher among African Americans than among Whites (Silverman et al., 2003). Rates for native Hawaiians are slightly higher than for Whites, whereas rates for Hispanics and Asian Americans are generally lower (Miller et al.). Increased incidence occurs with advancing age (ACS).

Risk Factors and Prevention

A family history of pancreatic cancer and inherited syndromes (e.g., Peutz-Jeghers syndrome, nonpolyposis colon cancer, BRCA2 mutations, familial atypical multiple mole melanoma, hereditary pancreatitis) increase the risk of developing this malignancy (Klein, Hruban, Brune, Petersen, & Goggins, 2001). Cigarette and cigar smoking consistently have been identified as important risk factors for pancreatic cancer evidenced by incidence rates that are twice as high for smokers compared with nonsmokers (ACS, 2005).

Diabetes mellitus also is an established risk factor, with long-standing disease of five years or more increasing the risk of death from pancreatic cancer by twofold (Fisher, 2001). Although carbohydrate and sucrose intake have no association with overall pancreatic cancer risk (Michaud et al., 2002), abnormal glucose metabolism has been shown to increase risk (Gapstur et al., 2000; Michaud et al., 2002). This association is stronger in men and is independent of other known risk factors, such as smoking, age, race, and body mass index (Gapstur et al.). The role of obesity alone has been questioned in the development of pancreatic cancer, but a recent meta-analysis (Berrington de Gonzalez, Sweetland, & Spencer, 2003) showed only a weak association. However, positive energy balance (high caloric intake and frequent meals per day) and activity level may play a role related to their influence on weight status and insulin resistance (Michaud et al., 2001). Further investigation to identify the link among glucose metabolism, insulin resistance, and pancreatic cancer is needed.

In women, extended periods of regular aspirin use (> 14 tablets per week) appear to be associated with increased risk of developing pancreatic cancer (Schernhammer et al., 2004). However, parity appears to decrease risk (Skinner et al., 2003). Researchers also have investigated the association between intake of meat, dairy products, fat, and cholesterol and pancreatic cancer risk in women and found no relationship (Michaud, Giovannucci, Willett, Colditz, & Fuchs, 2003). Gallstones and cholecystectomy do not appear to be significant risk factors for pancreatic cancer in women (Schernhammer et al., 2002).

To reduce the risk of developing pancreatic cancer, individuals are advised to follow the American Institute for Cancer Research's health guidelines (2004). These recommendations include lifestyle modifications, such as increasing the intake of plant-based foods and selecting foods low in fat and salt. The guidelines also suggest maintaining a healthy weight, being physically active, quitting smoking, and limiting alcohol consumption.

Treatment Modalities

More than 95% of pancreatic cancers are adenocarcinomas. Islet cell, carcinoid tumors, and sarcomas may arise in the pancreas but are exceedingly rare. The latter have distinct biologic behaviors and prognoses and unique therapeutic and nutritional challenges. This chapter is limited to a discussion of pancreatic adenocarcinoma.

The treatment of pancreatic cancer depends on how advanced it is at initial diagnosis. The 2002 revision of the American Joint Committee on Cancer's (2002) TNM staging system designates four stages based on the characteristics of the primary tumor (T), involvement of regional lymph nodes (N), and presence or absence of distant metastatic disease (M). The treatment and prognosis of adenocarcinoma of the pancreas are determined by its resectability at the time of diagnosis. Only 10%–20% of patients present with resectable disease (Redlich, Ahrendt, & Pitt, 2001). The five-year survival for those that can be resected with free margins is 18%–24% and is < 5% for those with nonresectable disease.

Resectable Disease

The surgical procedure depends on the location of the tumor. Most pancreatic cancers occur in the head of the pancreas, often presenting with obstructive jaundice, which is accompanied by anorexia, steatorrhea caused by digestive exocrine pancreatic insufficiency, glucose intolerance, and pruritus. Presenting jaundice increases the potential for malabsorption, malnutrition, and consequent immune dysfunction (Spanknebel & Conlon, 2001). Biliary drainage often is performed prior to definitive surgery to maximize liver function (Redlich et al., 2001). Four surgical procedures are used to resect tumors occurring in the head of the pancreas: pancreaticoduodenectomy (PD), also known as the Whipple procedure, pylorus preserving pancreaticoduodenectomy (PPPD), regional pancreatectomy (RP), and total pancreatectomy (TP). All surgical approaches compromise the gastrointestinal tract, either by excising anatomic portions of it (e.g., the gastric antrum [PD]), delaying gastric emptying (PPPD and RP), or obliterating pancreatic function (TP). For body or tail pancreatic cancers, both PD and distal partial pancreatectomy are employed. How the gastrointestinal tract is reconstructed, pancreaticojejunostomy or pancreaticogastrostomy, continues to be controversial (Spanknebel & Conlon).

Adjuvant Therapy

The role of postoperative adjuvant therapy in patients who have had a successful resection remains ill defined. In the 1980s, one study showed marginally improved survival with adjuvant 5-fluorouracil (5-FU) and radiation therapy (Gastrointestinal Tumor Study Group, 1987). Other studies have refuted the need for radiation therapy. In 2004, the European Study Group for Pancreatic Cancer published results of its adjuvant study that attempted to quantitate the value of adjuvant treatment and also determine the relative impact of chemotherapy versus radiation therapy. The trial accrued 289 patients. Postsurgical adjuvant treatment with chemotherapy alone was superior to chemoradiotherapy and superior to surgery alone. The chemotherapy alone patients had an estimated five-year survival of 20% versus 10% for the chemoradiotherapy group (Neoptolemos et al., 2004). The results of an adjuvant study by the Radiation Therapy Oncology Group using the newer agent gemcitabine in combination with 5-FU and radiation therapy are anxiously awaited to shed light on the value of chemotherapy in combination with current radiotherapy techniques. Today, in the United States, postoperative adjuvant therapy with concurrent 5-FU and radiation therapy or chemotherapy alone is acceptable adjuvant treatment.

Unresectable Disease

Because preoperative staging of pancreatic cancer does not always accurately identify resectable disease, some patients undergo incomplete resection (Brand, 2001). These patients are treated with postoperative 5-FU and local radiation therapy to manage residual disease. Studies using gemcitabine in combination with radiation are in progress.

Management of obviously unresectable disease is aimed at managing ongoing complications of disease and controlling tumor growth. Patients presenting with obstructive jaundice most often are managed with either endoscopic stenting or radiologically directed percutaneous drainage procedures and less frequently with surgical biliary bypass. Prophylactic gastric bypass procedures are sometimes performed to avoid later gastric outlet obstruction. Zervos, Rosemurgy, Al-Saif, and Durkin (2004) noted that as systemic therapy improves survival rates of unresected patients, the need for proactive gastric bypass procedures might increase.

Standard therapy for locally advanced, nonmetastatic cancer of the pancreas consists of systemic 5-FU with external beam radiation therapy. The use of gemcitabine-containing regimens with radiation, radioactive implants, and the value of intraoperative radiotherapy are under investigation. Neoadjuvant treatment, the use of preoperative chemotherapy and radiation, in locally advanced disease also is being evaluated.

Metastatic Disease

Chemotherapy with gemcitabine- or 5-FU–based regimens is the standard for first-line treatment of metastatic pancreatic adenocarcinoma. Gemcitabine as a single agent has improved survival over 5-FU alone (18% versus 2% at one year) (Burris et al., 1997). Because the prognosis for metastatic pancreatic cancer is dismal with or without current chemotherapeutic interventions, patients should be encouraged to participate in clinical trials evaluating new drugs and regimens.

Palliative Care

In addition to the nutritional challenges caused by pancreatic cancer, infection and pain are major problems. The location of the pancreas and the growth characteristics of the tumor (diffuse, infiltrative) result in extension to the multiple nerves located in anatomic proximity. Controlling pain is of paramount importance. In addition to the administration of scheduled opioids, chemical splanchnicectomy with 50% alcohol can be performed. This procedure may be done prophylactically at the time of initial surgical exploration. Radiation therapy with or without chemotherapy, the administration of gemcitabine alone or in combination, and intrathecal or epidural analgesics can palliate pain. Neurosurgical procedures such as percutaneous celiac plexus blocks result in pain control in most cases (Brescia, 2004).

Ascending cholangitis frequently occurs because of obstruction of the biliary tree. This may result when stents/drainage devices become occluded and require replacement. Prophylactic antibiotics are not effective. Because mortality from ascending cholangitis can be high, patient education about its signs and symptoms, early intervention to relieve obstruction, and prompt institution of antibiotic therapy are imperative (Muir, 2004).

Future Directions

Significant optimism exists about improving outcomes in pancreatic cancer. Preliminary results of multidrug chemoimmunotherapy combined with radiation administered after PD show five-year survival rates as high as 55% (Zervos et al., 2004). New molecularly targeted agents recently have entered clinical practice and offer potential efficacy in this malignancy, as do the use of novel combinations and sequences in the adjuvant and neoadjuvant purviews (El-Rayes & Philip, 2003; El-Rayes, Shields, Vaitkevicius, & Philip, 2003; McGinn & Zalupski, 2001; Saad & Hoff, 2004).

Nutritional Implications

Pancreatic cancer has a profound effect on nutritional status. Upon diagnosis, patients have most likely lost weight, with a majority experiencing significant ($\leq 10\%$ loss from baseline) or severe ($> 10\%$ loss from baseline) weight loss (DeWys, Begg, & Larvin, 1980). Patients with weight loss have reduced chemotherapy tolerance, increased chemotherapy-related complications, and reduced quality of life as compared to those who do not lose weight (Andreyev, Norman, Oates, & Cunningham, 1998). Severe weight loss, known as cancer cachexia, is implicated in the death of 30%–50% of all patients with cancer (Bruera & Higginson, 1996).

Cancer cachexia results not only in loss of weight but, more importantly, loss of lean body mass, which leads to altered skeletal muscle metabolism and function (Tisdale, 1997). Loss of lean body mass impacts multiple organ systems and can lead to reduced cardiac mass and contractility, impaired respiratory muscle function, and atrophy of smooth muscle of the intestinal tract (Daly, Vars, & Dudrick, 1972; Heymsfield et al., 1978). The progress of cancer cachexia in patients with pancreatic cancer correlates positively with markers of the acute phase protein response, including increased resting energy expenditure (Falconer, Fearon, Plester, Ross, & Carter, 1994), increased C-reactive protein (Barber, Ross, Preston, Shenkin, & Fearon, 1999), and increased pro-inflammatory cytokines (Falconer et al.). Studies suggest that pro-inflammatory cytokines may affect appetite and food intake in addition to stimulating the acute phase protein response. In addition, certain tumor-specific factors, such as a proteolysis-inducing factor (PIF), appear to accelerate the loss of lean body mass in these patients (Fearon, Barber, & Moses, 2001).

Anorexia and fat malabsorption are major clinical features that contribute to malnutrition seen in these patients (Ottery, 1996). When biliary duct obstruction reduces pancreatic enzyme output to below 10% of normal, steatorrhea occurs (Wigmore et al., 1997). When fat malabsorption is severe, absorption of the fat-soluble vitamins A, D, E, and K is affected and may lead to deficiency of these vitamins (Bruno, Haverkort, Tijssen, Tytgat, & van Leeuwen, 1998). Deficiencies of trace minerals also may occur (Bank, 1986). Malnutrition is associated with dysfunction of the immune system, increasing the risk of postoperative complications.

Altered macronutrient metabolism occurs because of the acute phase protein response and because of insulin deficiency. Both disease-induced and surgically related hyperglycemia occur in pancreatic cancer. The degree of derangement of glucose metabolism must be determined and interventions tailored to control blood sugar.

Chemotherapy and radiation therapy for pancreatic cancer cause side effects that interfere with nutritional intake and contribute to malnutrition. These side effects include stomatitis/mucositis, dysgeusia, nausea, vomiting, abdominal cramping, and diarrhea. Which side effects occur and their severity depends on the antineoplastic agents used and the area irradiated.

A collaborative effort between the oncology nurse and an oncology dietitian optimizes the assessment of the nutritional status and needs of the patient with pancreatic cancer. Assessment is based upon the following four categories of data: (a) pancreatic cancer extent and proposed treatment, (b) nutrition history, dietary intake, and influencing factors, (c) interview, observation, and physical examination of the patient, and (d) anthropometric and biochemical measurements. The Patient-Generated Subjective Global Assessment (PG-SGA) serves as a rapid, easily administered assessment tool that describes the patient's perception of his or her nutritional status (McMahon, Decker, & Ottery, 1998) (see Appendix A). It is a useful guide for the nurse and dietitian in completing a more detailed nutrition assessment (see Figure 10-1).

Special Considerations for Nutrition

Once the nutrition assessment has been completed, a nutrition care plan can be developed. The goal of the nutrition care plan is to avoid or reverse the catabolic effects of pancreatic cancer and its treatment on body composition and function. Optimizing nutrition can enhance the response to treatment, minimize complications, foster immune function, decrease fatigue, and improve quality of life (Wilson, 2000). The nutrition care plan must be individualized and fluid. Although the course of pancreatic cancer is short for most patients, the changes in disease status and therapeutic and palliative interventions are many, and each represents specific nutritional challenges.

Surgical Considerations

Most patients with pancreatic cancer present with weight loss. For those undergoing initial surgical intervention, consideration should be given to preoperative nutritional interventions, especially if weight loss exceeds 10% of usual body weight (Redlich et al., 2001). Because many patients may require preoperative biliary drainage procedures to optimize liver function, there should be ample opportunity to intervene preoperatively. Surgically induced delayed gastric emptying requires attention to nutritional fat content. When gastric or duodenal obstruction occurs, enteral or parenteral nutrition should be considered, with or without surgical bypass, depending on the patient's overall prognosis and anticipated duration of survival.

Alterations of Glucose Metabolism and Malabsorption

If TP is planned, preoperative diabetic counseling should be done. All patients with hyperglycemia may benefit from consultation with a diabetes nurse educator. A social service consultation facilitates the patient's procurement of diabetic supplies. Oral pancreatic enzymes may be used to correct pancreatic insufficiency (Lopez & Tehrani, 2001).

Chemotherapy and Radiation Therapy

Interventions to control side effects must be instituted and tailored to the individual patient. These range from practical approaches (minimizing exposure to cooking odors to reduce nausea) to pharmacologic interventions (administering antiemetics 30 minutes prior to meals).

Figure 10-1. Assessment of Nutritional Status in Pancreatic Cancer

Pancreatic Cancer Data
- Resectable versus nonresectable disease
- Biliary obstruction with or without invasive or noninvasive biliary drainage
- Current or potential for gastric/duodenal obstruction
- Planned surgery (PD, PPD, RP, RT) with or without proactive gastric bypass
- Chemotherapy and/or radiotherapy and/or immunotherapy, simultaneously or concurrently, preoperatively or postoperatively
- Prognosis

Objective Measurements
- Diet history and recall of current food intake
- Anthropometric measurements: height, weight, skin fold thickness, arm muscle circumference
- Medication evaluation—impact of medicine on nutrition, such as inducing constipation, diarrhea, taste changes, mucositis, mentation changes, nausea or vomiting, muscle weakness, or decreased gastrointestinal motility. (Note: Consultation with a pharmacist may be very helpful here.) Include alternative therapies (e.g., nutritional supplements) in the assessment.
- Biochemical data—albumin, prealbumin, total protein, hemoglobin, hematocrit, transferrin, fasting glucose with two-hour postprandial blood sugar if elevated

Patient Interview/Observation/Examination
- Performance status (e.g., Karnofsky, Eastern Cooperative Oncology Group)
- Patient-Generated Subjective Global Assessment (PG-SGA)
- Medical and social history: comorbid conditions (e.g., cardiac, pulmonary, thyroid, or musculoskeletal disease, other gastrointestinal pathology [ulcers, Crohn's], tobacco, alcohol, or illicit drug use [inquire about marijuana]) influencing overall nutrition and nutritional interventions
- Nutrition impact signs and symptoms
  - *Global physical problems*—anorexia, fever/infection, fatigue, pain, muscle weakness, depression, anxiety, food aversions
  - *Gastrointestinal-specific problems*—stomatitis, dentition, sensory changes, dysphagia, esophagitis, epigastric pain, nausea, vomiting, delayed gastric emptying, diarrhea, constipation, steatorrhea, jaundice, gastric/duodenal obstruction
- Physical examination—general appearance, skin turgor, muscle wasting, fat loss, skin/nail/hair texture and tone, mucous membrane characteristics, dentition, sensory changes, presence of edema, ascites, or other fluid collections, mobility, physical signs of comorbidities (e.g., labored respirations, clubbing)
- Socioeconomic data—living situation, support system, understanding of current situation and therapy, ability to obtain/prepare adequate food functionally and economically

Calculated Data
- Optimal body weight
- Percentage of weight loss
- Body mass index
- Protein, calorie, and micronutrient needs
- Percentage of lean body mass

Pharmacologic Appetite Stimulation

Because of the decrease in appetite induced by both the disease and its treatment, pharmacologic agents to correct metabolic abnormalities and stimulate appetite should be considered. Progestational agents, cannabinoids, and glucocorticoids can improve appetite but generally result in gains in fat, not lean body mass, in addition to having potentially significant side effects (Walker, 2001). Anabolic steroids, growth hormone, and cytokine inhibitors (nonsteroidal anti-inflammatory agents, thalidomide) are purported to increase anabolism and/or improve appetite but remain under investigation (Nelson, 2000). Anabolic steroids have significant side effects, and growth hormone is very expensive.

Nutritional Modulation of Cachexia

Eicosapentaenoic acid is a long-chain polyunsaturated omega-3 fatty acid found in fatty fish, such as salmon and mackerel, and has been shown to slow tumor growth and attenuate cachexia in a variety of cell cultures and animal and clinical studies. Studies have shown that eicosapentaenoic acid inhibits severe weight loss and reduces production of proinflammatory cytokines caused by cancer (Falconer et al., 1994; Tisdale & Dhesi, 1990). Eicosapentaenoic acid reduces arachidonic acid in the cell membrane (Pratt et al., 2002) and induces a significant anti-inflammatory effect (Goldman, Pickett, & Goetzl, 1983). Several studies demonstrate the benefits of dietary supplementation with eicosapentaenoic acid (fish oil) in the management of cancer cachexia (Gogos et al., 1998; Pratt et al.; Wigmore, Barber, Ross, Tisdale, & Fearon, 2000; Wigmore et al., 1996). These studies indicate that approximately 2 grams per day of eicosapentaenoic acid can stabilize weight by attenuating some of the metabolic abnormalities seen in these patients. Further studies showed that consumption of additional calories and protein in a nutritionally dense eicosapentaenoic acid–containing formula leads to gains in weight and lean body mass (Barber, Ross, Voss, Tisdale, & Fearon, 1999; Fearon et al., 2003), reduction in resting energy expenditure, improved appetite and dietary intake, and improvement in the acute phase protein response (Barber, Ross, Preston, et al., 1999). Furthermore, patients consuming the eicosapentaenoic acid–containing formula increased their physical activity level (Moses, Slater, Preston, Barber, & Fearon, 2004) and reported improvements in quality of life (Fearon et al., 2003).

Ongoing Evaluation and Intervention

Because of the disease trajectory of pancreatic cancer, the nutrition care plan must be established upon diagnosis, implemented, and constantly evaluated and revised in light of the patient's changing disease status and therapies and the resultant nutritional challenges. Early intervention for identified nutritional deficits and proactive intervention for anticipated nutritional difficulties will have a greater impact than either approach alone (McMahon & Brown, 2000). When hospice and terminal care become appropriate, the focus of nutritional intervention changes from one of maximizing nutrition to that of emphasizing the comforting aspects of food, nutrition, and hydration.

Expected Outcomes of Therapy

The expected outcomes of nutrition therapy in patients with pancreatic cancer are restoring a positive nitrogen balance, thereby stopping weight loss and other adverse catabolic effects; inducing a gain in lean body mass; and restoring nutritional homeostasis. Meeting metabolic needs in the face of the challenges of pancreatic cancer and its treatment will restore and maintain body composition and function. Outcomes can be divided into short-term and long-term improvements in nutritional status.

Short-Term Outcomes

Increasing nutritional intake is the initial, immediate goal of nutritional intervention (Wilson, 2000). This requires intervening to control side effects of treatment as well as disease. Examples include managing appetite loss, bowel function, blood glucose, pancreatic insufficiency, delayed gastric emptying, and mucositis or esophagitis induced by chemotherapy and radiation therapy and the side effects of concomitant medications.

Because most nonsurgical management of cancer of the pancreas is performed in the outpatient setting, patients must be encouraged to be conscious of food, fluid, and medical nutritional product intake to ensure comprehensive data. By having the patient recall current dietary intake, the dietitian can document improvements in the nutritional composition of the diet. Laboratory parameters such as total protein, albumin, and prealbumin and weekly weight measurements can verify improved nutritional status.

Long-Term Outcomes

The ultimate goal of nutritional intervention in patients with cancer of the pancreas is the restoration of anabolic metabolism that maximizes the patient's ability to undergo treatment (Wilson, 2000). Desired outcomes of successful nutritional management include (a) maintenance of weight, (b) increase in lean body mass, (c) normalization of objective measures of nutritional status, (d) restoration or improvement in strength and energy, (e) maximized immune function and fewer infectious complications, (f) decreased or controlled treatment side effects, (g) completion of recommended treatments, and (h) improved quality of life and functional status.

Meeting these long-term goals requires active collaboration among all members of the healthcare team: physicians (surgeon, radiation therapist, medical oncologist), nurses, dietitians, psychologists, social workers, and pharmacists (Inui, 2002). Physicians must communicate changes in the disease status and treatment plan as soon as they are identified. Nurses should recognize changes in the nutrition assessment and potential toxicities of disease and treatment changes and anticipate their impact on nutritional status. The pharmacist identifies the influence of medications on the patient's symptoms and projects the development of side effects as medications change. Psychologists can manage mental health status, which will influence appetite. Social workers intervene to solve family and economic problems that interfere with compliance with therapeutic and nutrition recommendations. All members of the team need to rapidly communicate data to the dietitian so that revisions of the nutrition care plan can be accomplished proactively. Early, proactive nutritional intervention can maximize the patient's ability to tolerate the next phase of the pancreatic cancer challenge. The overall goal in managing the patient with pancreatic cancer is improving quality of life. If quality of life improves for the patient, the nutrition and therapeutic care plans are ultimately successful.

References

American Cancer Society. (2005). *Cancer facts and figures, 2005*. Atlanta, GA: Author.

American Institute for Cancer Research. (2004). *Diet and health guidelines for cancer prevention*. Retrieved March 17, 2004, from http://www.aicr.org/guides.htm

American Joint Committee on Cancer. (2002). Exocrine pancreas. In *AJCC cancer staging manual* (6th ed., pp. 157–164). New York: Springer-Verlag.

Andreyev, H.J.N., Norman, A.R., Oates, J., & Cunningham, D. (1998). Why do patients with weight loss have a worse outcome when undergoing chemotherapy for gastrointestinal malignancies? *European Journal of Cancer, 34*, 503–509.

Bank, S. (1986). Chronic pancreatitis: Clinical features and medical management. *American Journal of Gastroenterology, 81*, 153–167.

Barber, M.D., Ross, J.A., Preston, T., Shenkin, A., & Fearon, K.C.H. (1999). A fish oil-enriched nutritional supplement changes the acute phase response in weight-losing patients with advanced pancreatic cancer. *American Society for Nutritional Sciences, 129*, 120–125.

Barber, M.D., Ross, J.A., Voss, A.C., Tisdale, M.J., & Fearon, K.C.H. (1999). The effect of an oral nutritional supplement enriched with fish oil on weight loss in patients with pancreatic cancer. *British Journal of Cancer, 81*(1), 80–86.

Berrington de Gonzalez, A., Sweetland, S., & Spencer, E. (2003). A meta-analysis of obesity and the risk of pancreatic cancer. *British Journal of Cancer, 89*, 519–523.

Brand, R. (2001). The diagnosis of pancreatic cancer. *Cancer Journal, 7*, 287–297.

Brescia, F.J. (2004). Palliative care in pancreatic cancer. *Cancer Control: Journal of the Moffitt Cancer Center, 11*, 39–45.

Bruera, E., & Higginson, I. (1996). *Cachexia-anorexia in cancer patients*. New York: Oxford University Press.

Bruno, M.J., Haverkort, E.B., Tijssen, G.P., Tytgat, G.N., & van Leeuwen, D.J. (1998). Placebo controlled trial of enteric coated pancreatin microsphere treatment in patients with unresectable cancer of the pancreatic head region. *Gut, 42*, 92–96.

Burris, H.A., III, Moore, M.J., Andersen, J., Green, M.R., Rothenberg, M.L., Modiano, M.R., et al. (1997). Improvements in survival and clinical benefit with gemcitabine as first-line therapy for patients with advanced pancreas cancer: A randomized trial. *Journal of Clinical Oncology, 15*, 2403–2413.

Daly, J., Vars, H., & Dudrick, S. (1972). Effects of protein depletion on strength of colonic anastomosis. *Surgery, Gynecology and Obstetrics, 13,* 415–421.

DeWys, W., Begg, C., & Larvin, P. (1980). Prognostic effect of weight loss prior to chemotherapy in cancer patients. *American Journal of Medicine, 68,* 683–690.

DiMango, E.P., Reber, H.A., & Tempero, M.A. (1999). AGA technical review on the epidemiology, diagnosis, and treatment of pancreatic ductal adenocarcinoma. *Gastroenterology, 117,* 1464–1484.

El-Rayes, B.F., & Philip, P.A. (2003). A review of systemic therapy for advanced pancreatic cancer. *Clinical Advances in Hematology and Oncology, 1,* 430–434.

El-Rayes, B.F., Shields, A.F., Vaitkevicius, V., & Philip, P.A. (2003). Developments in the systemic therapy of pancreatic cancer. *Cancer Investigation, 21,* 73–86.

Falconer, J.S., Fearon, K.C.H., Plester, C.E., Ross, J.A., & Carter, D.C. (1994). Cytokines, the acute phase protein response, and resting energy expenditure in cachectic patients with pancreatic cancer. *Cancer, 75,* 2077–2082.

Fearon, K.C.H., Barber, M.D., & Moses, A.G.W. (2001). The cancer cachexia syndrome. *Surgical Oncology Clinics of North America, 10,* 109–126.

Fearon, K.C.H., von Meyenfeldt, M.F., Moses, A.G.W., van Geenen, R., Roy, A., Gouma, D.J., et al. (2003). Effect of a protein and energy dense N-3 fatty acid enriched oral supplement on loss of weight and lean tissue in cancer cachexia: A randomized double blind trial. *Gut, 52,* 1479–1486.

Fisher, W.E. (2001). Diabetes: Risk factor for the development of pancreatic cancer or manifestation of the disease? *World Journal of Surgery, 25,* 503–508.

Gapstur, S., Gann, P., Lowe, W., Liv, K., Colangelo, L., & Dyer, A. (2000). Abnormal glucose metabolism and pancreatic cancer mortality. *JAMA, 283,* 2552–2558.

Gastrointestinal Tumor Study Group. (1987). Further evidence of effective adjuvant combined radiation and chemotherapy following curative resection of pancreatic cancer. *Cancer, 59,* 2006–2010.

Gogos, C.A., Ginopoulos, P., Salsa, B., Apostolidou, E., Zoumbos, N.C., & Kalfarentzos, F. (1998). Dietary omega-3 polyunsaturated fatty acids plus vitamin E restore immunodeficiency and prolong survival for severely ill patients with generalized malignancy: A randomized control trial. *Cancer, 82,* 395–402.

Goldman, D.W., Pickett, W.C., & Goetzl, E.J. (1983). Human neutrophil chemotactic and degranulating activities of leukotriene B5 (LTB5) derived from eicosapentaenoic acid. *Biochemistry and Biophysiology Research Communication, 117,* 282–288.

Heymsfield, S., Bethel, R., Ansley, J., Gibbs, D.M., Felner, J.M., & Nutter, D.O. (1978). Cardiac abnormalities in cachetic patients before and during nutritional repletion. *American Heart Journal, 95,* 584–594.

Inui, A. (2002). Cancer anorexia-cachexia syndrome: Current issues in research and management. *CA: A Cancer Journal for Clinicians, 52,* 72–91.

Jemal, A., Murray, T., Ward, E., Samuels, A., Tiwari, R.C., Ghafoor, A., et al. (2005). Cancer statistics, 2005. *CA: A Cancer Journal for Clinicians, 55,* 10–30.

Klein, A.P., Hruban, R.H., Brune, K.A., Petersen, G.M., & Goggins, M. (2001). Familial pancreatic cancer. *Cancer Journal, 7,* 266–273.

Lopez, M.J., & Tehrani, H.Y. (2001). Nutrition and the cancer patient. In R.E. Lenhard, R.T. Oteen, & T. Gansler (Eds.), *American Cancer Society textbook of clinical oncology* (4th ed., pp. 811–822). Atlanta, GA: American Cancer Society.

McGinn, C.J., & Zalupski, M.M. (2001). Combined-modality therapy in pancreatic cancer: Current status and future directions. *Cancer Journal, 7,* 338–348.

McMahon, K., & Brown, J.K. (2000). Nutritional screening and assessment. *Seminars in Oncology Nursing, 16,* 106–112.

McMahon, K., Decker, G., & Ottery, F.D. (1998). Integrating proactive nutritional assessment in clinical practices to prevent complications and cost. *Seminars in Oncology, 25*(Suppl. 6), 20–27.

Michaud, D.S., Giovannucci, E., Willett, W.C., Colditz, G.A., & Fuchs, C.S. (2003). Dietary meat, dairy products, fat, and cholesterol and pancreatic cancer risk in a prospective study. *American Journal of Epidemiology, 157,* 1115–1125.

Michaud, D.S., Giovannucci, E., Willett, W.C., Colditz, G.A., Stamfer, M.J., & Fuchs, C.S. (2001). Physical activity, obesity, height, and the risk of pancreatic cancer. *JAMA, 286,* 921–929.

Michaud, D.S., Lui, S., Giovannucci, E., Willett, W.C., Colditz, G.A., & Fuchs, C.S. (2002). Dietary sugar, glycemic load, and pancreatic cancer risk in a prospective study. *Journal of the National Cancer Institute, 94,* 1293–1300.

Miller, B.A., Kolonel, L.N., Bernstein, L., Young, J.L., Swanson, G.M., West, D., et al. (Eds.). (1996). *Racial/ethnic patterns of cancer in the United States, 1988–1992.* NIH Pub. No. 96-4104. Bethesda, MD: National Cancer Institute.

Moses, A.W., Slater, C., Preston, T., Barber, M.D., & Fearon, K.C. (2004). Reduced total energy expenditure and physical activity in cachectic patients with pancreatic cancer can be modulated by an energy dense oral supplement enriched with n-3 fatty acids. *British Journal of Cancer, 90,* 996–1002.

Muir, C.A. (2004). Acute ascending cholangitis. *Clinical Journal of Oncology Nursing, 8,* 157–160.

Nelson, K.A. (2000). The cancer anorexia-cachexia syndrome. *Seminars in Oncology, 27,* 64–68.

Neoptolemos, J.P., Stocken, D.D., Friess, H., Bassi, C., Dunn, J.A., Hickey, H., et al. (2004). A randomized trial of chemoradiotherapy and chemotherapy after resection of pancreatic cancer. *New England Journal of Medicine, 350,* 1200–1210.

Ottery F. (1996). Supportive nutritional management of the patient with pancreatic cancer. *Oncology, 10,* 26–32.

Pratt, V.C., Watanabe, S., Bruera, E., Mackey, J., Clandinin, M.T., Baracos, V.E., et al. (2002). Plasma and neutrophil fatty acid composition in advanced cancer patients and response to fish oil supplementation. *British Journal of Cancer, 87,* 1370–1378.

Redlich, P.N., Ahrendt, S.A., & Pitt, H.A. (2001). Tumors of the pancreas, gallbladder, and bile ducts. In R.E. Lenhard, R.T. Oteen, & T. Gansler (Eds.), *American Cancer Society textbook of clinical oncology* (4th ed., pp. 373–382). Atlanta, GA: American Cancer Society.

Saad, E.D., & Hoff, P.H. (2004). Molecular-targeted agents in pancreatic cancer. *Cancer Control: Journal of the Moffitt Cancer Center, 11,* 32–38.

Schernhammer, E.S., Kang, J.H., Chan, A.T., Michaud, D.S., Skinner, H.G., Giovannucci, E., et al. (2004). A prospective study of aspirin use and the risk of pancreatic cancer in women. *Journal of the National Cancer Institute, 96,* 22–28.

Schernhammer, E.S., Michaud, D.S., Leitzmann, M.F., Giovannucci, E., Colditz, G.A., & Fuchs, C.S. (2002). Gallstones, cholecystectomy, and the risk for developing pancreatic cancer. *British Journal of Cancer, 86,* 1081–1084.

Silverman, D.T., Hoover, R.N., Brown, L.M., Swanson, G.M., Schiffman, M., Greenberg, R.S., et al. (2003). Why do Black Americans have a higher risk of pancreatic cancer than White Americans? *Epidemiology, 14*(1), 45–54.

Skinner, H.G., Michaud, D.S., Colditz, G.A., Giovannucci, E.L., Stampfer, M.J., Willett, W.C., et al. (2003). Parity, reproductive factors, and the risk of pancreatic cancer in women. *Cancer Epidemiology, Biomarkers and Prevention, 12,* 433–438.

Spanknebel, K., & Conlon, K.C.P. (2001). Advances in the surgical management of pancreatic cancer. *Cancer Journal, 7,* 312–323.

Tisdale, M.J. (1997). Biology of cachexia—A review. *Journal of the National Cancer Institute, 89,* 1763–1773.

Tisdale, M.J., & Dhesi, J.K. (1990). Inhibition of weight loss by n-3 fatty acids in an experimental cachexia model. *Cancer Research, 50,* 5022–5026.

Walker, P.W. (2001). The anorexia/cachexia syndrome. *Primary Care and Cancer, 21*(8), 13–17.

Wigmore, S., Barber, M.D., Ross, J.A., Tisdale, M.J., & Fearon, K.C. (2000). Effect of oral eicosapentaenoic acid on weight loss in patients with pancreatic cancer. *Nutrition and Cancer, 36*(2), 177–184.

Wigmore, S., Plester, C., Richardson, R., & Fearon, K. (1997). Changes in nutritional status associated with unresectable pancreatic cancer. *British Journal of Cancer, 75,* 106–109.

Wigmore, S., Ross, J., Falconer, S., Plester, C., Tisdale, M., Carter, D., et al. (1996). The effect of polyunsaturated fatty acids on the progress of cachexia in patients with pancreatic cancer. *Nutrition, 12*(Suppl.), 27–30.

Wilson, R.L. (2000). Optimizing nutrition for patients with cancer. *Clinical Journal of Oncology Nursing, 4,* 23–28.

Zervos, E.E., Rosemurgy, A.S., Al-Saif, O., & Durkin, A.J. (2004). Surgical management of early-stage pancreatic cancer. *Cancer Control: Journal of the Moffitt Cancer Center, 11,* 23–31.

CHAPTER 11

Prostate Cancer

Natalie Lagomarcino Ledesma, MS, RD
Jamie S. Myers, RN, MN, AOCN®

Overview

Cancer of the prostate is a disease that primarily affects older men. The median age at diagnosis is 72 (National Cancer Institute [NCI], 2003b; O'Rourke, 2001). Most prostate cancers are adenocarcinomas (95%) and occur in the peripheral zone of the prostate gland (NCI, 2003b). Early detection and improved treatment modalities have increased the five-year survival rate of prostate cancer from 67% to 98%. Diagnosis in a local or regional stage of the disease is associated with a five-year survival rate of 100% (American Cancer Society [ACS], 2005). Once prostate cancer advances, cure is no longer expected. The median survival with distant metastases is one to three years (NCI, 2003b). The most common site of distant metastases is bone (NCI, 2003b).

ACS (2005) recommends annual prostate-specific antigen (PSA) testing and digital rectal examination (DRE) beginning at age 50 for men with at least a 10-year life expectancy. Men in high-risk groups are recommended to begin screening at age 45.

Early-stage prostate cancer is asymptomatic. As the disease progresses, symptoms may include difficulty with urination, urinary frequency (particularly at night), hematuria, pain or burning with urination, or pain in the back, pelvis, or upper thighs (ACS, 2005). An elevated PSA and/or abnormalities noted on a DRE lead to a prostatic biopsy (transrectal ultrasound may facilitate needle biopsy) for tissue diagnosis. Further staging of the disease may be accomplished through computed tomography, magnetic resonance imaging, surgical lymph node dissection, and radionuclide bone scans. Two staging systems are commonly used today: the Jewett system (stages A through D) and the American Joint Committee on Cancer's TNM system (tumor-node-metastasis stages I–IV). The Gleason score is used to define the grade of the tumor.

Incidence

Prostate cancer is the most common cancer in men and the second leading cause of cancer-related death in men. An estimated 232,090 new cases and 30,350 deaths will occur in 2005 (ACS, 2005). The highest incidence of prostate cancer in the world occurs in African American males (NCI, 2003a). In the United States, the incidence in African Americans is 60% higher than Whites, and the death rate is more than twice the rate for Whites (ACS). The lowest incidence of prostate cancer exists in Asia. Epidemiologic studies, however, show that Chinese or Japanese males who move to the United States or southern Europe subsequently exhibit a similar incidence as American males within a few generations (Djavan et al., 2004).

Risk Factors and Prevention

The primary risk factors for prostate cancer are age, family history and genetics, and ethnicity. Risk increases with age. Prostate cancer is rare for people younger than age 40. Men aged 40–59 have a 1 in 45 risk of developing prostate cancer. This risk increases to 1 in 7 for those aged 60–70 and a 1 in 6 overall lifetime risk (Ruijter et al., 1999).

An estimated 5%–10% of prostate cancers are attributed to inherited genetic factors or prostate cancer susceptibility genes (NCI, 2003a). The following genetic susceptibility loci have been identified: HPC1, HPCX, and PCAP (NCI, 2003a). A family history of a first-degree relative (father or brother) with prostate cancer is related to a two- to threefold increase in risk. Diagnosis in younger relatives is associated with greater risk (NCI, 2003a). Controversy exists regarding the relationship between history of breast cancer and prostate cancer within families. There is some indication that the *BRCA1* and *BRCA2* genes may be associated with an increased risk of prostate cancer in families at risk for breast cancer (Gayther et al., 2000).

Ethnic differences in incidence have yet to be explained. One hypothesis relates to dietary consumption (see the Nutritional Implications section in this chapter). Another hypothesis relates to the amount of circulating testosterone. Hypogonadal males or those with castration levels of testosterone do not develop prostate cancer (NCI, 2003a). African American men have been noted to have higher total and free testosterone levels than Whites (O'Rourke, 2001).

An overexpression of cyclooxygenase (COX-2) also has been associated with an increased risk of prostate cancer. Nonsteroidal anti-inflammatory drugs, such as celecoxib and rofecoxib, are being evaluated (Barqawi, Thompson, & Crawford, 2003; Basler & Piazza, 2004; Mahmud, Franco, & Aprikian, 2004). Potential mechanisms of action for these drugs include antiangiogenesis and the repression of androgen receptors (Barqawi et al.). Studies also are being conducted to evaluate the potential role of chronic inflammation in the development of prostate cancer (Lucia & Torkko, 2004; Platz & De Marzo, 2004).

A variety of clinical trials have been and currently are being conducted to evaluate various strategies for the prevention of prostate cancer. Furthermore, NCI hosts an excellent Web site (www.cancer.gov) that provides a current summary of prevention trials sponsored by the National Institutes of Health.

Prostate Cancer Prevention Trial

This randomized, placebo-controlled trial, funded by NCI and the Southwest Oncology Group (SWOG), evaluated the use of finasteride (Proscar®, Merck & Co., Inc., Whitehouse Station, NJ) in men age 55 and older. The study was halted early and the results published because of the statistically significant (25%) decrease in prostate cancer risk for the men taking finasteride (Thompson et al., 2003). Finasteride blocks the action of the enzyme 5-alpha reductase, which is needed to convert testosterone into dihydrotestosterone (DHT). DHT is involved in the development of prostate cancer. One confounding result of the study was that men taking finasteride who developed prostate cancer had more aggressive disease as measured by a higher Gleason score (NCI, 2003c).

Reduction by Dutasteride in Prostate Cancer

This commercially sponsored phase II randomized, placebo-controlled trial will evaluate daily dutasteride in the prevention of biopsy-proven prostate cancer in men age 50–75 with increased PSA levels and recent negative prostate biopsy after two and four years of treatment. Similar to finasteride, dutasteride is a 5-alpha reductase inhibitor (Djavan et al., 2004).

Alpha-Tocopherol, Beta-Carotene Cancer Prevention Trial

NCI and the National Public Health Institute of Finland developed this trial to evaluate if vitamin E (50 mg) and beta-carotene (20 mg) would prevent lung cancer and other cancers in a group of male smokers. Results showed that vitamin E consumption was associated with a 32% reduction in the risk of prostate cancer. Follow-up after the trial showed that prostate cancer rates returned to normal soon after participants completed the study and stopped taking vitamin E (NCI, 2003a).

Selenium and Vitamin E Chemoprevention Trial

NCI and SWOG currently are conducting a phase III randomized, placebo-controlled trial to evaluate the use of selenium (200 mcg) and vitamin E (400 IU) in the prevention of prostate cancer. Patients will be randomized to receive selenium alone, vitamin E alone, a combination of the two, or two placebos.

Treatment Modalities

Treatment of prostate cancer depends on several factors: the stage of the disease, the patient's life expectancy and performance status, and the patient's choice regarding expected side effects and toxicities and the effects on quality of life. In general, men with early-stage prostate cancer are offered the choice between surgery and radiation therapy. Men with advanced disease are offered hormonal therapy. "Expectant management" or "watchful waiting" are terms for observation only. Men with early-stage, low-grade, low-volume prostate cancer often die from other causes. Elderly men with early-stage disease or men with a more advanced stage of disease in conjunction with a short life expectancy because of comorbidities may choose to refrain from treatment until symptoms or signs of disease progression develop (Holmberg et al., 2002; Steineck et al., 2002). Clinical trials are ongoing to investigate chemotherapeutic regimens. Chemotherapy typically is reserved for advanced and/or refractory disease.

Surgery

Radical prostatectomy is used for stage I and II prostate cancer. Both retropubic and perineal approaches currently are used. Men in good health without evidence of lymphatic spread or distant metastases are candidates. Development of the nerve-sparing procedure has reduced the incidence of impotence related to surgery. Improved surgical techniques also have increased the preservation of postoperative urinary continence to approximately 92%. Cryosurgical ablation of the prostate (CSAP) is a procedure that involves freezing the prostate gland and the seminal vesicles using gas-driven probes. As a modality, CSAP is considered third generation. Current research indicates a good safety profile with low incidence of tissue sloughing, incontinence, urinary retention, and pain (Han et al., 2003). Further trials are needed to determine long-term efficacy (Donnelly et al., 2002; Fahmy & Bissada, 2003; Han et al.).

Radiation Therapy

Radiation therapy may be used as the primary treatment for stage I and II prostate cancer. Available techniques include external beam radiation therapy (EBRT), three-dimensional conformal radiation therapy, intensity-modulated radiation therapy, and brachytherapy or seed implant. Radiation also may be used for stage III disease, recurrent disease, or palliation in stage IV disease. In these instances, it commonly is used in conjunction with other modalities, such as hormonal therapy. Sexual potency is maintained in 73%–82% of patients receiving EBRT (Miaskowski, 1999). Ten-year survival and five-year biochemical relapse-free survival data for brachytherapy are associated with results that are comparable with EBRT and radical prostatectomy (Kupelian,

Potters, Khuntia, Ciezki, & Reddy, 2004; Potters, 2003). Brachytherapy is associated with a lower incidence of long-term risk for urinary incontinence and erectile dysfunction than other modalities (Woolsey, Miller, & Theodorescu, 2003). Research indicates that sildenafil citrate (Viagra®, Pfizer Inc., Cambridge, MA) may improve sexual function in men who have been treated with radiation therapy (NCI, 2003b) and radical retropubic prostatectomy (Schwartz, Wong, & Graydon, 2004).

Hormonal Therapy

The goal of hormonal therapy is to suppress the levels of testosterone in the body. Most prostate cancers are hormone dependent and stimulated by circulating androgens. Orchiectomy, the surgical removal of the testes, achieves a 90%–95% reduction in testosterone very rapidly (Miaskowski, 1999). This is the treatment of choice for men who have severe pain or impending paralysis from spinal cord compression. Hormonal therapy also is being studied in men with localized disease, such as bulky stage IIb tumors, and has shown favorable results when given in combination with radiation therapy (NCI, 2003b).

Medical androgen ablation can be achieved by the use of luteinizing hormone releasing hormone (LHRH) agonists (e.g., leuprolide, goserelin, buserelin) alone or in combination with antiandrogens (e.g., flutamide, bicalutamide). Combined androgen blockade (CAB) employs the combination of LHRH agonists and antiandrogens or the addition of an antiandrogen to orchiectomy. CAB has been shown to be superior in terms of disease progression and survival rates (Miaskowski, 1999). Side effects of LHRH agonists include impotence, decreased libido, and hot flashes. Flutamide may cause nausea, diarrhea, and breast tenderness. Bicalutamide may cause nausea, breast tenderness, hot flashes, loss of libido, and impotence (NCI, 2003b). Androgen deprivation therapy (ADT) also results in osteoporosis, as evidenced by decreased bone mineral density (BMD) and increased fracture risk (NCI, 2003b; Smith, 2002). Prostate cancer that is no longer responsive to ADT may respond to the withdrawal of antiandrogens. Flutamide withdrawal from the CAB regimen has produced short-term responses, including symptom improvement and decreases in PSA (Paul & Breul, 2000).

Chemotherapy

The use of chemotherapy for treatment of prostate cancer usually is reserved for disease that is refractory to hormonal manipulation. A variety of regimens has been used. To date, most of the results have been palliative in nature. Activity has been seen in combinations of vinca alkaloids and taxanes with estramustine. Mitoxantrone also has shown activity and provided improvement in pain and quality of life (Autorino, DiLorenzo, Damioano, De Placido, & D'Armiento, 2003). Clinical trials continue to search for agents and combinations that will be effective.

Supportive Care

The most common site of metastases in prostate cancer is the bone. Bony disease leads to a variety of complications referred to as skeletal-related events (SREs). These include pain, pathologic fracture, hypercalcemia, and spinal cord compression. Painful bony metastases can be treated with EBRT as well as with the use of radiopharmaceuticals, such as strontium. Regular use of the IV bisphosphonate zoledronic acid (Zometa®, Novartis Oncology, East Hanover, NJ) has been shown to significantly decrease the incidence of SREs in patients with bone metastases (Body, 2003; Saad et al., 2002; Saad & Shulman, 2004).

Men receiving ADT also are at risk for osteoporosis (Chang, 2003). Studies suggest that ADT results in a 5%–10% decrease in BMD per year, and this correlates with higher levels of markers of bone resorption (Daniell et al., 2000; Kiratli, Srinivas, Perkash, & Terris, 2001; Maillefert et al., 1999; Mittan et al., 2002; Stoch et al., 2001; Wei et al., 1999). Research findings show that IV bisphosphonates pamidronate and zoledronic acid prevent decreases in BMD during ADT (Saad & Schulman, 2004). A recent trial showed an increase in BMD during ADT for men receiving zoledronic acid versus placebo (Saad & Schulman; Smith et al., 2003). Trials are ongoing to further validate these results.

Complementary Therapy

Until February 2002, the herbal combination PC-SPES (stated to contain eight herbs: chrysanthemum, isatis, licorice, lucid ganoderma, pseudo-ginseng, rubescens, saw palmetto, and scute) was available as a nutritional supplement for "prostate health" (NCI, 2003b). Early clinical trials documented some estrogen-like activity, including reduction in PSA, decreased libido, impotence, gynecomastia, and thromboembolism (NCI, 2003b). The U.S. Food and Drug Administration issued a warning to consumers to stop using PC-SPES when it was found to be contaminated with diethylstilbestrol, indomethacin, and warfarin (Sovak, Seligson, Konas, Jahduch, & Dolezal, 2002).

Investigational Therapy

Patients who have become refractory to standard therapies may be eligible for a variety of trials. Immunotherapy, genetic therapy, and targeted therapy with novel agents are being investigated.

Nutritional Implications

According to Heber, Fair, and Ornish (1999), "scientific evidence suggests that differences in diet and lifestyle may account in large part for the variability of prostate cancer rates in different countries" (p. 3). Good nutrition may reduce the incidence of prostate cancer and help to reduce the risk of prostate cancer progression. Many studies currently are being conducted to aid in further understanding how diet and prostate cancer are related. An estimated one-third of cancer deaths in the United States can be attributed to diet in adulthood, including diet's effect on obesity (Byers et al., 2002).

Fruits and Vegetables

Fruits and vegetables are rich sources of vitamins, minerals, dietary fiber, and a variety of cancer-fighting phytochemicals. Vibrant, intense color in fruits and vegetables is one indicator of phytochemical content. There is extensive and consistent evidence that high fruit and vegetable intakes are associated with decreased risks of many cancers (Eastwood, 1999; Freudenheim et al., 1996; Khaw et al., 2001; Rock, Saxe, Ruffin, August, & Schottenfeld, 1996; Steinmetz & Potter, 1996; U.S. Department of Agriculture, 1995; Voorrips et al., 2000; Willett, 2000; World Cancer Research Fund & American Institute for Cancer Research, 1997; Zhang et al., 1999, 2000), and although results for prostate cancer risk are not yet conclusive, they are promising (Cohen, Kristal, & Stanford, 2000; Deneo-Pellegrini, De Stefani, Ronco, & Mendilaharsu, 1999; Hodge et al., 2004; Jain, Hislop, Howe, & Ghadirian, 1999). A case-control study found that men who consumed 28 or more servings of vegetables weekly had a 35% reduced risk of prostate cancer compared to men who consumed fewer than 14 servings weekly (Cohen et al.) (a serving is equivalent to ½ cup fruit or vegetable, 1 cup raw leafy vegetable, ¼ cup dried fruit or vegetable, or 6 fl oz. of fruit or vegetable juice). Although some studies (Key et al., 2004; Shike et al., 2002) have observed no relationship between fruits and vegetables and prostate cancer, none of those studies has recorded fruit and vegetable consumption at levels recommended by many nutrition professionals. It may be that a minimum of 8–10 servings of fruit and vegetables are needed to provide the greatest protection against cancer (Pierce et al., 2002).

Some research indicates that the amount of fruits and vegetables may be less important than certain compounds found in specific fruit and vegetable families. Evidence indicates that certain carotenoids, namely lycopene and beta-carotene, may be of particular significance. Lycopene acts as an antioxidant that scavenges free radicals to reduce tissue damage. Higher blood levels of lycopene are associated with reduced risk of prostate cancer (Gann et al., 1999; Hwang & Bowen, 2002; Lu et al., 2001; Wu et al., 2004). Furthermore, lycopene inhibits the proliferation of prostate cancer cells (Kim et al., 2003; Kucuk et al., 2002). Various studies have observed a protective effect for tomatoes, a rich dietary source of lycopene (Bosetti et al., 2000; Jain et al., 1999; Mills, Beeson, Phillips, & Fraser, 1989; Norrish, Jackson, Sharpe, & Skeaff, 2000b; Tzonou et al., 1999). Mucci et al. (2001) reported a significant inverse association between the consumption of cooked tomatoes and insulin-like growth factor (IGF-I), a component that has been implicated in risk of prostate cancer.

The largest prospective study to date observed that men who consumed tomato sauce two to four times weekly had a 34% lower risk of prostate cancer (Giovannucci et al., 1995). Men with prostate cancer who consumed 30 mg lycopene (equivalent to ¾ cup tomato sauce, 12 fl oz. tomato juice, 4½ tablespoons tomato paste, 8 raw tomatoes, or 4 cups watermelon) daily in the form of tomato sauce for three weeks increased their lycopene concentration in serum and prostate tissue, experienced a 28% reduction in oxidative DNA damage, and decreased PSA values by approximately 18% (Bowen et al., 2002; Chen et al., 2001; Kucuk et al., 2002). Researchers later reported that the prostate cells of men who consumed tomato sauce (30 mg lycopene) daily for three weeks expressed greater apoptotic cell death (Kim et al., 2003). As a fat-soluble compound, lycopene-rich foods are best absorbed in the presence of fat (such as a small amount of olive oil) (Weisberger, 1998). There appear to be other protective compounds found in the tomato in addition to lycopene; thus, lycopene is best obtained from food sources (Boileau et al., 2003).

Dietary beta-carotene may reduce prostate cancer risk if combined with a diet rich in fruits and vegetables and low in fat (Key, Silcocks, Davey, Appleby, & Bishop, 1997; Kolonel et al., 2000; Ohno et al., 1988; Wu et al., 2004) (see Table 11-1). The protective effect of beta-carotene may be especially pronounced in younger men (Wu et al.). Other researchers, however, have observed no effect (Daviglus et al., 1996; Norrish et al., 2000b). Nonetheless, beta-carotene supplements have not offered protection against prostate cancer (Hennekens et al., 1996; Omenn et al., 1996; Schuurman, Goldbohm, Brants, & van den Brandt, 2002). Findings from an alpha-tocepherol, beta-carotene trial revealed a 23% increased risk of prostate cancer incidence in men who consumed 20 mg of beta-carotene supplements (Heinonen et al., 1998).

Some evidence exists that vegetable consumption, particularly cruciferous vegetables (broccoli, cauliflower, cabbage, kale, brussels sprouts, bok choy), may be associated with a reduced risk of prostate cancer (Chinni, Li, Upadhyay, Koppolu, & Sarkar, 2001; Cohen et al., 2000; Jain et al., 1999; Kolonel et al., 2000; Wang et al., 2004). A study by Cohen et al. reported that men who ate three or more servings of cruciferous vegetables per week had a 41% decreased risk of prostate cancer compared with men who ate less than one serving per week. Two primary components in cruciferous vegetables, isothiocyanates and indole-3-carbinol (I3C), are likely related to the protective effect. Sulforaphane, one of the isothiocyanates, may inhibit both the initiation and progression of prostate cancer via apoptosis (Chiao et al., 2002; Frydoonfar, McGrath, & Spigelman, 2003; Singh, Xiao, Lew, Dhir, & Singh, 2004; Wang et al., 2004). Sulforaphane (Brooks, Paton, & Vidanes, 2001), I3C, and 3'-diindolylmethane (DIM) (Li, Li, & Sarkar, 2003) upregulate phase II detoxifying enzymes, which may further explain the anticancer effects of cruciferous vegetables. I3C appears to induce apoptosis in prostate cancer cells (Chinni et al.; Frydoonfar et al.; Jeon et al., 2003; Li, Li, et al.; Nachshon-Kedmi, Yannai, Haj, & Fares, 2003; Zhang, Hsu, Kinseth, Bjeldanes, & Firestone, 2003). Furthermore, DIM, a metabolite of I3C, has been observed to exert antip-

Table 11-1. Dietary Sources of Nutrients and Food Compounds

Nutrient or Compound	Dietary Sources
Lycopene	Tomato products[a] (tomato juice, vegetable juice cocktail, spaghetti sauce, ketchup), guava, grapefruit, papaya, watermelon
Beta-carotene	Carrots, sweet potatoes, winter squash, cantaloupe, mango
Whole grains	Oats, barley, quinoa, amaranth, bulgur, millet, soba noodles
Saturated fats	Fatty meats, whole milk dairy products (cheese, sour cream, ice cream, whole milk), butter, baked goods, mayonnaise
Trans fatty acids	Margarine, fried foods, various processed foods (breads, crackers, cookies, cereals)
Omega-6 fatty acids	Corn oil, safflower oil, sunflower oil, cottonseed oil, soybean oil, other polyunsaturated oils
Omega-3 fatty acids	Cold-water fish (salmon, trout, herring, sardines, mackerel), flaxseeds, walnuts, soybeans, canola oil
Selenium	Brazil nuts, seafood, enriched brewer's yeast, grains (content depends somewhat on amount in soil)
Vitamin E	Vegetable oils, wheat germ, nuts, seeds, soybeans, sweet potatoes, avocado
Soy	Soybeans, edamame, tofu, soymilk, tempeh, miso, soy nuts
Vitamin D	Cold-water fish (salmon, trout, sardines, herring), fortified products (soymilk, cereals), sunlight

[a] Cooked tomato products or juices, however, contain higher amounts of lycopene, as the cellular wall can be broken down with heat and absorption enhanced.

roliferative and antiandrogenic properties in androgen-dependent human prostate cancer cells (Le, Schaldach, Firestone, & Bjeldanes, 2003; Li, Li, et al.; Nachshon-Kedmi et al.).

Additionally, recent evidence indicates that the allium family, which includes onions, garlic, shallots, scallions, chives, and leeks, may offer protection against prostate cancer (Hodge et al., 2004; Hsing et al., 2002; Key et al., 1997; Pinto & Rivlin, 2001). These allium vegetables are rich in flavonoids and organosulfur compounds that have anticancer properties, which may act to detoxify carcinogens and stimulate cytochrome P450 enzymes (Lamm & Riggs, 2001). A recent Chinese study found that men who consumed one-third of an ounce or more of one of the allium-rich foods mentioned above had approximately a 50% reduction in prostate cancer risk compared to men who consumed lesser amounts (Hsing et al., 2002). One study reported a reduced risk of prostate cancer when subjects consumed natural garlic at least twice weekly (Key et al., 1997). Garlic supplements do not appear to have the same beneficial effects as real garlic (raw or cooked) in regard to prostate cancer (Fleischauer & Arab, 2001).

Dietary Fiber

Fiber is important in the diet for a variety of reasons, including bowel regularity and cholesterol-lowering effects, as well as its potentially anticancer effects. Fiber may function to bind to toxic compounds and carcinogens circulating in the body, which later can be eliminated from the body (Harris, Roberton, Watson, Triggs, & Ferguson, 1993). Additionally, a high-fiber diet works to reduce hormone levels that may be involved in the progression of prostate cancer (Slavin, 2000; Tariq et al., 2000; Tymchuk, Barnard, Heber, & Aronson, 2001). Fiber intake may (Tariq et al.) or may not (Shike et al., 2002) lead to a reduction in PSA values. Some research indicates an inverse relationship between prostate cancer and dietary intake of fiber (Pelucchi et al., 2004; Tymchuk et al.) or fiber-rich foods, such as whole grains (La Vecchia, Chatenoud, Negri, & Franceschi, 2003), legumes, nuts, and seeds (Jain et al., 1999; Kolonel et al., 2000) (see Table 11-1). Prostate cancer mortality is inversely associated with consumption of cereals and nuts and seeds, according to an NCI study (Hebert et al., 1998). A diet rich in natural fiber obtained from fruits, vegetables, legumes, and whole grains may reduce cancer risk and reduce the risk of prostate cancer progression. Patients may want to aim for 25–35 grams of fiber daily (Williams, Williams, & Weisberger, 1999).

Dietary Fat

The increased cancer risk observed in developed countries may be, in part, because a high-fat diet stimulates increased testosterone levels, which are associated with prostate cancer growth (Habito & Ball, 2001; Spentzos et al., 2003). A comprehensive review reported that 20 of 30 studies found positive, although not all statistically significant, associations between dietary fat intake and prostate cancer risk (Fleshner, Bagnell, Klotz, & Venkateswaran, 2004). Although a positive association between prostate cancer and fat intake was not observed in all studies (Veierod, Laake, & Thelle, 1997), some prospective studies reported significant findings (Bairati, Meyer, Fradet, & Moore, 1998; Giovannucci et al., 1993; Le Marchand, Kolonel, Wilkens, Myers, & Hirohata, 1994; Meyer, Bairati, Shadmani, Fradet, & Moore, 1999). Most researchers agree to aim for 20% of total calories from fat, with less than 10% of total calories from saturated fat (Williams et al., 1999). The type of fat is significant and may, in fact, be of greater importance than total fat.

Saturated Fat

Several studies indicate a positive association between saturated fat intake from meat and dairy products (animal sources) and prostate cancer (Bosetti et al., 2000; Fradat, Meyer, Bairati, Shadmani, & Moore, 1999; Kushi & Giovannucci, 2002; Lee et al., 1998; Meyer, Bairati, Fradet, & Moore, 1997). Intake of red meat (Bairati et al., 1998; Chan et al., 1998; Giovannucci et al., 1993; Michaud et al., 2001; Ramon et al., 2000) and dairy products (Bairati et al.; Bosetti et al.; Chan et al.; Michaud et al.; Ramon et al.) also may increase risk of metastatic prostate cancer.

Trans Fatty Acids

Preliminary research indicates that trans fatty acids, or hydrogenated oils, may be associated with increased cancer risk (Bakker, Van't Veer, & Zock, 1997; Slattery, Benson, Ma, Schaffer, & Potter, 2001; Voorrips et al., 2000). A recent prostate cancer trial reported a 30% increased cancer risk in men who used margarine once or more daily (Hodge et al., 2004).

Omega-6 Fatty Acids

Research indicated that omega-6 fatty acids (linoleic acid, which can be converted to arachidonic acid) may stimulate growth of prostate cancer cells (Ghosh & Meyers, 1997; Godley et al., 1996; Hughes-Fulford, Chen, & Tjandrawinata, 2001; Newcomer, King, Wicklund, & Stanford, 2001). Other studies, however, have reported no association (Gann et al., 1994; Giovannucci et al., 1993; Harvei et al., 1997; Mannisto et al., 2003). Alternatively, olive oil and canola oil, which are rich in omega-9 fats, have not been shown to increase cancer risk (Hodge et al., 2004; Hughes-Fulford et al.; Norrish, Jackson, Sharpe, & Skeaff, 2000a; Veierod et al., 1997).

Omega-3 Fatty Acids

Omega-3 fatty acids may reduce risk for prostate cancer as well as reduce the risk of cancer progression (Augustsson et al., 2003; Hodge et al., 2004; Hughes-Fulford et al., 2001; Norrish, Skeaff, Arribas, Sharpe, & Jackson, 1999; Terry, Lichtenstein, Feychting, Ahlbom, & Wolk, 2001). In vitro and animal studies consistently have reported reduced cell proliferation and decreased rate of cancer progression with intake of omega-3 fatty acids (Chung, Mitchell, Zhang, & Young, 2001; Terry, Rohan, & Wolk, 2003). These fats appear to induce apoptosis, suppress cancer cell initiation, and compete with arachidonic acid (Bartsch, Nair, & Owen, 1999; Norrish, Skeaff, et al., 1999). Recent studies reported that men who consumed cold-water fish three or more times per week had a 44% lower risk of prostate cancer, especially for metastatic prostate cancer, where the effect was even greater (Augustsson et al.). Conversely, a 30-year follow-up study found that men who ate no fish had a two- to threefold higher frequency of prostate cancer than those who ate moderate or high amounts of fish (Terry et al., 2001). Researchers in New Zealand reported that men with high levels of eicosapentaenoic acid (EPA) and docosahexaenoic acid (DHA), the omega-3 fats found in fish, had a 40% lower risk of prostate cancer than those with low blood levels (Norrish, Skeaff, et al., 1999). A case-control study, however, observed no effect between serum EPA and DHA and prostate cancer (Kristal, Cohen, Qu, & Stanford, 2002).

Flaxseed, the richest plant source of omega-3 fatty acids, contains alpha-linolenic acid (ALA). Flax may work to block tumor growth, inhibit angiogenesis, and enhance immune system function (Dabrosin, Chen, Wang, & Thompson, 2002). The lignans, phytoestrogens found in flax, appear to bind with testosterone, lowering circulating levels of testosterone (Demark-Wahnefried et al., 2001; Denis, Morton, & Griffiths, 1999). This action may act as one of the protective mechanisms of flax. Preliminary data suggest reduced tumor growth and spread with the use of flaxseed (Demark-Wahnefried et al.; Lin et al., 2002; Moyad, 2000). One study reported that patients with prostate cancer following a 20% fat diet and consuming 30 grams of flax daily resulted in reduced cancer growth rates the more days patients followed the above diet (Demark-Wahnefried et al.). Animal data indicate the consumption of flax may lead to less aggressive tumors and a lower risk of metastasis (Lin et al.). Ground flaxseed has greater bioavailability than whole flaxseed, but because of its instability, it is best to store flax in the refrigerator or freezer. Flaxseed oil is highly concentrated and lacks the protein, fiber, vitamins, minerals, and lignans that are found in ground flaxseed.

Although not all studies agree (Andersson et al., 1996; Mannisto et al., 2003), some research indicates a positive association between ALA and prostate cancer (De Stefani, Deneo-Pellegrini, Boffetta, Ronco, & Mendilaharsu, 2000; Gann et al., 1994; Giovannucci et al., 1993; Newcomer et al., 2001; Ramon et al., 2000). The primary source of ALA in these studies, however, was red meat, milk, butter, mayonnaise, and margarine (De Stefani et al.; Giovannucci et al., 1993; Ramon et al.). Although De Stefani et al. observed a strong association with ALA from both animal and plant sources, ALA from vegetables comprised approximately 10% of the ALA intake. Although flax is rich in ALA, it may be compounds in these other foods that explain the association observed between ALA and prostate cancer.

Simple Sugars

High-sugar foods usually are highly processed and refined, low in nutrient value, and low in dietary fiber. Additionally, refined cereals (primarily breads and pasta) have been reported to increase cancer risk (Chatenoud et al., 1999). Deneo-Pellegrini et al. (1999) noted that consumption of desserts, in particular, increased risk of prostate cancer. Furthermore, these foods appear to increase serum insulin and serum IGF-I levels and contribute to insulin resistance (Hsing, Gao, Chua, Deng, & Stanczyk, 2003; Manolio et al., 1991; Reiser et al., 1981; Snyder, Clemmons, & Underwood, 1989). Elevated serum insulin and IGF-I levels (Aksoy, Aksoy, Bakan, Atmaca, & Akcay, 2004; Barnard, Ngo, Leung, Aronson, & Golding, 2003; Cardillo et al., 2003; Giovannucci, 2003; Hsing et al., 2001; Kaaks & Lukanova, 2001; Li, Yu, Schumacher, Casey, &

Witte, 2003; Moyad, 2003; Ngo, Barnard, Tymchuk, Cohen, & Aronson, 2002; Yu & Berkel, 1999) as well as insulin resistance (Hsing et al., 2003) appear to lead to both the development and promotion of cancer. Various mechanisms have been proposed regarding how IGF-I signaling may contribute to each stage of cancer progression. IGF-I may promote tumor development by inhibiting apoptosis, stimulating cell proliferation, stimulating synthesis of sex steroids, and inhibiting the synthesis of sex hormone-binding globulin (SHBG) (Grimberg, 2003; Kaaks & Lukanova). Sugars to be consumed in limited amounts include products made with refined flours or refined grains, alcohol, and sweets, such as candy, cookies, cakes, and pies.

Caloric Restriction

Substantial evidence indicates that a high caloric intake increases risk of various cancers, including prostate cancer (Andersson et al., 1996; Deneo-Pellegrini et al., 1999; Hsieh et al., 2003; Kristal et al., 2002; Meyer et al., 1997; Rohan, Howe, Burch, & Jain, 1995). The Netherlands Cohort Study (Schuurman, van den Brandt, Dorant, Brants, & Goldbohm, 1999), however, found no association between prostate carcinoma and energy intake. Recently, a large cohort study reported no association between total energy intake with prostate cancer incidence, but a modest increase in metastatic and fatal disease was observed (Platz, Leitzmann, Michaud, Willett, & Giovannucci, 2003). An earlier study found that caloric intake was positively associated with preclinical prostate cancer risk; as caloric intake increased, cancer risk rose significantly (Meyer et al., 1997). The mechanism involved may be related to the decrease in IGF-I observed when caloric intake is restricted (Meyer et al., 1997; Sonntag et al., 1999).

Body Mass and Physical Activity

Higher body mass and physical inactivity may contribute to prostate cancer risk. A large prospective study observed a significant positive association between body mass index (BMI) (see Appendix B) and prostate cancer risk (Veierod et al., 1997). The study by Calle, Rodriguez, Walker-Thurmond, and Thun (2003) reported obese men to have a 20% increased risk of dying from prostate cancer, and men who were severely obese had a 34% elevated risk. This research was further supported by recent evidence that obesity is a risk factor for aggressive prostate cancer (Amling et al., 2004; Freedland et al., 2004).

Selenium

Selenium acts as an antioxidant, which appears to inhibit cellular changes that may lead to prostate cancer. Selenium also may work to inhibit angiogenesis (Corcoran, Najdovska, & Costello, 2004) and induce apoptosis (Sinha & El-Bayou, 2004). Selenium consistently has been reported to reduce risk of prostate cancer (Clark et al., 1998; Combs, Clark, & Turnbull, 1997; Giovannucci et al., 1998; Yoshizawa et al., 1998) and inhibit its progression (Corcoran et al.). Low plasma selenium levels are associated with a four- to fivefold increased risk of prostate cancer (Brooks, Metter, et al., 2001). Additionally, selenium supplements have been shown to decrease the recurrence of prostate cancer by 63% (Clark et al.). Some research indicates that the combination of selenium and vitamin E may work synergistically in reducing risk for prostate cancer (Venkateswaran, Fleshner, & Klotz, 2004).

Vitamin E

Studies show that vitamin E intake may reduce the risk of prostate cancer (Deneo-Pellegrini et al., 1999; Heinonen et al., 1998; Helzlsouer et al., 2000; Huang et al., 2003; Kristal, Stanford, Cohen, Wicklund, & Patterson, 1999; Nomura, Stemmermann, Lee, & Craft, 1997) and inhibit prostate cancer cell growth (Fleshner, Fair, Huryk, & Heston, 1999; Galli et al., 2004). In a six-year follow-up study where men consumed 50–100 IU vitamin E (Heinonen et al.), cancer incidence was reduced by 33%, and death from prostate cancer was reduced by 41%. Results suggested that long-term vitamin E (α-tocopherol) supplementation decreases serum androgen concentrations, which is related to a reduced incidence of and mortality from prostate cancer (Hartman et al., 2001). Other researchers have found γ-tocopherol to offer a protective effect against prostate cancer (Huang et al.; Moyad, Brumfield, & Pienta, 1999; Nomura et al.). Large doses of α-tocopherol appear to suppress γ-tocopherol levels (Chopra & Bhagavan, 1999; Handelman et al., 1994; Handelman, Machlin, Fitch, Weiter, & Dratz, 1985).

The most provocative study found that, unlike α-tocopherol, men with the highest plasma γ-tocopherol concentrations had a fivefold lower risk of prostate cancer compared to men in the lowest quintile (Helzlsouer et al., 2000). Although the protective mechanism remains to be determined, scientists suggest that γ-tocopherol may possess an ability to detoxify nitrogen dioxide as well as inhibit COX-2 activity (Campbell, Stone, Whaley, Qui, & Krishnan, 2003).

Because of the high fat content of many dietary sources of vitamin E, a supplement may be beneficial. Natural forms of vitamin E (γ-tocopherol, d-α-tocopherol) appear to be better absorbed by the body but are more expensive (Jiang, Christen, Shigenaga, & Ames, 2001; Zu & Ip, 2003). The combination of γ- and α-tocopherol may offer greater protection from DNA damage than α-tocopherol alone (Galli et al., 2004). Many of the studies on vitamin E and prostate cancer have used synthetic forms of vitamin E (dl-α-tocopherol) (Hartman et al., 2001; Heinonen et al., 1998; Sigounas, Anagnostou, & Steiner, 1997; Zu & Ip).

Green Tea

Green tea contains phytochemicals known as polyphenols that provide antioxidant and anticancer properties, which may act by blocking the formation of cancer-causing compounds, such as nitrosamines (Leone et al., 2003). Many studies indicate a lower risk of cancer with green tea consumption (Gupta, Hussain, & Mukhtar, 2003; Jian, Xie, Lee, & Binns, 2004; Saleem, Adhami, Siddiqui, & Mukhtar, 2003), but more research is needed for conclusive evidence. Green tea catechins, a phytochemical, suppress cell growth and induce cell death in human prostate cancer cells (Brusselmans, De Schrijver, Heyns, Verhoeven, & Swinnen, 2003; Chung, Cheung, et al., 2001; Gupta et al., 2003; Hastak et al., 2003; Yu, Yin, & Shen, 2004).

Animal studies have observed inhibition of prostate cancer development, lower serum testosterone concentrations, and increased survival (Gupta, Hastak, Ahmad, Lewin, & Mukhtar, 2001). The combination of soy and green tea synergistically inhibited final tumor weight and metastasis and significantly reduced serum concentrations of both testosterone and DHT in vivo (Zhou, Yu, Zhong, & Blackburn, 2003). A case-control study observed heightened protective effects of green tea with increasing frequency, duration, and quantity of green tea consumption (Jian et al., 2004).

Soy

Soy is rich in various nutrients, including antioxidants known as isoflavones, namely genistein and daidzein. Among other benefits, soy appears to offer protection against prostate cancer (Arliss & Biermann, 2002; Aronson et al., 1999; Hebert et al., 1998; Jacobsen, Knutsen, & Fraser, 1998; Kolonel et al., 2000; Messina, 2003; Messina, Persky, Setchell, & Barnes, 1994; Pollard & Wolter, 2000; Zhou et al., 2002). Soy has been one diet component thought to play a role in the lower rate of prostate cancer in the Asian countries.

Research shows that phytoestrogens, such as soy, also may prevent prostate cancer by decreasing blood androgen levels, increasing SHBG concentration, binding to hormone receptors, inhibiting 5-alpha reductase, restricting other enzymes associated with cell growth, causing direct tumor destruction that essentially starves the tumor, and/or decreasing IGF-I (Yi et al., 2002; Zhou et al., 2002). Although the majority of research has reported soy to decrease IGF-I activity (McCarty, 1999; Wang, DeGroff, & Clinton, 2003; Zhou et al., 1999), one study observed no relationship (Nagata et al., 2003), and Spentzos et al. (2003) found that soy protein supplements actually increased IGF-I activity.

A prospective study reported that consuming soymilk more than once a day resulted in a 70% reduction of prostate cancer risk (Jacobsen et al., 1998). Research indicates that soy foods (Gardner-Thorpe, O'Hagen, Young, & Lewis, 2003; Habito & Ball, 2001) and soy supplements (Zhou et al., 2002) may decrease serum testosterone and DHT levels. A low-fat diet combined with soy has been shown to decrease PSA values significantly in a three-month period (Tsutsumi, Suzuki, Shiga, Ishikawa, & Ishikawa, 2002). A different study, however, found no significant decrease in PSA values in men who consumed 44 grams of soy protein daily for one month (Jenkins et al., 2003).

Vitamin D and Calcium

Vitamin D is known to inhibit prostate cancer in animals (Blutt, Polek, Stewart, Kattan, & Weigel, 2000; Getzenberg et al., 1997; Lokeshwar et al., 1999; Schwartz, Oeler, Uskokovic, & Bahnson, 1994; Vegesna et al., 2003), and although human research remains unclear, vitamin D appears to be of benefit (Ahonen, Tenkanen, Teppo, Hakama, & Tuohimaa, 2000; Giovannucci et al., 1998; Peehl, Krishnan, & Feldman, 2003; Tuohimaa et al., 2004). Vitamin D is believed to be important in the protection of human prostate cells (Chen, Wang, Whitlatch, Flanagan, & Holick, 2003; Gross, Stamey, Hancock, & Feldman, 1998; Peehl et al.; Studzinski & Moore, 1995). Epidemiologic studies indicate that sunlight exposure, a significant source of vitamin D, is inversely proportional to prostate cancer mortality and that prostate cancer risk is greater in men with lower levels of vitamin D (Ahonen et al.; Corder et al., 1993; Hanchette & Schwartz, 1992; Studzinski & Moore; Tuohimaa et al.). Tuohimaa et al. observed elevated cancer risk in men with both low (≤ 19 nmol/l) and high (≥ 80 nmol/l) serum 25 (OH)-vitamin D levels. Men with the lowest risk had normal serum 25(OH)-vitamin D levels ranging between 40–60 nmol/l. A recent study on advanced prostate cancer reported that the combination of vitamin D and the chemotherapy agent docetaxel was twice as effective as docetaxel alone based on PSA responses (Beer, 2003). Current research is investigating the potential use of 25 (OH), 1,25-dihydroxyvitamin D3 (1,25(OH)2D3), and other analogs as therapy or chemotherapeutic agents for prostate cancer (Bauer, Thompson, Church, Ariazi, & Wilding, 2003; Gross et al.; Johnson, Hershberger, & Trump, 2002; Krishnan, Peehl, & Feldman, 2003; Peehl et al.). Excessive doses of vitamin D (> 2,000 IU daily), however, can be toxic and lead to hypercalcemia.

Epidemiologic studies (12 of 14) have reported increased prostate cancer incidence with high calcium intakes (Giovannucci et al., 1998). One theory is that high amounts of calcium (> 2,000 mg daily) suppress circulating vitamin D blood levels (Giovannucci et al., 1998; Grant, 1999). The relationship between dairy foods and increased prostate cancer risk may be because of the high calcium content in dairy and/or to the animal fats in dairy. Some studies found that consumption of skim or low-fat milk resulted in an increased association with prostate cancer, supporting the calcium connection (Grant; Veierod et al., 1997). One analysis identified a four- to fivefold risk elevation of advanced prostate cancer with very high (> 2,000 mg/day) or very low (< 500 mg/day) calcium intakes (Giovannucci et al., 1998). A recent study found that higher calcium intakes resulted in a modest 7% increased risk of localized prostate cancer but more than a 200% increased risk for advanced prostate cancer compared to men with the lowest calcium intake (Kristal et al., 2002). Additionally, Gunnell et al. (2003) reported a positive association between IGF-I and intake of milk, dairy products, and calcium.

It is advisable for patients to consume adequate amounts of vitamin D and calcium but to avoid high calcium intakes. Ten to 15 minutes of sunlight three to four times per week typically provides one with adequate vitamin D (Holick, 1995). Vitamin D absorption declines with age, and vitamin D deficiency is common among older adults (Ebeling et al., 1992; Rasmussen et al., 2000; Silverberg et al., 1989; Thomas et al., 1998; Webb, Pilbeam, Hanafin, & Holick, 1990). Thus, patients, especially those on ADT, may benefit from a serum vitamin D blood test (25-OH; 1,25-OH).

Assessment Guidelines

Quality of life, activities of daily living, and functional status are important areas of assessment. Additionally, patients' use of complementary therapies and dietary supplements should be included in a successful nutrition assessment. The possible risks/benefits of a given therapy must be discussed with the patient. Based on the assessment, nutrition counseling can focus on developing an individualized dietary plan for a patient to help to achieve nutrition goals and desired health outcomes. Appendix E lists components included in a nutrition assessment.

Special Considerations for Nutrition

Most patients with prostate cancer complete their cancer treatment with relative ease. The predominant nutrition-related issue to prostate cancer treatment is diarrhea when undergoing radiation therapy, primarily only observed with full pelvic radiation therapy. If a patient has advanced cancer and is undergoing chemotherapy, he may face additional challenges. Additionally, if a patient is on hormone therapy, managing hot flashes, maintaining lean body mass, and preserving bone mass may become important concerns.

Diarrhea

Various nutrition steps should be followed if a patient suffers from diarrhea. Some patients, however, can undergo cancer treatment without any gastrointestinal distress, in which case, the dietary modifications that follow would be unnecessary.

Nutritional Options for Diarrhea
- Drink six to eight cups of room-temperature fluids to help to prevent dehydration. These might include water, tea, fluid replacement drinks, ginger ale, or apple juice. Limit consumption of alcohol and caffeinated beverages.
- Allow carbonated beverages to lose their fizz, or stir before drinking.

- Foods high in soluble fiber, including bananas, white rice, applesauce, oatmeal, and barley, act as binding agents to produce a more solid bowel movement.
- Consider the BRAT diet: bananas, rice, applesauce, and toast.
- Try breads made from oats, barley, millet, or refined flours without seeds or nuts.
- Foods rich in insoluble fiber may worsen diarrhea. These foods include whole wheat breads and cereals, raw vegetables (cooked vegetables are generally okay), fruit peels (the flesh of fruit is generally okay), beans, peas, and popcorn. Patients can resume consumption of higher fiber foods, fruits, and vegetables once the diarrhea stops.
- Consume potassium-rich foods such as orange juice, tomato juice, bananas, and potatoes.
- Avoid greasy and spicy foods.
- If lactose intolerant, use dairy products sparingly. Consider Lactaid® (McNeil Nutritionals, Fort Washington, PA), yogurt, or soymilk.
- Avoid sugar-free foods that contain sorbitol, mannitol, or maltitol. These compounds are sugar alcohols that may worsen diarrhea.
- Eat frequent, small meals.
- Consider rice congee: combine one cup long-cooking white rice with six to seven cups of water and one tablespoon of salt; cook rice according to package directions; patients can eat and drink this sticky, soupy mixture; broth may be substituted for water (omit salt if using broth).
- Try clove tea: simmer six to eight whole cloves with one tea bag of herbal, non-caffeinated tea (try ginger or chamomile) and one cup of water; simmer this mixture until the volume is reduced by half; let cool until lukewarm and drink.
- The use of probiotics and/or l-glutamine may help to improve symptoms. Probiotics are healthy bacteria that aid in the health of the digestive tract. Glutamine is an amino acid that is essential to the integrity of the intestinal cells. Glutamine powder can be taken 10 grams one to three times daily to help to reduce diarrhea.

Antioxidant Supplements

Patients often are instructed to NOT consume high-dose antioxidant supplements during chemotherapy or radiation treatment because of a lack of current human research. It has been hypothesized that high doses of antioxidants may decrease the effectiveness of chemotherapy or radiation therapies (Labriola & Livingston, 1999). Other researchers, however, disagree and find that antioxidants may enhance an individual's response to chemotherapy or radiation therapy in addition to mitigating various side effects of these treatments (Conklin, 2000; Lamson & Brignall, 1999).

Nonetheless, to date, consuming a diet rich in antioxidants seems to be the most prudent advice when confronted with the issue of antioxidant supplementation during cancer therapy.

Hormone Therapy

Patients who undergo hormone therapy may experience various side effects, notably hot flashes, night sweats, weight gain, and possibly a decline in BMD. The pathophysiology of hot flashes is complex but not yet well understood (Thompson, Shanafelt, & Loprinzi, 2003). Although studies involving men are lacking, many studies have found that dietary and supplemental strategies do not appear to significantly affect hot flashes when compared to a placebo in women. The placebo effect, however, has been considerable in various studies.

No studies have assessed the effects of red clover and hot flashes in men, but four double-blind, placebo-controlled studies in women have been conducted (Baber, Templeman, Morton, Kelly, & West, 1999; Knight, Howes, & Eden, 1999; Tice et al., 2003; van de Weijer & Barentsen, 2002). Three of these studies observed no benefit for the women receiving red clover when compared to women receiving a placebo (Baber et al.; Knight et al.; Tice et al.). One study, however, reported that red clover helped to reduce the occurrence of hot flashes by nearly 50% (van de Weijer & Barentsen). Research findings regarding the use of black cohosh for hot flashes are somewhat mixed. Although not all studies are in agreement (Jacobson et al., 2001; Borrelli & Ernst, 2002), the majority of studies have found black cohosh to be effective for reducing hot flashes ("*Cimicifuga racemosa*," 2003; Hernandez & Pluchino, 2003; Kronenberg & Fugh-Berman, 2002; Lieberman, 1998). A recent review of 13 studies evaluating the effects of soy and isoflavone supplements on hot flashes reported a statistically significant association between initial hot flash frequency and treatment efficacy (Messina & Hughes, 2003). Nonetheless, current research evidence is insufficient to support or refute these compounds' effects on hot flashes (North American Menopause Society, 2004).

Similarly to women in menopause, men often report increased fat mass accompanied with a decrease in lean body mass while on ADT (Basaria et al., 2002; Berruti et al., 2002; Nowicki, Bryc, & Kokot, 2001; Smith, 2002, 2004). This change is of concern considering the evidence regarding increased body mass and prostate cancer risk.

Multiple prospective studies have examined the relationship between ADT for prostate cancer and BMD. Collectively, these studies suggest that significant bone loss is clearly observed within the first year of ADT (Berruti et al., 2002; Daniell et al., 2000; Kiratli et al., 2001; Maillefert et al., 1999; Mittan et al., 2002; Stoch et al., 2001; Wei et al., 1999). Clinical trials are needed to evaluate the role of vitamin D, calcitonin, and oral bisphosphonates for the prevention and treatment of osteoporosis in patients undergoing ADT (Basaria et al., 2002). Nonetheless, dual-energy x-ray absorptiometry screening for osteoporosis is recommended prior to ADT, again at one year, and then at appropriate intervals thereafter. Additionally, serum vitamin D (25-OH; 1,25-OH) levels should be assessed with these patients. Patients should be encouraged to maintain adequate, yet not excessive, amounts of dietary calcium and vitamin D intake. Furthermore, exercise, particularly resistance training, may reduce the risk of osteoporosis and increase muscle mass (Basaria et al.).

Expected Outcomes of Therapy

For patients who experience side effects from cancer treatment that may be mitigated with diet, the primary focus is to alleviate those symptoms, such as diarrhea, fatigue, hot flashes, and/or a decline in bone mass. The nutrition care plan for the majority of patients with prostate cancer, however, will simply be to optimize a patient's diet and lifestyle. A healthy diet helps to increase energy levels, facilitate recovery, and enhance the immune system, all of which would facilitate a patient's journey with cancer. Ultimately, the hope is that good nutrition and specific dietary supplements, when clinically appropriate, would help to reduce PSA levels, inhibit prostate cancer cell growth, and reduce risk of cancer recurrence.

References

Ahonen, M.H., Tenkanen, L., Teppo, L., Hakama, M., & Tuohimaa, P. (2000). Prostate cancer risk and prediagnostic serum 25-hydroxyvitamin D levels (Finland). *Cancer Causes and Control, 11,* 847–852.

Aksoy, Y., Aksoy, H., Bakan, E., Atmaca, A.F., & Akcay, F. (2004). Serum insulin-like growth factor-I and insulin-like growth factor-binding protein-3 in localized, metastasized prostate cancer and benign prostatic hyperplasia. *Urologia Internationalis, 72*(1), 62–65.

American Cancer Society. (2005). *Cancer facts and figures, 2005.* Atlanta, GA: Author.

Amling, C.L., Riffenburgh, R.H., Sun, L., Moul, J.W., Lance, R.S., Kusuda, L., et al. (2004). Pathologic variables and recurrence rates as related to obesity and race in men with prostate cancer undergoing radical prostatectomy. *Journal of Clinical Oncology, 22,* 439–445.

Andersson, S.O., Wolk, A., Bergstrom, R., Giovannucci, E., Lindgren, C., Baron, J., et al. (1996). Energy, nutrient intake and prostate cancer risk: A population-based case-control study in Sweden. *International Journal of Cancer, 68,* 716–722.

Arliss, R.M., & Biermann, C.A. (2002). Do soy isoflavones lower cholesterol, inhibit atherosclerosis, and play a role in cancer prevention? *Holistic Nursing Practice, 16*(5), 40–48.

Aronson, W.J., Tymchuk, C.N., Elashoff, R.M., McBride, W.H., McLean, C., Wang, H., et al. (1999). Decreased growth of human prostate LNCaP tumors in SCID mice fed a low-fat, soy protein diet with isoflavones. *Nutrition and Cancer, 35*(2), 130–136.

Augustsson, K., Michaud, D.S., Rimm, E.B., Leitzmann, M.F., Stampfer, M.J., Willett, W.C., et al. (2003). A prospective study of intake of fish and marine fatty acids and prostate cancer. *Cancer Epidemiology, Biomarkers and Prevention, 12*(1), 64–67.

Autorino, R., DiLorenzo, G., Damioano, R., De Placido, S., & D'Armiento, M. (2003). Role of chemotherapy in hormone-refractory prostate cancer: Old issues, recent advances and new perspectives. *Urology International, 70*(1), 1–14.

Baber, R.J., Templeman, C., Morton, T., Kelly, G.E., & West, L. (1999). Randomized placebo-controlled trial of an isoflavone supplement and menopausal symptoms in women. *Climacteric, 2,* 85–92.

Bairati, I., Meyer, F., Fradet, Y., & Moore, L. (1998). Dietary fat and advanced prostate cancer. *Journal of Urology, 159,* 1271–1275.

Bakker, N., Van't Veer, P., & Zock, P.L. (1997). Adipose fatty acids and cancers of the breast, prostate and colon: An ecological study. EURAMIC Study Group. *International Journal of Cancer, 72,* 587–591.

Barnard, R.J., Ngo, T.H., Leung, P.S., Aronson, W.J., & Golding, L.A. (2003). A low-fat diet and/or strenuous exercise alters the IGF axis in vivo and reduces prostate tumor cell growth in vitro. *Prostate, 56*(3), 201–206.

Barqawi, A., Thompson, I.M., & Crawford, E.D. (2003). Prostate cancer chemoprevention: An overview of United States trials. *Journal of Urology, 171*(2 Pt. 2), S5–S9.

Bartsch, H., Nair, J., & Owen, R.W. (1999). Dietary polyunsaturated fatty acids and cancers of the breast and colorectum: Emerging evidence for their role as risk modifiers. *Carcinogenesis, 20,* 2209–2218.

Basaria, S., Lieb, J., II, Tang, A.M., DeWeese, T., Carducci, M., Eisenberger, M., et al. (2002). Long-term effects of androgen deprivation therapy in prostate cancer patients. *Clinical Endocrinology, 56,* 779–786.

Basler, J.W., & Piazza, G.A. (2004). Nonsteroidal anti-inflammatory drugs and cyclooxygenase-2 selective inhibitors for prostate cancer chemoprevention. *Journal of Urology, 171*(2 Pt. 2), S59–S62.

Bauer, J.A., Thompson, T.A., Church, D.R., Ariazi, E.A., & Wilding, G. (2003). Growth inhibition and differentiation in human prostate carcinoma cells induced by the vitamin D analog 1alpha, 24-dihydroxyvitamin D2. *Prostate, 55*(3), 159–167.

Beer, T.M. (2003). Development of weekly high-dose calcitriol based therapy for prostate cancer. *Urologic Oncology, 21,* 399–405.

Berruti, A., Dogliotti, L., Terrone, C., Cerutti, S., Isaia, G., Tarabuzzi, R., et al. (2002). Changes in bone mineral density, lean body mass and fat content as measured by dual energy x-ray absorptiometry in patients with prostate cancer without apparent bone metastases given androgen deprivation therapy. *Journal of Urology, 167,* 2361–2367.

Blutt, S.E., Polek, T.C., Stewart, L.V., Kattan, M.W., & Weigel, N.L. (2000). A calcitriol analogue, EB1089, inhibits the growth of LNCaP tumors in nude mice. *Cancer Research, 60,* 779–782.

Body, J.J. (2003). Rationale for the use of bisphosphonates in osteoblastic and osteolytic bone lesions. *Breast, 12*(Suppl. 2), S37–S44.

Boileau, T.W., Liao, Z., Kim, S., Lemeshow, S., Erdman, J.W., Jr., Clinton, S.K., et al. (2003). Prostate carcinogenesis in N-methyl-N-nitrosourea (NMU) testosterone treated rats fed tomato powder, lycopene, or energy-restricted diets. *Journal of the National Cancer Institute, 95,* 1578–1586.

Borrelli, F., & Ernst, E. (2002). Cimicifuga racemosa: A systematic review of its clinical efficacy. *European Journal of Clinical Pharmacology, 58,* 235–241.

Bosetti, C., Tzonou, A., Lagiou, P., Negri, E., Trichopoulos, D., Hsieh, C.C., et al. (2000). Fraction of prostate cancer incidence attributed to diet in Athens, Greece. *European Journal of Cancer Prevention, 9*(2), 119–123.

Bowen, P., Chen, L., Stacewicz-Sapuntzakis, M., Duncan, C., Sharifi, R., Ghosh, L., et al. (2002). Tomato sauce supplementation and prostate cancer: Lycopene accumulation and modulation of biomarkers of carcinogenesis. *Experimental Biology and Medicine, 227,* 886–893.

Brooks, J.D., Metter, E.J., Chan, D.W., Sokoll, L.J., Landis, P., Nelson, W.G., et al. (2001). Plasma selenium level before diagnosis and the risk of prostate cancer development. *Journal of Urology, 166,* 2034–2038.

Brooks, J.D., Paton, V.G., & Vidanes, G. (2001). Potent induction of phase 2 enzymes in human prostate cells by sulforaphane. *Cancer Epidemiology, Biomarkers and Prevention, 10,* 949–954.

Brusselmans, K., De Schrijver, E., Heyns, W., Verhoeven, G., & Swinnen, J.V. (2003). Epigallocatechin-3-gallate is a potent natural inhibitor of fatty acid synthase in intact cells and selectively induces apoptosis in prostate cancer cells. *International Journal of Cancer, 106,* 856–862.

Byers, T., Nestle, M., McTiernan, A., Doyle, C., Currie-Williams, A., Gansler, T., et al. (2002). American Cancer Society guidelines on nutrition and physical activity for cancer prevention: Reducing the risk of cancer with healthy food choices and physical activity. *CA: A Cancer Journal for Clinicians, 52,* 92–119.

Calle, E., Rodriguez, C., Walker-Thurmond, K., & Thun, M.J. (2003). Overweight, obesity, and mortality from cancer in a prospectively studied cohort of U.S. adults. *New England Journal of Medicine, 348,* 1625–1638.

Campbell, S.E., Stone, W.L., Whaley, S.G., Qui, M., & Krishnan, K. (2003). Gamma (γ) tocopherol upregulates peroxisome proliferator activated receptor (PPAR) gamma (γ) expression in SW 480 human colon cancer cell lines. *BioMed Central Cancer, 3*(1), 25.

Cardillo, M.R., Monti, S., Di Silverio, F., Gentile, V., Sciarra, F., Toscano, V., et al. (2003). Insulin-like growth factor (IGF)-I, IGF-II and IGF type I receptor (IGFR-I) expression in prostatic cancer. *Anticancer Research, 23*(5A), 3825–3835.

Chan, J.M., Giovannucci, E., Andersson, S.O., Yuen, J., Adami, H.O., Wolk, A., et al. (1998). Dairy products, calcium, phosphorous, vitamin D, and risk of prostate cancer (Sweden). *Cancer Causes and Control, 9,* 559–566.

Chang, S.S. (2003). Exploring the effects of luteinizing hormone-releasing hormone agonist therapy on bone health: Implications in the management of prostate cancer. *Urology, 62*(6 Suppl. 1), 29–35.

Chatenoud, L., La Vecchia, C., Franceschi, S., Tavani, A., Jacobs, D.R.J., Parpinel, M.T., et al. (1999). Refined-cereal intake and risk of selected cancers in Italy. *American Journal of Clinical Nutrition, 70,* 1107–1110.

Chen, L., Stacewicz-Sapuntzakis, M., Duncan, C., Sharifi, R., Ghosh, L., van Breemen, R., et al. (2001). Oxidative DNA damage in prostate cancer patients consuming tomato sauce-based entrees as a whole-food intervention. *Journal of the National Cancer Institute, 93,* 1872–1879.

Chen, T.C., Wang, L., Whitlatch, L.W., Flanagan, J.N., & Holick, M.F. (2003). Prostatic 25-hydroxyvitamin D-1alpha-hydroxylase and its implication in prostate cancer. *Journal of Cell Biochemistry, 88,* 315–322.

Chiao, J.W., Chung, F.L., Kancherla, R., Ahmed, T., Mittelman, A., Conaway, C.C., et al. (2002). Sulforaphane and its metabolite mediate growth arrest and apoptosis in human prostate cancer cells. *International Journal of Oncology, 20,* 631–636.

Chinni, S.R., Li, Y., Upadhyay, S., Koppolu, P.K., & Sarkar, F.H. (2001). Indole-3-carbinol (I3C) induced cell growth inhibition, G1 cell cycle arrest and apoptosis in prostate cancer cells. *Oncogene, 20,* 2927–2936.

Chopra, R.K., & Bhagavan, H.N. (1999). Relative bioavailabilities of natural and synthetic vitamin E formulations containing mixed tocopherols in human subjects. *International Journal of Vitamin Nutrition Research, 69*(2), 92–95.

Chung, B.H., Mitchell, S.H., Zhang, J.S., & Young, C.Y. (2001). Effects of docosahexaenoic acid and eicosapentaenoic acid on androgen-mediated cell growth and gene expression in LNCaP prostate cancer cells. *Carcinogenesis, 22,* 1201–1206.

Chung, L.Y., Cheung, T.C., Kong, S.K., Fung, K.P., Choy, Y.M., Chan, Z.Y., et al. (2001). Induction of apoptosis by green tea catechins in human prostate cancer DU145 cells. *Life Sciences, 68,* 1207–1214.

Cimicifuga racemosa [Monograph]. (2003). *Alternative Medicine Review, 8*(2), 186–189.

Clark, L.C., Dalkin, B., Krongrad, A., Combs, G.F., Jr., Turnbull, B.W., Slate, E.H., et al. (1998). Decreased incidence of prostate cancer with selenium supplementation: Results of a double-blind cancer prevention trial. *British Journal of Urology, 81,* 730–734.

Cohen, J.H., Kristal, A.R., & Stanford, J.L. (2000). Fruit and vegetable intakes and prostate cancer risk. *Journal of the National Cancer Institute, 92*, 61–68.

Combs, G.F., Jr., Clark, L.C., & Turnbull, B.W. (1997). Reduction of cancer risk with an oral supplement of selenium. *Biomedical Environmental Sciences, 10*(2–3), 227–234.

Conklin, K.A. (2000). Dietary antioxidants during cancer chemotherapy: Impact on chemotherapeutic effectiveness and development of side effects. *Nutrition and Cancer, 37*(1), 1–18.

Corcoran, N.M., Najdovska, M., & Costello, A.J. (2004). Inorganic selenium retards progression of experimental hormone refractory prostate cancer. *Journal of Urology, 171*(2 Pt. 1), 907–910.

Corder, E.H., Guess, H.A., Hulka, B.S., Friedman, G.D., Sadler, M., Vollmer, R.T., et al. (1993). Vitamin D and prostate cancer: A prediagnostic study with stored sera. *Cancer Epidemiology, Biomarkers and Prevention, 2*, 467–472.

Dabrosin, C., Chen, J., Wang, L., & Thompson, L.U. (2002). Flaxseed inhibits metastasis and decreases extracellular vascular endothelial growth factor in human breast cancer xenografts. *Cancer Letters, 185*(1), 31–37.

Daniell, H.W., Dunn, S.R., Ferguson, D.W., Lomas, G., Niazi, Z., Stratte, P.T., et al. (2000). Progressive osteoporosis during androgen deprivation therapy for prostate cancer. *Journal of Urology, 163*, 181–186.

Daviglus, M.L., Dyer, A.R., Persky, V., Chavez, N., Drum, M., Goldberg, J., et al. (1996). Dietary beta-carotene, vitamin C, and risk of prostate cancer: Results from the Western Electric Study. *Epidemiology, 7*, 472–477.

Demark-Wahnefried, W., Price, D.T., Polascik, T.J., Robertson, C.N., Anderson, E.E., Paulson, D.F., et al. (2001). Pilot study of dietary fat restriction and flaxseed supplementation in men with prostate cancer before surgery: Exploring the effects on hormonal levels, prostate-specific antigen, and histopathologic features. *Urology, 58*(1), 47–52.

Deneo-Pellegrini, H., De Stefani, E., Ronco, A., & Mendilaharsu, M. (1999). Foods, nutrients and prostate cancer: A case-control study in Uruguay. *British Journal of Cancer, 80*, 591–597.

Denis, L., Morton, M.S., & Griffiths, K. (1999). Diet and its preventive role in prostatic disease. *European Urology, 35*, 377–387.

De Stefani, E., Deneo-Pellegrini, H., Boffetta, P., Ronco, A., & Mendilaharsu, M. (2000). Alpha-linolenic acid and risk of prostate cancer: A case-control study in Uruguay. *Cancer Epidemiology, Biomarkers and Prevention, 9*, 335–338.

Djavan, B., Zlotta, A., Schulman, C., Teillac, P., Iversen, P., Boccon, B.L., et al. (2004). Chemotherapeutic prevention studies of prostate cancer. *Journal of Urology, 171*(2 Pt. 2), S10–S13.

Donnelly, B.J., Saliken, J.C., Ernst, D.S., Ali-Ridha, N., Brasher, P.M., Robinson, J.W., et al. (2002). Prospective trial of cryosurgical ablation of the prostate: Five-year results. *Urology, 60*, 645–649.

Eastwood, M.A. (1999). Interaction of dietary antioxidants in vivo: How fruits and vegetables prevent disease? *Quarterly Journal of Medicine, 92*, 527–530.

Ebeling, P.R., Sandgren, M.E., DiMagno, E.P., Lane, A.W., DeLuca, H.F., Riggs, B.L., et al. (1992). Evidence of an age-related decrease in intestinal responsiveness to vitamin D: Relationship between serum 1,25-dihydroxyvitamin D-3 and intestinal vitamin D receptor concentrations in normal women. *Journal of Clinical Endocrinology Metabolism, 75*, 176–182.

Fahmy, W.E., & Bissada, N.K. (2003). Cryosurgery for prostate cancer. *Archives of Andrology, 49*, 397–407.

Fleischauer, A.T., & Arab, L. (2001). Garlic and cancer: A critical review of the epidemiologic literature. *Journal of Nutrition, 131*(Suppl. 3), 1032S–1040S.

Fleshner, N., Bagnell, P.S., Klotz, L., & Venkateswaran, V. (2004). Dietary fat and prostate cancer. *Journal of Urology, 171*(2 Pt. 2), S19–S24.

Fleshner, N., Fair, W.R., Huryk, R., & Heston, W.D. (1999). Vitamin E inhibits the high-fat diet promoted growth of established human prostate LNCaP tumors in nude mice. *Journal of Urology, 161,* 1651–1654.

Fradet, Y., Meyer, F., Bairati, I., Shadmani, R., & Moore, L. (1999). Dietary fat and prostate cancer progression and survival. *European Urology, 35,* 388–391.

Freedland, S.J., Aronson, W.J., Kane, C.J., Presti, J.C., Jr., Amling, C.L., Elashoff, D., et al. (2004). Impact of obesity on biochemical control after radical prostatectomy for clinically localized prostate cancer: A report by the Shared Equal Access Regional Cancer Hospital database study group. *Journal of Clinical Oncology, 22,* 446–453.

Freudenheim, J.L., Marshall, J.R., Vena, J.E., Laughlin, R., Brasure, J.R., Swanson, M.K., et al. (1996). Premenopausal breast cancer risk and intake of vegetables, fruits, and related nutrients. *Journal of the National Cancer Institute, 88,* 340–348.

Frydoonfar, H.R., McGrath, D.R., & Spigelman, A.D. (2003). The effect of indole-3-carbinol and sulforaphane on a prostate cancer cell line. *ANZ Journal of Surgery, 73*(3), 154–156.

Galli, F., Stabile, A.M., Betti, M., Conte, C., Pistilli, A., Rende, M., et al. (2004). The effect of alpha- and gamma-tocopherol and their carboxyethyl hydroxychroman metabolites on prostate cancer cell proliferation. *Archives of Biochemistry and Biophysics, 423*(1), 97–102.

Gann, P.H., Hennekens, C.H., Sacks, F.M., Grodstein, F., Giovannucci, E.L., Stampfer, M.J., et al. (1994). Prospective study of plasma fatty acids and risk of prostate cancer. *Journal of the National Cancer Institute, 86,* 281–286.

Gann, P.H., Ma, J., Giovannucci, E., Willett, W., Sacks, F.M., Hennekens, C.H., et al. (1999). Lower prostate cancer risk in men with elevated plasma lycopene levels: Results of a prospective analysis. *Cancer Research, 59,* 1225–1230.

Gardner-Thorpe, D., O'Hagen, C., Young, I., & Lewis, S.J. (2003). Dietary supplements of soya flour lower serum testosterone concentrations and improve markers of oxidative stress in men. *European Journal of Clinical Nutrition, 57*(1), 100–106.

Gayther, S.A., de Foy, K.A., Harrington, P., Pharoah, P., Dunsmuir, W.D., Edwards, S.M., et al. (2000). The frequency of germ-line mutations in the breast cancer predisposition genes BRCA1 and BRCA2 in familial prostate cancer. *Cancer Research, 60,* 4513–4518.

Getzenberg, R.H., Light, B.W., Lapco, B.W., Konety, B.R., Nangia, A.K., Acierno, J.S., et al. (1997). Vitamin D inhibition of prostate adenocarcinoma growth and metastasis in the Dunning rat prostate model system. *Urology, 50,* 999–1006.

Ghosh, J., & Myers, C.E. (1997). Arachidonic acid stimulates prostate cancer cell growth: Critical role of 5-lipoxygenase. *Biochemical and Biophysical Research Communications, 235,* 418–423.

Giovannucci, E. (2003). Nutrition, insulin, insulin-like growth factors and cancer. *Hormone and Metabolic Research, 35,* 694–704.

Giovannucci, E., Ascherio, A., Rimm, E.B., Stampfer, M.J., Colditz, G.A., Willett, W.C., et al. (1995). Intake of carotenoids and retinol in relation to risk of prostate cancer. *Journal of the National Cancer Institute, 87,* 1767–1776.

Giovannucci, E., Rimm, E.B., Colditz, G.A., Stampfer, M.J., Ascherio, A., Chute, C.C., et al. (1993). A prospective study of dietary fat and risk of prostate cancer. *Journal of the National Cancer Institute, 85,* 1571–1579.

Giovannucci, E., Rimm, E.B., Wolk, A., Ascherio, A., Stampfer, M.J., Colditz, G.A., et al. (1998). Calcium and fructose intake in relation to risk of prostate cancer. *Cancer Research, 58,* 442–447.

Godley, P.A., Campbell, M.K., Gallagher, P., Martinson, F.E., Mohler, J.L., Sandler, R.S., et al. (1996). Biomarkers of essential fatty acid consumption and risk of prostatic carcinoma. *Cancer Epidemiology, Biomarkers and Prevention, 5,* 889–895.

Grant, W.B. (1999). An ecologic study of dietary links to prostate cancer. *Alternative Medicine Reviews, 4*(3), 162–169.

Grimberg, A. (2003). Mechanisms by which IGF-I may promote cancer. *Cancer Biology and Therapy, 2,* 630–635.

Gross, C., Stamey, T., Hancock, S., & Feldman, D. (1998). Treatment of early recurrent prostate cancer with 1,25-dihydroxyvitamin D3 (calcitriol). *Journal of Urology, 159,* 2035–2039.

Gunnell, D., Oliver, S.E., Peters, T.J., Donovan, J.L., Persad, R., Maynard, M., et al. (2003). Are diet-prostate cancer associations mediated by the IGF axis? A cross-sectional analysis of diet, IGF-I and IGFBP-3 in healthy middle-aged men. *British Journal of Cancer, 88,* 1682–1686.

Gupta, S., Hastak, K., Ahmad, N., Lewin, J.S., & Mukhtar, H. (2001). Inhibition of prostate carcinogenesis in TRAMP mice by oral infusion of green tea polyphenols. *Proceedings of the National Academy of Sciences of the United States of America, 98,* 10350–10355.

Gupta, S., Hussain, T., & Mukhtar, H. (2003). Molecular pathway for (-)-epigallocatechin-3-gallate-induced cell cycle arrest and apoptosis of human prostate carcinoma cells. *Archives of Biochemistry and Biophysics, 410*(1), 177–185.

Habito, R.C., & Ball, M.J. (2001). Postprandial changes in sex hormones after meals of different composition. *Metabolism, 50,* 505–511.

Han, K.R., Cohen, J.K., Miller, R.J., Pantuck, A.J., Feitas, D.G., Cuevas, C.A., et al. (2003). Treatment of organ confined prostate cancer with third generation cryosurgery: Preliminary multicenter experience. *Journal of Urology, 170*(4 Pt. 1), 1126–1131.

Hanchette, C.L., & Schwartz, G.G. (1992). Geographic patterns of prostate cancer mortality. Evidence for a protective effect of ultraviolet radiation. *Cancer, 70,* 2861–2869.

Handelman, G.J., Epstein, W.L., Peerson, J., Spiegelman, D., Machlin, L.J., & Dratz, E.A. (1994). Human adipose alpha-tocopherol and gamma-tocopherol kinetics during and after 1 y of alpha-tocopherol supplementation. *American Journal of Clinical Nutrition, 59,* 1025–1032.

Handelman, G.J., Machlin, L.J., Fitch, K., Weiter, J.J., & Dratz, E.A. (1985). Oral alpha-tocopherol supplements decrease plasma gamma-tocopherol levels in humans. *Journal of Nutrition, 115,* 807–813.

Harris, P.J., Roberton, A.M., Watson, M.E., Triggs, C.M., & Ferguson, L.R. (1993). The effects of soluble-fiber polysaccharides on the adsorption of a hydrophobic carcinogen to an insoluble dietary fiber. *Nutrition and Cancer, 19*(1), 43–54.

Hartman, T.J., Dorgan, J.F., Woodson, K., Virtamo, J., Tangrea, J.A., Heinonen, O.P., et al. (2001). Effects of long-term alpha-tocopherol supplementation on serum hormones in older men. *Prostate, 46*(1), 33–38.

Harvei, S., Bjerve, K.S., Tretli, S., Jellum, E., Robsahm, T.E., Vatten, L., et al. (1997). Prediagnostic level of fatty acids in serum phospholipids: Omega-3 and omega-6 fatty acids and the risk of prostate cancer. *International Journal of Cancer, 71,* 545–551.

Hastak, K., Gupta, S., Ahmad, N., Agarwal, M.K., Agarwal, M.L., Mukhtar, H., et al. (2003). Role of p53 and NF-kappaB in epigallocatechin-3-gallate-induced apoptosis of LNCaP cells. *Oncogene, 22,* 4851–4859.

Heber, D., Fair, W., & Ornish, D. (1999). *Nutrition and prostate cancer: A monograph from the CaP CURE Nutrition Project* (2nd ed.). Retrieved January 18, 2004, from http://www.capcure.org.il/abstracts/pub-pdf/nutrition.pdf

Hebert, J.R., Hurley, T.G., Olendzki, B.C., Teas, J., Ma, Y., Hampl, J.S., et al. (1998). Nutritional and socioeconomic factors in relation to prostate cancer mortality: A cross-national study. *Journal of the National Cancer Institute, 90,* 1637–1647.

Heinonen, O.P., Albanes, D., Virtamo, J., Taylor, P.R., Huttunen, J.K., Hartman, A.M., et al. (1998). Prostate cancer and supplementation with alpha-tocopherol and beta-carotene: Incidence and mortality in a controlled trial. *Journal of the National Cancer Institute, 90,* 440–446.

Helzlsouer, K.J., Huang, H.Y., Alberg, A.J., Hoffman, S., Burke, A., Norkus, E.P., et al. (2000). Association between alpha-tocopherol, gamma-tocopherol, selenium, and subsequent prostate cancer. *Journal of the National Cancer Institute, 92,* 2018–2023.

Hennekens, C.H., Buring, J.E., Manson, J.E., Stampfer, M., Rosner, B., Cook, N.R., et al. (1996). Lack of effect of long-term supplementation with beta-carotene on the incidence of malignant neoplasms and cardiovascular disease. *New England Journal of Medicine, 334*, 1145–1149.

Hernandez, M.G., & Pluchino, S. (2003). Cimicifuga racemosa for the treatment of hot flushes in women surviving breast cancer. *Maturitas, 44*(Suppl. 1), S59–S65.

Hodge, A.M., English, D.R., McCredie, M.R., Severi, G., Boyle, P., Hopper, J.L., et al. (2004). Foods, nutrients and prostate cancer. *Cancer Causes and Control, 15*, 11–20.

Holick, M.F. (1995). Defects in the synthesis and metabolism of vitamin D. *Experimental and Clinical Endocrinology and Diabetes, 103*(4), 219–227.

Holmberg, L., Bill-Axelson, A., Helgesen, G., Salo, J.O., Folmerz, P., Haggman, M., et al. (2002). A randomized trial comparing radical prostatectomy with watchful waiting in early prostate cancer. *New England Journal of Medicine, 347*, 781–789.

Hsieh, L.J., Carter, H.B., Landis, P.K., Tucker, K.L., Metter, E.J., Newschaffer, C.J., et al. (2003). Association of energy intake with prostate cancer in a long-term aging study: Baltimore Longitudinal Study of Aging (United States). *Urology, 61*, 297–301.

Hsing, A.W., Chokkalingam, A.P., Gao, Y.T., Madigan, M.P., Deng, J., Gridley, G., et al. (2002). Allium vegetables and risk of prostate cancer: A population-based study. *Journal of the National Cancer Institute, 94*, 1648–1651.

Hsing, A.W., Chua, S., Jr., Gao, Y.T., Gentzschein, E., Chang, L., Deng, J., et al. (2001). Prostate cancer risk and serum levels of insulin and leptin: A population-based study. *Journal of the National Cancer Institute, 93*, 783–789.

Hsing, A.W., Gao, Y.T., Chua, S., Jr., Deng, J., & Stanczyk, F.Z. (2003). Insulin resistance and prostate cancer risk. *Journal of the National Cancer Institute, 95*(1), 67–71.

Huang, H.Y., Alberg, A.J., Norkus, E.P., Hoffman, S.C., Comstock, G.W., Helzlsouer, K.J., et al. (2003). Prospective study of antioxidant micronutrients in the blood and the risk of developing prostate cancer. *American Journal of Epidemiology, 157*, 335–344.

Hughes-Fulford, M., Chen, Y., & Tjandrawinata, R.R. (2001). Fatty acid regulates gene expression and growth of human prostate cancer PC-3 cells. *Carcinogenesis, 22*, 701–707.

Hwang, E.S., & Bowen, P.E. (2002). Can the consumption of tomatoes or lycopene reduce cancer risk? *Integrative Cancer Therapies, 1*(2), 121–132.

Jacobsen, B.K., Knutsen, S.F., & Fraser, G.E. (1998). Does high soymilk intake reduce prostate cancer incidence? The Adventist Health Study (United States). *Cancer Causes and Control, 9*, 553–557.

Jacobson, J.S., Troxel, A.B., Evans, J., Klaus, L., Vahdat, L., Kinne, D., et al. (2001). Randomized trial of black cohosh for the treatment of hot flashes among women with a history of breast cancer. *Journal of Clinical Oncology, 19*, 2739–2745.

Jain, M.G., Hislop, G.T., Howe, G.R., & Ghadirian, P. (1999). Plant foods, antioxidants, and prostate cancer risk: Findings from case-control studies in Canada. *Nutrition and Cancer, 34*(2), 173–184.

Jenkins, D.J., Kendall, C.W., D'Costa, M.A., Jackson, C.J., Vidgen, E., Singer, W., et al. (2003). Soy consumption and phytoestrogens: Effect on serum prostate specific antigen when blood lipids and oxidized low-density lipoprotein are reduced in hyperlipidemic men. *Journal of Urology, 169*, 507–511.

Jeon, K.I., Rih, J.K., Kim, H.J., Lee, Y.J., Cho, C.H., Goldberg, I.D., et al. (2003). Pretreatment of indole-3-carbinol augments TRAIL-induced apoptosis in a prostate cancer cell line. *FEBS Letters, 544*, 246–251.

Jian, L., Xie, L.P., Lee, A.H., & Binns, C.W. (2004). Protective effect of green tea against prostate cancer: A case-control study in southeast China. *International Journal of Cancer, 108*(1), 130–135.

Jiang, Q., Christen, S., Shigenaga, M.K., & Ames, B.N. (2001). Gamma-tocopherol, the major form of vitamin E in the U.S. diet, deserves more attention. *American Journal of Clinical Nutrition, 74*, 714–722.

Johnson, C.S., Hershberger, P.A., & Trump, D.L. (2002). Vitamin D-related therapies in prostate cancer. *Cancer Metastasis Reviews, 21*(2), 147–158.

Kaaks, R., & Lukanova, A. (2001). Energy balance and cancer: The role of insulin and insulin-like growth factor-I. *Proceedings of the Nutrition Society, 60*(1), 91–106.

Key, T.J., Allen, N., Appleby, P., Overvad, K., Tjonneland, A., Miller, A., et al. (2004). Fruits and vegetables and prostate cancer: No association among 1,104 cases in a prospective study of 130,544 men in the European Prospective Investigation into Cancer and Nutrition (EPIC). *International Journal of Cancer, 109*(1), 119–124.

Key, T.J., Silcocks, P.B., Davey, G.K., Appleby, P.N., & Bishop, D.T. (1997). A case-control study of diet and prostate cancer. *British Journal of Cancer, 76,* 678–687.

Khaw, K.T., Bingham, S., Welch, R.L.A., Wareham, N., Oakes, S., Day, N., et al. (2001). The European Prospective Investigation into Cancer and Nutrition. Relation between plasma ascorbic acid and mortality in men and women in EPIC—Norfolk prospective study: A prospective population study. *Lancet, 357,* 657–663.

Kim, H.S., Bowen, P., Chen, L., Duncan, C., Ghosh, L., Sharifi, R., et al. (2003). Effects of tomato sauce consumption on apoptotic cell death in prostate benign hyperplasia and carcinoma. *Nutrition and Cancer, 47*(1), 40–47.

Kiratli, B.J., Srinivas, S., Perkash, I., & Terris, M.K. (2001). Progressive decrease in bone density over 10 years of androgen deprivation therapy in patients with prostate cancer. *Urology, 57,* 127–132.

Knight, D.C., Howes, J.B., & Eden, J.A. (1999). The effect of Promensil, an isoflavone extract, on menopausal symptoms. *Climacteric, 2,* 79–84.

Kolonel, L.N., Hankin, J.H., Whittemore, A.S., Wu, A.H., Gallagher, R.P., Wilkens, L.R., et al. (2000). Vegetables, fruits, legumes and prostate cancer: A multiethnic case-control study. *Cancer Epidemiology, Biomarkers and Prevention, 9,* 795–804.

Krishnan, A.V., Peehl, D.M., & Feldman, D. (2003). The role of vitamin D in prostate cancer. *Recent Results in Cancer Research, 164,* 205–221.

Kristal, A.R., Cohen, J.H., Qu, P., & Stanford, J.L. (2002). Associations of energy, fat, calcium, and vitamin D with prostate cancer risk. *Cancer Epidemiology, Biomarkers and Prevention, 11,* 719–725.

Kristal, A.R., Stanford, J.L., Cohen, J.H., Wicklund, K., & Patterson, R.E. (1999). Vitamin and mineral supplement use is associated with reduced risk of prostate cancer. *Cancer Epidemiology, Biomarkers and Prevention, 8,* 887–892.

Kronenberg, F., & Fugh-Berman, A. (2002). Complementary and alternative medicine for menopausal symptoms: A review of randomized, controlled trials. *Annals of Internal Medicine, 137,* 805–813.

Kucuk, O., Sarkar, F.H., Djuric, Z., Sakr, W., Pollak, M.N., Khachik, F., et al. (2002). Effects of lycopene supplementation in patients with localized prostate cancer. *Experimental Biology and Medicine, 227,* 881–885.

Kupelian, P.A., Potters, L., Khuntia, D., Ciezki, J.P., & Reddy, C.A. (2004). Radical prostatectomy, external beam radiotherapy < 72 Gy, external beam radiotherapy > or +72 Gy, permanent seed implantation, or combined seeds/external beam radiotherapy for sage T1-T2 prostate cancer. *International Journal of Radiation Oncology, Biology, Physics, 58*(1), 25–33.

Kushi, L., & Giovannucci, E. (2002). Dietary fat and cancer. *American Journal of Medicine, 113*(Suppl. 9B), 63S–70S.

Labriola, D., & Livingston, R. (1999). Possible interactions between dietary antioxidants and chemotherapy. *Oncology, 13,* 1003–1012.

Lamm, D.L., & Riggs, D.R. (2001). Enhanced immunocompetence by garlic: Role in bladder cancer and other malignancies. *Journal of Nutrition, 131*(Suppl. 3), 1067S–1070S.

Lamson, D., & Brignall, M. (1999). Antioxidants in cancer therapy; their actions and interactions with oncologic therapies. *Alternative Medicine Review, 4,* 304–329.

La Vecchia, C., Chatenoud, L., Negri, E., & Franceschi, S. (2003). Session: Whole cereal grains, fibre and human cancer wholegrain cereals and cancer in Italy. *Proceedings of the Nutrition Society, 62*(1), 45–49.

Le, H.T., Schaldach, C.M., Firestone, G.L., & Bjeldanes, L.F. (2003). Plant-derived 3,3'-diindolylmethane is a strong androgen antagonist in human prostate cancer cells. *Journal of Biological Chemistry, 278,* 21136–21145.

Le Marchand, L., Kolonel, L.N., Wilkens, L.R., Myers, B.C., & Hirohata, T. (1994). Animal fat consumption and prostate cancer: A prospective study in Hawaii. *Epidemiology, 5,* 276–282.

Lee, M.M., Wang, R.T., Hsing, A.W., Gu, F.L., Wang, T., Spitz, M., et al. (1998). Case-control study of diet and prostate cancer in China. *Cancer Causes and Control, 9,* 545–552.

Leone, M., Zhai, D., Sareth, S., Kitada, S., Reed, J.C., & Pellecchia, M. (2003). Cancer prevention by tea polyphenols is linked to their direct inhibition of antiapoptotic Bcl-2-family proteins. *Cancer Research, 63,* 8118–8121.

Li, L., Yu, H., Schumacher, F., Casey, G., & Witte, J.S. (2003). Relation of serum insulin-like growth factor-I (IGF-I) and IGF binding protein-3 to risk of prostate cancer (United States). *Cancer Causes and Control, 14,* 721–726.

Li, Y., Li, X., & Sarkar, F.H. (2003). Gene expression profiles of I3C- and DIM-treated PC3 human prostate cancer cells determined by cDNA microarray analysis. *Journal of Nutrition, 133,* 1011–1019.

Lieberman, S. (1998). A review of the effectiveness of Cimicifuga racemosa (black cohosh) for the symptoms of menopause. *Journal of Women's Health, 7,* 525–529.

Lin, X., Gingrich, J.R., Bao, W., Li, J., Haroon, Z.A., Demark-Wahnefried, W., et al. (2002). Effect of flaxseed supplementation on prostatic carcinoma in transgenic mice. *Urology, 60,* 919–924.

Lokeshwar, B.L., Schwartz, G.G., Selzer, M.G., Burnstein, K.L., Zhuang, S.H., Block, N.L., et al. (1999). Inhibition of prostate cancer metastasis in vivo: A comparison of 1,23-dihydroxyvitamin D (calcitriol) and EB1089. *Cancer Epidemiology, Biomarkers and Prevention, 8,* 241–248.

Lu, Q.Y., Hung, J.C., Heber, D., Go, V.L., Reuter, V.E., Cordon-Cardo, C., et al. (2001). Inverse associations between plasma lycopene and other carotenoids and prostate cancer. *Cancer Epidemiology, Biomarkers and Prevention, 10,* 749–756.

Lucia, M.S., & Torkko, K.C. (2004). Inflammation as a target for prostate cancer chemoprevention: Pathological and laboratory rationale. *Journal of Urology, 171*(2 Pt. 2), S30–S34.

Mahmud, S., Franco, E., & Aprikian, A. (2004). Prostate cancer and use of nonsteroidal anti-inflammatory drugs: Systematic review and meta-analysis. *British Journal of Cancer, 90,* 93–99.

Maillefert, J.F., Sibilia, J., Michel, F., Saussine, C., Javier, R.M., Tavernier, C., et al. (1999). Bone mineral density in men treated with synthetic gonadotropin-releasing hormone agonists for prostatic carcinoma. *Journal of Urology, 161,* 1219–1222.

Mannisto, S., Pietinen, P., Virtanen, M.J., Salminen, I., Albanes, D., Giovannucci, E., et al. (2003). Fatty acids and risk of prostate cancer in a nested case-control study in male smokers. *Cancer Epidemiology, Biomarkers and Prevention, 12,* 1422–1428.

Manolio, T.A., Savage, P.J., Burke, G.L., Hilner, J.E., Liu, K., Orchard, T.J., et al. (1991). Correlates of fasting insulin levels in young adults: The CARDIA study. *Journal of Clinical Epidemiology, 44,* 571–578.

McCarty, M.F. (1999). Vegan proteins may reduce risk of cancer, obesity, and cardiovascular disease by promoting increased glucagon activity. *Medical Hypotheses, 53,* 459–485.

Messina, M.J. (2003). Emerging evidence on the role of soy in reducing prostate cancer risk. *Nutrition Reviews, 61,* 117–131.

Messina, M.J., & Hughes, C. (2003). Efficacy of soyfoods and soybean isoflavone supplements for alleviating menopausal symptoms is positively related to initial hot flush frequency. *Journal of Medicinal Food, 6*(1), 1–11.

Messina, M.J., Persky, V., Setchell, K.D., & Barnes, S. (1994). Soy intake and cancer risk: A review of the in vitro and in vivo data. *Nutrition and Cancer, 21,* 113–131.

Meyer, F., Bairati, I., Fradet, Y., & Moore, L. (1997). Dietary energy and nutrients in relation to preclinical prostate cancer. *Nutrition and Cancer, 29*(2), 120–126.

Meyer, F., Bairati, I., Shadmani, R., Fradet, Y., & Moore, L. (1999). Dietary fat and prostate cancer survival. *Cancer Causes and Control, 10,* 245–251.

Miaskowski, C. (1999). Prostate cancer. In C. Miaskowski & P. Buchsel (Eds.), *Oncology nursing: Assessment and clinical care* (pp. 1471–1501). St. Louis, MO: Mosby.

Michaud, D.S., Augustsson, K., Rimm, E.B., Stampfer, M.J., Willett, W.C., Giovannucci, E., et al. (2001). A prospective study on intake of animal products and risk of prostate cancer. *Cancer Causes and Control, 12,* 557–567.

Mills, P.K., Beeson, W.L., Phillips, R.L., & Fraser, G.E. (1989). Cohort study of diet, lifestyle, and prostate cancer in Adventist men. *Cancer, 64,* 598–604.

Mittan, D., Lee, S., Miller, E., Perez, R.C., Basler, J.W., Bruder, J.M., et al. (2002). Bone loss following hypogonadism in men with prostate cancer treated with GnRH analogs. *Journal of Clinical Endocrinology and Metabolism, 87,* 3656–3661.

Moyad, M.A. (2000). *The ABCs of nutrition and supplements for prostate cancer.* Ann Arbor, MI: J.W. Edwards.

Moyad, M.A. (2003). The use of complementary/preventive medicine to prevent prostate cancer recurrence/progression following definitive therapy: Part I—lifestyle changes. *Current Opinion in Urology, 13*(2), 137–145.

Moyad, M.A., Brumfield, S.K., & Pienta, K.J. (1999). Vitamin E, alpha- and gamma-tocopherol, and prostate cancer. *Seminars in Urologic Oncology, 17*(2), 85–90.

Mucci, L.A., Tamimi, R., Lagiou, P., Trichopoulou, A., Benetou, V., Spanos, E., et al. (2001). Are dietary influences on the risk of prostate cancer mediated through the insulin-like growth factor system? *BJU International, 87,* 814–820.

Nachshon-Kedmi, M., Yannai, S., Haj, A., & Fares, F.A. (2003). Indole-3-carbinol and 3,3'-diindolylmethane induce apoptosis in human prostate cancer cells. *Food and Chemical Toxicology, 41,* 745–752.

Nagata, C., Shimizu, H., Takam, R., Hayashi, M., Takeda, N., Yasuda, K., et al. (2003). Dietary soy and fats in relation to serum insulin-like growth factor-1 and insulin-like growth factor-binding protein-3 levels in premenopausal Japanese women. *Nutrition and Cancer, 45*(2), 185–189.

National Cancer Institute. (2003a). *Alpha-Tocopherol, Beta-Carotene (ATBC) cancer prevention trial.* Retrieved January 19, 2004, from http://cancer.gov/newscenter/pressreleases/ATBCfollowup

National Cancer Institute. (2003b). *Prostate cancer (PDQ): treatment.* Retrieved January 18, 2004, from http://cancer.gov/cancerinfo/pdq/treatment/prostate/healthprofessional/

National Cancer Institute. (2003c). *Prostate Cancer Prevention Trial (PCPT): Questions and answers.* Retrieved January 19, 2004, from http://cancer.gov/templates/content_nav_print.aspx?viewid=5a904165-870e-4ale-ala5-f92

Newcomer, L.M., King, I.B., Wicklund, K.G., & Stanford, J.L. (2001). The association of fatty acids with prostate cancer risk. *Prostate, 47,* 262–268.

Ngo, T.H., Barnard, R.J., Tymchuk, C.N., Cohen, P., & Aronson, W.J. (2002). Effect of diet and exercise on serum insulin, IGF-I, and IGFBP-1 levels and growth of LNCaP cells in vitro (United States). *Cancer Causes and Control, 13,* 929–935.

Nomura, A.M., Stemmermann, G.N., Lee, J., & Craft, N.E. (1997). Serum micronutrients and prostate cancer in Japanese Americans in Hawaii. *Cancer Epidemiology, Biomarkers and Prevention, 6,* 487–491.

Norrish, A.E., Jackson, R.T., Sharpe, S.J., & Skeaff, C.M. (2000a). Men who consume vegetable oils rich in monounsaturated fat: Their dietary patterns and risk of prostate cancer (New Zealand). *Cancer Causes and Control, 11,* 609–615.

Norrish, A.E., Jackson, R.T., Sharpe, S.J., & Skeaff, C.M. (2000b). Prostate cancer and dietary carotenoids. *American Journal of Epidemiology, 151*(2), 119–123.

Norrish, A.E., Skeaff, C.M., Arribas, G.L., Sharpe, S.J., & Jackson, R.T. (1999). Prostate cancer risk and consumption of fish oils: A dietary biomarker-based case-control study. *British Journal of Cancer, 81,* 1238–1242.

North American Menopause Society. (2004). Treatment of menopause-associated vasomotor symptoms: Position statement of the North American Menopause Society. *Menopause, 11*(1), 11–33.

Nowicki, M., Bryc, W., & Kokot, F. (2001). Hormonal regulation of appetite and body mass in patients with advanced prostate cancer treated with combined androgen blockade. *Journal of Endocrinological Investigation, 24*(1), 31–36.

Ohno, Y., Yoshida, O., Oishi, K., Okada, K., Yamabe, H., Schroeder, F.H., et al. (1998). Dietary beta-carotene and cancer of the prostate: A case-control study in Kyoto, Japan. *Cancer Research, 48,* 1331–1336.

Omenn, G.S., Goodman, G.E., Thornquist, M.D., Balmes, J., Cullen, M.R., Glass, A., et al. (1996). Risk factors for lung cancer and for intervention effects in CARET, the Beta-Carotene and Retinol Efficacy Trial. *Journal of the National Cancer Institute, 88,* 1550–1559.

O'Rourke, M.E. (2001). Genitourinary cancers. In S. Otto (Ed.), *Oncology nursing* (4th ed., pp. 213–247). St. Louis, MO: Mosby.

Paul, R., & Breul, J. (2000). Antiandrogen withdrawal syndrome associated with prostate cancer therapies: Incidence and clinical significance. *Drug Safety, 5,* 381–390.

Peehl, D.M., Krishnan, A.V., & Feldman, D. (2003). Pathways mediating the growth-inhibitory actions of vitamin D in prostate cancer. *Journal of Nutrition, 133*(Suppl. 7), 2461S–2469S.

Pelucchi, C., Talamini, R., Galeone, C., Negri, E., Franceschi, S., Dal Maso, L., et al. (2004). Fibre intake and prostate cancer risk. *International Journal of Cancer, 109,* 278–280.

Pierce, J.P., Faerber, S., Wright, F.A., Rock, C.L., Newman, V., Flatt, S.W., et al. (2002). A randomized trial of the effect of a plant-based dietary pattern on additional breast cancer events and survival: The Women's Healthy Eating and Living (WHEL) study. *Controlled Clinical Trials, 23,* 728–756.

Pinto, J.T., & Rivlin, R.S. (2001). Antiproliferative effects of allium derivatives from garlic. *Journal of Nutrition, 131*(Suppl. 3), 1058S–1060S.

Platz, E.A., & De Marzo, A.M. (2004). Epidemiology of inflammation and prostate cancer. *Journal of Urology, 171*(2 Pt. 2), S36–S40.

Platz, E.A., Leitzmann, M.F., Michaud, D.S., Willett, W.C., & Giovannucci, E. (2003). Interrelation of energy intake, body size, and physical activity with prostate cancer in a large prospective cohort study. *Cancer Research, 63,* 8542–8548.

Pollard, M., & Wolter, W. (2000). Prevention of spontaneous prostate-related cancer in Lobund-Wistar rats by a soy protein isolate/isoflavone diet. *Prostate, 45*(2), 101–105.

Potters, L. (2003). Permanent prostate brachytherapy in men with clinically localized prostate cancer. *Clinical Oncology, 6,* 301–315.

Ramon, J.M., Bou, R., Romea, S., Alkiza, M.E., Jacas, M., Ribes, J., et al. (2000). Dietary fat intake and prostate cancer risk: A case-control study in Spain. *Cancer Causes and Control, 11,* 679–685.

Rasmussen, L.B., Hansen, G.L., Hansen, E., Koch, B., Mosekilde, L., Molgaard, C., et al. (2000). Vitamin D: Should the supply in the Danish population be increased? *International Journal of Food Science Nutrition, 51*(3), 209–215.

Reiser, S., Bohn, E., Hallfrisch, J., Michaelis, O.E., Keeney, M., Prather, E.S., et al. (1981). Serum insulin and glucose in hyperinsulinemic subjects fed three different levels of sucrose. *American Journal of Clinical Nutrition, 34,* 2348–2358.

Rock, C.L., Saxe, G.A., Ruffin, M.T., August, D.A., & Schottenfeld, D. (1996). Carotenoids, vitamin A, and estrogen receptor status in breast cancer. *Nutrition and Cancer, 25,* 281–296.

Rohan, T.E., Howe, G.R., Burch, J.D., & Jain, M. (1995). Dietary factors and risk of prostate cancer: A case-control study in Ontario, Canada. *Cancer Causes and Control, 6,* 145–154.

Ruijter, E., van de Kaa, C., Miller, G., Ruiter, D., Debruyne, F., & Schalken, J. (1999). Molecular genetics and epidemiology of prostate carcinoma. *Endocrine Reviews, 20*(1), 22–45.

Saad, F., Gleason, D.M., Murray, R., Tchekmedyian, S., Venner, P., Lacombe, L., et al. (2002). A randomized, placebo-controlled trial of zoledronic acid in patients with hormone-refractory metastatic prostate carcinoma. *Journal of the National Cancer Institute, 94,* 1458–1468.

Saad, F., & Schulman, C.C. (2004). Role of bisphosphonates in prostate cancer. *European Urology, 45*(1), 26–34.

Saleem, M., Adhami, V.M., Siddiqui, I.A., & Mukhtar, H. (2003). Tea beverage in chemoprevention of prostate cancer: A mini-review. *Nutrition and Cancer, 47*(1), 13–23.

Schuurman, A.G., Goldbohm, R.A., Brants, H.A., & van den Brandt, P.A. (2002). A prospective cohort study on intake of retinol, vitamins C and E, and carotenoids and prostate cancer risk (Netherlands). *Cancer Causes and Control, 13,* 573–582.

Schuurman, A.G., van den Brandt, P.A., Dorant, E., Brants, H.A., & Goldbohm, R.A. (1999). Association of energy and fat intake with prostate carcinoma risk: Results from the Netherlands Cohort Study. *Cancer, 86,* 1019–1027.

Schwartz, E.J., Wong, P., & Graydon, R.J. (2004). Sildenafil preserves intracorporeal smooth muscle after radical retropubic prostatectomy. *Journal of Urology, 171*(2 Pt. 1), 771–774.

Schwartz, G.G., Oeler, T.A., Uskokovic, M.R., & Bahnson, R.R. (1994). Human prostate cancer cells: Inhibition of proliferation by vitamin D analogs. *Anticancer Research, 14,* 1077–1081.

Shike, M., Latkany, L., Riedel, E., Fleisher, M., Schatzkin, A., Lanza, E., et al. (2002). Lack of effect of a low-fat, high-fruit, -vegetable, and -fiber diet on serum prostate-specific antigen of men without prostate cancer: Results from a randomized trial. *Journal of Clinical Oncology, 20,* 3592–3598.

Sigounas, G., Anagnostou, A., & Steiner, M. (1997). dl-alpha-tocopherol induces apoptosis in erythroleukemia, prostate, and breast cancer cells. *Nutrition and Cancer, 28*(1), 30–35.

Silverberg, S.J., Shane, E., dela Cruz, L., Segre, C.V., Clemens, T.L., Bilezikian, J.P., et al. (1989). Vitamin D hydroxylation abnormalities in parathyroid hormone secretion and 1,25-dihydroxyvitamin D-3 formation in women with osteoporosis. *New England Journal of Medicine, 320,* 277–281.

Singh, A.V., Xiao, D., Lew, K.L., Dhir, R., & Singh, S.V. (2004). Sulforaphane induces caspase-mediated apoptosis in cultured PC-3 human prostate cancer cells and retards growth of PC-3 xenografts in vivo. *Carcinogenesis, 25*(1), 83–90.

Sinha, R., & El-Bayoumy, K. (2004). Apoptosis is a critical cellular event in cancer chemoprevention and chemotherapy by selenium compounds. *Current Cancer Drug Targets, 4*(1), 13–28.

Slattery, M.L., Benson, J., Ma, K.N., Schaffer, D., & Potter, J.D. (2001). Trans-fatty acids and colon cancer. *Nutrition and Cancer, 39*(2), 170–175.

Slavin, J.L. (2000). Mechanisms for the impact of whole grain foods on cancer risk. *Journal of the American College of Nutrition, 19*(Suppl. 3), 300S–307S.

Smith, M.R. (2002). Osteoporosis and other adverse body composition changes during androgen deprivation therapy for prostate cancer. *Cancer and Metastasis Reviews, 21*(2), 159–166.

Smith, M.R. (2004). Changes in fat and lean body mass during androgen-deprivation therapy for prostate cancer. *Urology, 63,* 742–745.

Smith, M.R., Eastham, J., Gleason, D.M., Shasha, D., Tchekmedyian, S., & Zinner, N. (2003). Randomized controlled trial of zoledronic acid to prevent bone loss in men receiving androgen deprivation therapy for nonmetastatic prostate cancer. *Journal of Urology, 69,* 2009–2012.

Snyder, D.K., Clemmons, D.R., & Underwood, L.E. (1989). Dietary carbohydrate content determines responsiveness to growth hormone in energy-restricted humans. *Journal of Clinical Endocrinology and Metabolism, 69,* 745–752.

Sonntag, W.E., Lynch, C.D., Cefalu, W.T., Ingram, R.L., Bennett, S.A., Thornton, P.L., et al. (1999). Pleiotropic effects of growth hormone and insulin-like growth factor (IGF)-1 on biological aging: Inferences from moderate caloric-restricted animals. *Journal of Gerontology. Biological Science and Medical Science, 54*(12), B521–B538.

Sovak, M., Seligson, A.L., Konas, M., Jahduch, M., & Dolezal, M. (2002). Herbal composition PC-SPES for management of prostate cancer: Identification of active principles. *Journal of the National Cancer Institute, 94,* 1275–1281.

Spentzos, D., Mantzoros, C., Regan, M.M., Morrissey, M.E., Duggan, S., Flickner-Garvey, S., et al. (2003). Minimal effect of a low-fat/high soy diet for asymptomatic, hormonally naive prostate cancer patients. *Clinical Cancer Research, 9,* 3282–3287.

Steineck, G., Helgesen, F., Adolfsson, J., Dickman, P.W., Hohansson, J.E., Norlen, B.J., et al. (2002). Quality of life after radical prostatectomy or watchful waiting. *New England Journal of Medicine, 347,* 790–796.

Steinmetz, K.A., & Potter, J.D. (1996). Vegetables, fruit, and cancer prevention: A review. *Journal of the American Dietetic Association, 96,* 1027–1039.

Stoch, S.A., Parker, R.A., Chen, L., Bubley, G., Ko, Y.J., Vincelette, A., et al. (2001). Bone loss in men with prostate cancer treated with gonadotropin-releasing hormone agonists. *Journal of Clinical Endocrinology and Metabolism, 86,* 2787–2791.

Studzinski, G.P., & Moore, D.C. (1995). Sunlight—can it prevent as well as cause cancer? *Cancer Research, 55,* 4014–4022.

Tariq, N., Jenkins, D., Vidgen, E., Fleshner, N., Kendall, C.W., Story, J.A., et al. (2000). Effect of soluble and insoluble fiber diets on serum prostate specific antigen in men. *Journal of Urology, 163,* 114–118.

Terry, P., Lichtenstein, P., Feychting, M., Ahlbom, A., & Wolk, A. (2001). Fatty fish consumption and risk of prostate cancer. *Lancet, 357,* 1764–1766.

Terry, P.D., Rohan, T.E., & Wolk, A. (2003). Intakes of fish and marine fatty acids and the risks of cancers of the breast and prostate and of other hormone-related cancers: A review of the epidemiologic evidence. *American Journal of Clinical Nutrition, 77,* 532–543.

Thomas, M.K., Lloyd-Jones, D.M., Thadhani, R.I., Shaw, A.C., Deraska, D.J., Kitch, B.T., et al. (1998). Hypovitaminosis D in medical inpatients. *New England Journal of Medicine, 338,* 777–778.

Thompson, C.A., Shanafelt, T.D., & Loprinzi, C.L. (2003). Andropause: Symptom management for prostate cancer patients treated with hormonal ablation. *Oncologist, 8,* 474–487.

Thompson, I.M., Goodman, P.J., Tangen, C.M., Lucia, M.S., Miller, M.S., Ford, L.G., et al. (2003). The influence of finasteride on the development of prostate cancer. *New England Journal of Medicine, 349,* 215–224.

Tice, J.A., Ettinger, B., Ensrud, K., Wallace, R., Blackwell, T., & Cummings, S.R. (2003). Phytoestrogen supplements for the treatment of hot flashes: The Isoflavone Clover Extract (ICE) study. *JAMA, 290,* 207–214.

Tsutsumi, M., Suzuki, K., Shiga, Y., Ishikawa, S., & Ishikawa, Y. (2002). A low-fat and high soybean protein diet for patients with elevated serum PSA level: Alteration of QOL and serum PSA level after the dietary intervention. *Hinyokika Kiyo, 48*(4), 207–211.

Tuohimaa, P., Tenkanen, L., Ahonen, M., Lumme, S., Jellum, E., Hallmans, G., et al. (2004). Both high and low levels of blood vitamin D are associated with a higher prostate cancer risk: A longitudinal, nested case-control study in the Nordic countries. *International Journal of Cancer, 108*(1), 104–108.

Tymchuk, C.N., Barnard, R.J., Heber, D., & Aronson, W.J. (2001). Evidence of an inhibitory effect of diet and exercise on prostate cancer cell growth. *Journal of Urology, 166,* 1185–1189.

Tzonou, A., Signorello, L.B., Lagiou, P., Wuu, J., Trichopoulos, D., & Trichopoulou, A. (1999). Diet and cancer of the prostate: A case-control study in Greece. *International Journal of Cancer, 80,* 704–708.

U.S. Deptartment of Agriculture. (1995). *Nutrition and your health: Dietary guidelines for Americans* (4th ed.). Washington, DC: U.S. Department of Health and Human Services.

van de Weijer, P.H., & Barentsen, R. (2002). Isoflavones from red clover (Promensil) significantly reduce menopausal hot flush symptoms compared with placebo. *Maturitas, 42*(3), 187–193.

Vegesna, V., O'Kelly, J., Said, J., Uskokovic, M., Binderup, L., Koeffle, H.P., et al. (2003). Ability of potent vitamin D3 analogs to inhibit growth of prostate cancer cells in vivo. *Anticancer Research, 23*(1A), 283–289.

Veierod, M.B., Laake, P., & Thelle, D.S. (1997). Dietary fat intake and risk of prostate cancer: A prospective study of 25,708 Norwegian men. *International Journal of Cancer, 73,* 634–638.

Venkateswaran, V., Fleshner, N.E., & Klotz, L.H. (2004). Synergistic effect of vitamin E and selenium in human prostate cancer cell lines. *Prostate Cancer and Prostatic Diseases, 7*(1), 54–56.

Voorrips, L.E., Goldbohm, R.A., Brants, H.A., van Poppel, G.A., Sturmans, F., Hermus, R.J., et al. (2000). A prospective cohort study on antioxidant and folate intake and male lung cancer risk. *Cancer Epidemiology, Biomarkers and Prevention, 9,* 357–365.

Wang, L., Liu, D., Ahmed, T., Chung, F.L., Conaway, C., Chiao, J.W., et al. (2004). Targeting cell cycle machinery as a molecular mechanism of sulforaphane in prostate cancer prevention. *International Journal of Oncology, 24*(1), 187–192.

Wang, S., DeGroff, V.L., & Clinton, S.K. (2003). Tomato and soy polyphenols reduce insulin-like growth factor-I-stimulated rat prostate cancer cell proliferation and apoptotic resistance in vitro via inhibition of intracellular signaling pathways involving tyrosine kinase. *Journal of Nutrition, 133,* 2367–2376.

Webb, A.R., Pilbeam, C., Hanafin, N., & Holick, M.F. (1990). An evaluation of the relative contributions of exposure to sunlight and of diet to the circulating concentrations of 25-hydroxyvitamin D in an elderly nursing home population in Boston. *American Journal of Clinical Nutrition, 51,* 1075–1081.

Wei, J.T., Gross, M., Jaffe, C.A. Gravlin, K., Lahaie, M., Faerber, G.J., et al. (1999). Androgen deprivation therapy for prostate cancer results in significant loss of bone density. *Urology, 54,* 607–611.

Weisburger, J.H. (1998). Evaluation of the evidence on the role of tomato products in disease prevention. *Proceedings of the Society for Experimental Biology and Medicine, 218*(2), 140–143.

Willett, W.C. (2000). Intakes of fruits, vegetables and related nutrients and the risk of non-Hodgkin's lymphoma among women. *Cancer Epidemiology, Biomarkers and Prevention, 9,* 477–485.

Williams, G.M., Williams, C.L., & Weisburger, J.H. (1999). Diet and cancer prevention: The fiber first diet. *Toxicological Sciences, 52*(Suppl. 2), 72–86.

Woolsey, J., Miller, N., & Theodorescu, D. (2003). Permanent intersitital brachytherapy for prostate cancer: A current review. *World Journal of Urology, 21*(4), 209–219.

World Cancer Research Fund & American Institute for Cancer Research. (1997). *Food, nutrition and the prevention of cancer: A global perspective.* Washington, DC: American Institute for Cancer Research.

Wu, K., Erdman, J.W., Jr., Schwartz, S.J., Platz, E.A., Leitzmann, M., Clinton, S.K., et al. (2004). Plasma and dietary carotenoids, and the risk of prostate cancer: A nested case-control study. *Cancer Epidemiology, Biomarkers and Prevention, 13,* 260–269.

Yi, M.A., Son, H.M., Lee, J.S., Kwon, C.S., Lim, J.K., Yeo, Y.K., et al. (2002). Regulation of male sex hormone levels by soy isoflavones in rats. *Nutrition and Cancer, 42*(2), 206–210.

Yoshizawa, K., Willett, W.C., Morris, S.J., Stampfer, M.J., Spiegelman, D., Rimm, E.B., et al. (1998). Study of prediagnostic selenium level in toenails and the risk of advanced prostate cancer. *Journal of the National Cancer Institute, 90,* 1219–1224.

Yu, H., & Berkel, H. (1999). Insulin-like growth factors and cancer. *Journal of the Louisiana State Medical Society, 151*(4), 218–223.

Yu, H.N., Yin, J.J., & Shen, S.R. (2004). Growth inhibition of prostate cancer cells by epigallocatechin gallate in the presence of Cu2+. *Journal of Agricultural Food Chemistry, 52,* 462–466.

Zhang, J., Hsu, J.C., Kinseth, M.A., Bjeldanes, L.F., & Firestone, G.L. (2003). Indole-3-carbinol induces a G1 cell cycle arrest and inhibits prostate-specific antigen production in human LNCaP prostate carcinoma cells. *Cancer, 98,* 2511–2520.

Zhang, S., Hunter, D.J., Forman, M.R., Rosner, B.A., Speizer, F.E., Colditz, G.A., et al. (1999). Dietary carotenoids and vitamins A, C, and E and risk of breast cancer. *Journal of the National Cancer Institute, 91,* 547–556.

Zhang, S.M., Hunter, D.J., Rosner, B.A., Giovannucci, E.L., Colditz, G.A., Speizer, F.E., et al. (2000). Intakes of fruits, vegetables, and related nutrients and the risk of non-Hodgkin's lymphoma among women. *Cancer Epidemiology, Biomarkers and Prevention, 9,* 477–485.

Zhou, J.R., Gugger, E.T., Tanaka, T., Guo, Y., Blackburn, G.L., Clinton, S.K., et al. (1999). Soybean phytochemicals inhibit the growth of transplantable human prostate carcinoma and tumor angiogenesis in mice. *Journal of Nutrition, 129,* 1628–1635.

Zhou, J.R., Yu, L., Zhong, Y., & Blackburn, G.L. (2003). Soy phytochemicals and tea bioactive components synergistically inhibit androgen-sensitive human prostate tumors in mice. *Journal of Nutrition, 133,* 516–521.

Zhou, J.R., Yu, L., Zhong, Y., Nassr, R.L., Franke, A.A., Gaston, S.M., et al. (2002). Inhibition of orthotopic growth and metastasis of androgen-sensitive human prostate tumors in mice by bioactive soybean components. *Prostate, 53*(2), 143–153.

Zu, K., & Ip, C. (2003). Synergy between selenium and vitamin E in apoptosis induction is associated with activation of distinctive initiator caspases in human prostate cancer cells. *Cancer Research, 63,* 6988–6995.

CHAPTER 12

Adult Leukemia

Gayle S. Jameson, RN, MSN, CRNP, AOCN®
Maria Petzel, RD, LD, CNSD

Overview

The diagnosis of leukemia can be a devastating event for any adult. It also can be a challenging group of life-threatening illnesses for the healthcare team to manage. Leukemia and/or the treatment of leukemia can result in many symptoms that will impact the patient's nutritional status. Optimal nutrition promotes health, healing, and a sense of well-being. However, to date, little research has been conducted regarding the impact of nutrition on the carcinogenesis, morbidity, and mortality of adults with leukemia.

Definition and Pathology of Leukemia

Leukemia is a malignant disease of the bone marrow or lymph nodes. It is characterized by a proliferation and accumulation of abnormal immature blood cells in the bone marrow and other tissues. Leukemogenesis, the development of leukemia, is thought to occur at the level of the pluripotent stem cell. Arrest of cell maturation results in an accumulation of immature cells in the marrow and eventual decreased production of normal blood cells (Leukemia and Lymphoma Society, 2004).

Types and Classification of Leukemia

Leukemias are categorized as acute or chronic, lymphoid or myeloid (see Figure 12-1) (Linet & Devesa, 2002). The acute leukemias demonstrate a more aggressive process, with rapid onset and predominance of very immature, nonfunctional malignant cells (blasts). In contrast, the chronic leukemias are of a slower, more insidious onset with more mature, somewhat functional, malignant cells. The leukemias are further classified as myeloid or lymphoid, based on the cell type of origin. The most commonly used system for classifying acute leukemias is the FAB (French, American, British) classification, which is based on differences in the leukemic cell morphology, cytogenetics, and immunophenotyping. The chronic leukemias are classified by phase, stage, and cell of origin. The three phases of chronic myelogenous leukemia (CML) are chronic, accelerated, and blastic. Two classification systems of chronic lymphocytic leukemia (CLL) are Binet, based on worsening prognosis, and Rai, based on extent of tissue involvement and bone marrow compromise (Wujcik, 2003).

Figure 12-1. Algorithm for Classification of Leukemia

Leukemia Classification			
Acute		**Chronic**	
Myeloid	**Lymphoid**	**Myeloid**	**Lymphoid**
(FAB)	(FAB)	Chronic phase	(Binet)
M0	L1	Accelerated phase	A
M1	L2	Blastic phase	B
M2	L3		C
M3			(Rai)
M4			I
M5			II
M6			III
M7			IV

FAB—French, American, British

Note. From "Molecular Biology of Leukemia," by D. Wujcik, 2003, *Seminars in Oncology Nursing, 19,* p. 85. Copyright 2003 by Elsevier. Reprinted with permission.

Incidence

In the United States, leukemia is a relatively uncommon diagnosis that accounts for approximately 3% of all cancers and 4% of all cancer deaths annually (see Table 12-1) (Miller & Grodman, 2001). Leukemia is predominantly a disease of adults (ratio of adults to children, 8:1), with more than 50% of cases occurring in those older than 64. Individuals of Caucasian/European descent have the highest incidence of leukemia, with lower rates seen among minority populations (Leukemia and Lymphoma Society, 2004).

Table 12-1. Incidence of Leukemia, United States, 2005

Type of Leukemia	Estimated Number of Cases
Lymphocytic	13,700
Myeloid	16,560
Other	4,550
Total new cases	34,810

Note. Based on information from Jemal et al., 2005.

Diagnosis

The diagnosis of leukemia is made through a thorough history and physical examination, analysis of the peripheral blood smear, and a bone marrow aspiration and biopsy, including cytogenetics (chromosome studies) and flow cytometry. Recurrent patterns of chromosome abnormalities are observed in more than 50% of all leukemia cases (Wujcik, 2003).

Prognostic Factors

Negative prognostic indicators at the time of diagnosis include advanced age, a white blood cell (WBC) count of > 100,000 myeloblasts, the presence of a serious infection, and detection of multiple chromosomal abnormalities. Favorable chromosomal abnormalities include translocation of chromosomes 15 and 17, t(15;17), and t(8;21) (Murphy-Ende & Chernecky, 2002).

Clinical Presentation—Acute Leukemia

Patients diagnosed with acute leukemia may be asymptomatic at the time of diagnosis. However, more commonly, the patient will present with symptoms related to bone marrow infiltration of leukemic cells and decreased production of normal bone marrow cells, resulting in anemia, thrombocytopenia, and leukopenia (Dorfman & Skarin, 2003). Infection, fatigue, and bleeding are common. Nutritional deficiencies, such as weight loss and hypoalbuminemia, may not be immediately apparent because of the rapid onset of illness. However, the patient's nutritional status can become quickly compromised from the disease, treatment, and expected side effects of therapy. Acute leukemia without treatment most often is fatal within weeks to months (Miller & Grodman, 2001).

Clinical Presentation—Chronic Leukemia

Chronic leukemias generally are slow in onset and frequently are diagnosed incidentally when an individual is noted to have an unexplained elevation in the WBC count. Significant weight loss (> 10% of body weight) is an uncommon finding at the time of diagnosis of chronic leukemia. CLL frequently is not treated until the patient develops symptoms of progressive disease (Breed, 2003), such as bulky adenopathy, anemia, thrombocytopenia, anorexia, early satiety, and/or weight loss.

Risk Factors and Prevention

The cause of leukemia in most cases is unknown. However, radiation exposure in very high doses (e.g., atomic bombs of World War II) resulted in an increased incidence of leukemia, as well as other malignancies, in individuals who survived the exposure (Miller & Grodman, 2001). Chemicals such as toluene, benzene, and alkylating chemotherapeutic agents are associated with an increased risk of developing leukemia. Viruses such as HTLV-1 have been linked with an aggressive Burkitt's type acute lymphocytic leukemia (ALL) in Africa. Genetic abnormalities are also known to be a risk factor of leukemia. Down syndrome is associated with a 15-fold increase in risk of leukemia. Cigarette smoking is weakly linked to an increased risk of acute myelogenous leukemia (AML) (Linet & Devesa, 2002). Little data are available regarding the relationship of diet and nutrition to the development of leukemia. A retrospective analysis of data from the Iowa Women's Health Study suggested that increased vegetable consumption may decrease the risk of adult leukemia (Ross et al., 2002). However, additional confirmatory trials are needed to validate this conclusion.

Treatment Modalities

The goal of treatment in leukemia is to achieve a complete hematologic and cytogenetic remission. The specific treatment of leukemia varies widely based on the type and subclassification of disease. Patients receiving treatment for acute leukemia, both ALL and AML, are routinely hospitalized for induction (initial phase) of therapy. The standard treatment for ALL and AML differ but result in similar complications of intensive chemotherapy. Expected complications include severe granulocytopenia, anemia, and thrombocytopenia. Other probable complications of treatment include fevers, hypermetabolism, infections, mucositis, taste changes, anorexia, nausea and/or vomiting, diarrhea, constipation, or bleeding. It is often a great challenge for individuals receiving induction chemotherapy to meet their daily caloric demands. Weight loss, malnutrition, and electrolyte imbalances can occur rapidly. Proactive measures, prior to the initiation of therapy, can be helpful in minimizing weight loss. Nutrition therapy counseling regarding the importance of diet during therapy can motivate patients to see nutrition as equally important as the medications and chemotherapy in the restoration of health. Patients with chronic leukemia tend to be relatively well at the time of diagnosis. In CLL, treatment may not be indicated until the onset of symptoms, which occur because of bone marrow dysfunction, immune dysfunction, or bulky lymphadenopathy. CML in the chronic phase is now treated with oral imatinib mesylate (Gleevec®, Novartis, East Hanover, NJ), a well-tolerated enzyme blocker (Breed, 2003). CML that has progressed to the blastic phase is treated similarly to an acute leukemia.

Nutritional Implications

In general, people who are well nourished at the time of a cancer diagnosis have fewer problems related to the cancer and its treatment. Individuals with leukemia are at a lower risk for serious long-term nutrition problems compared with other cancers, such as upper and lower gastrointestinal malignancies (Foltz, 2000). However, especially in the treatment of acute leukemia, the patient's nutritional status can rapidly decline during induction therapy and not improve for several months after complete remission is achieved. During therapy and recovery, the patient's metabolic needs may increase, resulting in the need for an increase in calorie and protein intake. The increased need is because of mechanisms related to the disease process and treatment. The malignancy can initiate metabolic cellular change, and the treatment induces cellular damage requiring increased amounts of nutrients to repair tissues. Gastrointestinal side effects of chemotherapy may decrease the body's ability to absorb nutrients (Foltz).

Nutrition-related side effects that may be associated with the actual disease include nausea or anorexia, which often lead to weight loss. Chemotherapy can cause side effects such as stomatitis, electrolyte abnormalities, diarrhea, constipation, nausea, and/or vomiting. Patients with leukemia, whether in active treatment or not, are at a higher risk for infection. The use of antibiotics, antifungals, and antivirals may lead to nausea, vomiting, diarrhea, and electrolyte abnormalities. A severe drop in the number of white blood cells may render a patient neutropenic, increasing susceptibility to food-borne pathogens and other illnesses. Anorexia, early satiety, and/or weight loss all may continue or develop during treatment (Miller & Grodman, 2001). Other factors that may have nutritional implications are pain, anxiety, or depression (Bloch & Charuhas, 2001).

Assessment Guidelines

The American Dietetic Association's *Clinical Guide to Oncology Nutrition* states that "aggressive identification and treatment of nutrition-related symptoms can stabilize or reverse weight loss in 50% to 88% of oncology cases" (McCallum & Polisena, 2000, p. 11). The nurse plays an important role in the assessment of a patient's nutritional risk. A useful tool to assess the patient's nutritional status and risks is the Patient-Generated Subjective Global Assessment (PG-SGA) (Ottery, 1996) (see Appendix A). Patients at increased nutritional risk should be referred to the clinical dietitian for medical nutrition therapy. Factors to assess include (Ottery)

- Weight
    - What is the patient's current weight?
    - Has the patient lost or gained weight?
    - Over what period of time has the weight change occurred?
- Changes in food intake
    - How is the patient eating now in relation to how he or she has eaten in the past?
        - Is the patient eating about the same amount of food, more food, or less food?
        - Has the patient decreased his or her consumption of solid foods?
- Changes in activity
    - Does the patient continue to carry out his or her usual activities, or has the activity level declined?

Special Considerations for Nutrition

Optimal symptom management and patient participation in self-care can result in minimal weight loss and nutritional compromise in patients with leukemia (National Cancer Institute, 2004). In addition, nutrition screening and assessment tools and processes should comply with the current standards and elements of performance established by the Joint Commission on Accreditation of Healthcare Organizations in facilities that are accredited by that organization. The oral route is preferred for patients with adequate gastrointestinal functions. Based on current evidence, specialized nutritional support should be limited to specific clinical conditions (American Society for Parenteral and Enteral Nutrition Board of Directors, 2002). The following guidelines of the American Society for Enteral and Parenteral Nutrition may be applied to patients with leukemia.

- "SNS [specialized nutrition support] should not be used routinely as an adjunct to chemotherapy" (p. 83SA).
- "SNS is appropriate in patients receiving active anticancer treatment who are malnourished and who will be unable to absorb adequate nutrients for a prolonged period of time" (p. 83SA).

Controversy exists regarding the benefit of enteral or parenteral nutrition in patients with leukemia. Because of the profound pancytopenia that is present after induction chemotherapy in acute leukemia, the risk of infection and bleeding is great. Therefore, the current trend is to avoid enteral feedings and total parenteral nutrition unless the expected period of pancytopenia is prolonged. It may be appropriate to provide nutritional support if patients have prolonged severe stomatitis or prolonged diarrhea or vomiting. However, it would not be appropriate to use nutritional support simply because a patient has a poor appetite associated with chemotherapy.

Increased Risk of Infection

Patients with leukemia are at an increased susceptibility to infection. Therefore, as with all patients with cancer, those with leukemia should be following basic food safety guidelines to reduce their risk of food-borne illness. Guides for food safety for patients who are neutropenic are found in Appendix K. In addition to basic food safety, some patients may be instructed to follow a "neutropenic diet." There is a lack of strong data supporting its use. Neutropenic diet guidelines vary from institution to institution. Some institutions restrict consumption of all luncheon meats and raw fruits and vegetables. Other institutions restrict only those foods, such as alfalfa sprouts and cold luncheon meats, that are high risk for causing food-borne illness. With a lack of evidence supporting the benefit of the neutropenic diet, it is important to recognize that such dietary restrictions may further decrease the oral intake of patients already struggling to meet nutritional needs (Ladas, 2002; Shelton, 2003). Healthcare professionals should work together to develop a diet for patients with neutropenia.

Loss of Appetite and Weight Loss

The disease may cause a loss of appetite, or it may be treatment related. Regardless of cause, the management is the same. Tips for patients include
- Eat small, high-calorie, high-protein meals throughout the day.
- Keep snacks on hand.
- Plan meal times (may be difficult in hospital setting).
- Eat with friends or family.
- Sip on calorie- and protein-containing liquids, such as over-the-counter oral supplements.

The use of appetite-stimulating medications may be appropriate. It is important to ensure that the recommended effective dose is prescribed. Three medications used for appetite stimulation are megestrol acetate (Megace®, Bristol-Myers Squibb, New York, NY), dronabinol (Marinol®, Unimed Pharmaceuticals, Marietta, GA), and mirtazapine (Remeron®, Organon, Roseland, NJ). Selection of the appropriate agent can be determined by review of the side effect profiles (Cunningham, 2004).

Mucositis/Stomatitis

Nutrition modifications along with aggressive pain management can help to maximize the patient's tolerance of oral intake. Tips for patients include
- Avoid fruits and juices high in acid (e.g., orange, lime, lemon, grapefruit, tomato, pineapple).

- Avoid salty foods.
- Avoid spicy foods.
- Eat and drink foods at room temperature.
- Eat soft foods, including foods that can be smashed with a fork or foods that have been blended.
- Avoid rough-textured foods, such as raw vegetables, crackers, granola, and popcorn.

Topical medications may be beneficial for mild mouth or throat pain and discomfort. Moderate to severe mucositis or systemic pain may be better managed by use of a narcotic patient-controlled analgesic 10–15 minutes prior to eating.

Nausea and Vomiting

Nausea and/or vomiting may be a result of chemotherapeutic agents or other medications prescribed for the treatment or prophylaxis of infection. Tips for patients include

- Eat and drink slowly.
- Eat small meals throughout the day (five to six per day).
- Drink fluids separate from meals.
- Chew food well.
- Eat foods at room temperature in an open area to avoid unpleasant aromas.
- Eat dry foods (toast, crackers, and cereal) after periods of rest.
- Try tart foods, such as lemons and pickles, to curb nausea.
- Avoid fried, high-fat, greasy, or spicy foods.
- Do not lie down flat for at least 30 minutes after a meal.
- Wear loose-fitting clothes.
- Breathe deeply.

In addition to nutritional management for nausea and vomiting, antiemetic medication often is necessary. A variety of prescription antiemetics are available. Patient teaching should include the importance of early intervention; medication should be taken at the first sign of nausea. Around-the-clock dosing also may be beneficial until stimulus of nausea is removed or resolved.

Diarrhea

Medicinal treatment of diarrhea depends upon the causation of the symptom. Nutritional management is uniform regardless of the cause of diarrhea. Tips for patients include

- Increase fluid intake.
- Avoid high-fiber, high-fat, and highly spiced foods.
- Eat small amounts of food throughout the day.
- Avoid hot or very cold liquids.
- Avoid beverages with caffeine or alcohol.

Constipation

Constipation not only causes discomfort or pain but also may contribute to loss of appetite or nausea. Resolution of constipation may be difficult to achieve with nutrition alone. The use of laxatives or stool softeners may be required to relieve constipation. Tips for patients include

- Drink plenty of fluids (2–2.5 l/day).
- Drink warm or hot fluids.
- Drink prune juice or eat prunes.
- Eat high-fiber foods.
- Exercise.

Electrolyte Abnormalities

Patients receiving certain chemotherapeutic agents or antibiotics are at risk for developing hypomagnesemia and/or hypokalemia. A diet that includes high-magnesium or high-potassium foods may prevent the need for oral supplementation. Tables 12-2 and 12-3 list foods that are high in magnesium and potassium. Avoidance of oral supplementation can reduce the risk of additional medication-induced side effects.

Table 12-2. Selected Magnesium-Rich Foods

Food	Portion Size	Magnesium (mg)
Pumpkin seeds, roasted	1 oz (about 142 seeds)	151
All bran cereal	½ cup	114
Brazil nuts	1 oz	107
Halibut, cooked	3 oz	91
Oat bran muffin	1	89
Spinach, canned or cooked	½ cup	79
Almonds	1 oz	78
Cashews	1 oz	74–77
Artichoke, cooked	1	72
Soybeans, cooked	½ cup	54–74
White beans, cooked	½ cup	67
Nuts, mixed	1 oz	64–67
Black beans, cooked	½ cup	60
Navy beans, cooked	½ cup	54
Tuna, cooked	3 oz	54
Crab meat (Alaskan King), cooked	3 oz	54
Lima beans, cooked	½ cup	41–50
Peanuts	1 oz	50
Flounder, cooked	3 oz	49

(Continued on next page)

Table 12-2. Selected Magnesium-Rich Foods *(Continued)*

Food	Portion Size	Magnesium (mg)
Beet greens, cooked	½ cup	49
Salmon, cooked	3 oz	48
Okra (frozen), boiled	½ cup	47
Soymilk	1 cup	47
Black-eyed peas, boiled	½ cup	34–46
Hazelnuts	1 oz	46
Baked beans	½ cup	41–44
Great northern beans, cooked	½ cup	44
Walnuts	1 oz	45
Oat bran, cooked	½ cup	44
Haddock, cooked	3 oz	43
Refried beans	½ cup	42
Raisin bran cereal	½ cup	20–42
Sunflower seeds	1 oz or ¼ cup	37–41
Kidney beans, cooked	½ cup	36–40
Chickpeas/garbanzo beans	½ cup	35–40
Lentils, cooked	½ cup	36
Split peas, cooked	½ cup	35
Pinto beans, cooked	½ cup	35

Note. Based on information from the U.S. Department of Agriculture, Agricultural Research Service, 2004.

Table 12-3. Selected Potassium-Rich Foods

Food	Portion Size	Potassium (mg)
Beet greens, cooked	½ cup	654
White beans, canned	½ cup	595
Raisins, seedless	½ cup	543
Baked potato, with skin	½ potato	540
Molasses, blackstrap	1 tbsp	498
Halibut, cooked	3 oz	490
Soybeans, cooked	½ cup	443–485
Tuna, yellowfin, cooked	3 oz	484
Lima beans, cooked	½ cup	370–478
Cod, cooked	3 oz	439
Winter squash, cooked	½ cup	448
Chocolate milk	1 cup	418–425

(Continued on next page)

Table 12-3. Selected Potassium-Rich Foods *(Continued)*

Food	Portion Size	Potassium (mg)
Artichoke	1 medium	425
Banana	1 medium	422
Spinach, cooked/canned	½ cup	370–419
Tomato sauce, canned	½ cup	406
Stewed prunes	½ cup	398
Papaya	½ papaya	391
Pork loin	3 oz	358–382
Baked beans	½ cup	376
Trout, rainbow, cooked	3 oz	375
Buttermilk, low fat	1 cup	340
Spaghetti/marinara sauce	½ cup	369
Milk, low fat and reduced fat	1 cup	366
Lentils, cooked	½ cup	365
Kidney beans, cooked	½ cup	357
Split peas, cooked	½ cup	355
Prune juice	½ cup	353
Yogurt, plain	1 cup	352
Whole milk	1 cup	349
Great northern beans, cooked	½ cup	346
Black-eyed peas	½ cup	319–345
Carrot juice	½ cup	345
Soymilk	1 cup	345
Beef, sirloin, cooked	3 oz	311–343
Mashed potatoes	½ cup	342
Bran cereal	½ cup	339
Haddock, cooked	3 oz	339
Refried beans	½ cup	336
Navy beans	½ cup	335
Kidney beans	½ cup	329
Orange roughy, cooked	3 oz	327
Salmon, cooked	3 oz	319
Ham, cooked	3 oz	298–317
Cabbage, cooked	½ cup	315
Black beans, cooked	½ cup	305
Lobster meat, cooked	3 oz	299
Perch (ocean), cooked	3 oz	298
Pistachio nuts	1 oz (47 nuts)	295
Flounder/sole, cooked	3 oz	292

(Continued on next page)

Table 12-3. Selected Potassium-Rich Foods *(Continued)*

Food	Portion Size	Potassium (mg)
Oat bran muffin	1 muffin	289
Spinach (frozen), cooked	½ cup	287
Tomato juice (with salt), canned	½ cup	278
Crab meat, cooked	3 oz	223–275
Nectarine	1 nectarine	273
Sunflower seed kernels	¼ cup	272
Lima beans	½ cup	258–265
Tomatoes, stewed	½ cup	264
Beets, cooked	½ cup	259
Turkey, cooked	3 oz	244–256
Orange juice	½ cup	218–248
Brussels sprouts, cooked	½ cup	225–247
Pinto beans, cooked	½ cup	247
Chocolate pudding	½ cup	237–247
Black-eyed peas	½ cup	206–239
Chickpeas/garbanzo beans	½ cup	206–239
Kiwi (fresh)	1 medium	237
Orange (fresh)	1 medium	237
Vegetable juice cocktail, canned	½ cup	234
Broccoli, cooked	½ cup	229
Pumpkin seed kernels	1 oz (142 seeds)	229
Tomatoes, whole, canned	½ cup	226
Tomato soup, prepared with milk	½ cup	224
Okra (frozen), cooked	½ cup	215
Cantaloupe	½ cup	214
Collard greens, cooked	½ cup	213
Tomato, fresh, ripe	½ cup	213
Celery, cooked	½ cup	213
Kale, cooked	½ cup	209
Egg substitute	¼ cup	207
Almonds	1 oz (24 nuts)	206
Peanuts	1 oz	206
Apricots, dried	5 halves	204
Grapefruit juice	½ cup	200–203
Apricots, canned	½ cup	201
Sauerkraut	½ cup	201
Tuna, canned	3 oz	201

Note. Based on information from the U.S. Department of Agriculture, Agricultural Research Service, 2004.

Care Planning

Developing the patient's plan of care should involve the patient, family, and multidisciplinary medical team. This team includes the physician, nurse, and dietitian. Other members of the team may include a nurse practitioner, physician's assistant, social worker, pharmacist, physical therapist, chaplain, or others, as needed. The patient and family must be actively involved in decisions and goal setting. Prior to the initiation of chemotherapy, nutrition goals must be developed (e.g., prevention of weight loss, achievement of prescribed calorie and protein intake, completion of daily calorie counts). These nutrition-related goals empower and enable the patient to play an active role in the treatment and recovery of leukemia. The care plan should be reviewed regularly, goals revised as agreed upon with the patient, and assessment goals attained. Involvement of the multidisciplinary team in this process is vital, including daily coaching and encouragement to facilitate achievement of the patient's nutrition goals.

Expected Outcomes of Therapy

Maintaining optimal nutrition during the treatment of leukemia may be quite challenging for the patient, family, and multidisciplinary team. Establishing nutrition goals with the patient and family prior to the initiation of therapy is recommended. Frequent encouragement, assessment, and prompt intervention of nutritional barriers by the multidisciplinary team will facilitate the patient's achievement of the defined nutrition goals. Optimal nutrition in leukemia will benefit the patient's quality of life. However, research is desperately needed to better define and quantify these benefits, as well as measure the impact of optimal nutrition on morbidity and mortality in adults living with leukemia.

References

American Society for Parenteral and Enteral Nutrition. (2002). Guidelines for the use of parenteral and enteral nutrition in adult and pediatric patients. *Journal of Parenteral and Enteral Nutrition, 26*(Suppl.), 82SA–83SA.

Bloch, A.S., & Charuhas, P.M. (2001). Cancer and cancer therapy. In M.M. Gottschlich, M.P. Fuhrman, K.A. Hammond, B.J. Holcombe, & D.L. Seidner (Eds.), *The science and practice of nutrition support: A case-based core curriculum.* Dubuque, IA: Kendall/Hunt.

Breed, C.D. (2003). Diagnosis, treatment, and nursing care of patients with chronic leukemia. *Seminars in Oncology Nursing, 19,* 109–117.

Cunningham, R.S. (2004). The anorexia-cachexia syndrome. In C.H. Yarbro, M.H. Frogge, & M. Goodman (Eds.), *Cancer symptom management* (3rd ed., pp. 137–155). Sudbury, MA: Jones and Bartlett.

Dorfman, D., & Skarin, A. (2003). Acute and chronic leukemias. In A.T. Skarin, K. Shaffer, T. Wieczorek, & G. Canellos (Eds.), *Dana-Farber Cancer Institute atlas of diagnostic oncology* (3rd ed., pp. 435–474). St. Louis, MO: Mosby.

Foltz, A.T. (2000). Nutritional disturbances. In C.H. Yarbro, M.H. Frogge, M. Goodman, & S.L. Groenwald (Eds.), *Cancer nursing: Principles and practice* (5th ed., pp. 754–775). Sudbury, MA: Jones and Bartlett.

Jemal, A., Murray, T., Ward, E., Samuels, A., Tiwari, R.C., Ghafoor, A., et al. (2005). Cancer statistics, 2005. *CA: A Cancer Journal for Clinicians, 55,* 10–30.

Ladas, E. (2002). The neutropenic diet: An examination of the evidence. *ON-LINE: A Publication of The Oncology Nutrition Dietetic Practice Group of the American Dietetic Association, 10*(2), 1–7.

Leukemia and Lymphoma Society. (2004). *Diseases information—Leukemia.* Retrieved April 17, 2004, from http://leukemia.org/all_page/item_id=9346

Linet, M.S., & Devesa, S.S. (2002). Epidemiology of leukemia: Overview and patterns of occurrence. In E.S. Henderson, T.A. Lister, & M.F. Greaves (Eds.), *Leukemia* (7th ed., pp. 131–151). Philadelphia: Saunders.

McCallum, P.D., & Polisena, C.G. (2000). *The clinical guide to oncology nutrition.* Chicago: American Dietetic Association.

Miller, K.B., & Grodman, H. (2001). Leukemia. In R. Lenhard, Jr., R. Osteen, & T. Gansler (Eds.), *American Cancer Society's clinical oncology* (pp. 527–551). Atlanta, GA: American Cancer Society.

Murphy-Ende, K., & Chernecky, C. (2002). Assessing adults with leukemia. *Nurse Practitioner, 27,* 49–60.

National Cancer Institute. (2004, March). *Nutrition in cancer care (PDQ®)—Health professionals.* Retrieved April 30, 2004, from http://www.cancer.gov/cancerinfo/pdq/supportivec-are/nutrition/healthprofessional/#section_153

Ottery, F.D. (1996). Oncology patient-generated SGA of nutritional status. *Nutritional Oncology, 1*(2), 9.

Rai, K.R., & Chiorazzi, N. (2003). Determining the clinical course and outcome in chronic lymphocytic leukemia. *New England Journal of Medicine, 348,* 1797–1799.

Ross, J.A., Kasum, C.M., Davies, S.M., Jacobs, D.R., Folsom, A.R., & Potter, J.D. (2002). Diet and risk of leukemia in the Iowa Women's Health Study. *Cancer Epidemiology, Biomarkers and Prevention, 11,* 777–781.

Shelton, B.K. (2003). Evidence-based care for the neutropenic patient with leukemia. *Seminars in Oncology Nursing, 19,* 133–141.

U.S. Department of Agriculture, Agricultural Research Service. (2004). *USDA national nutrient database for standard reference* (Release 16-1). Retrieved March 15, 2004, from http://www.nal.usda.gov/fnic/foodcomp/Data/SR16-1/sr16-1dc.pdf

Wujcik, D. (2003). Molecular biology of leukemia. *Seminars in Oncology Nursing, 19,* 83–89.

CHAPTER 13

Lymphoma

Kristen Baileys, MSN, CRNP, OCN®
Marcia Nahikian-Nelms, PhD, RD, LD

Overview

The term "lymphoma" encompasses Hodgkin disease (HD), also termed Hodgkin lymphoma, and non-Hodgkin lymphoma (NHL). The lymphomas are neoplasms involving the lymphatic system and often are referred to as lymphoproliferative malignancies.

The symptoms of HD and NHL are very similar. The most common presenting symptom associated with the lymphomas is persistent, painless swelling of the lymph nodes. Most often, the lymphadenopathy occurs in the cervical, axillary, or inguinal regions (National Cancer Institute, 2002). Once an infectious or inflammatory etiology for the lymphadenopathy is ruled out, the diagnosis of lymphoma should be entertained. HD and NHL can produce generalized symptoms that are referred to as B symptoms. B symptoms are fevers, chills, night sweats, and unexplained weight loss. More specific symptoms sometimes seen with HD include pruritus and pain involving a lymph node region following the consumption of alcohol (Cheson, 2001). Specific symptoms with NHL are associated with the lymphadenopathy itself (Cheson). Patients with NHL often have bone marrow involvement at presentation, therefore causing alterations in their blood counts.

HD and NHL can be differentiated by their pattern of spread throughout the body. HD usually is a unicentric disease, meaning it presents within a single lymph node group and spreads in a contiguous fashion from one lymph node group to another (Gutaj, 2000). In contrast, NHL is more multicentric, often involving several lymph node groups at presentation and having a less predictable pattern of spreading and far greater chance to seed through the bloodstream to extranodal sites (National Cancer Institute, 2003).

Incidence

Lymphomas account for 5% of all cancers diagnosed in the United States (Grossbard, 2002). In 2005, an estimated 7,350 new cases of HD and 1,410 deaths will occur (American Cancer Society, 2005). HD, however, has had the biggest decline in mortality of all cancers, largely related to excellent results with modern therapies (National Cancer Institute, 2003). HD is one of the most commonly occurring cancers among young adults. It has a bimodal age distribution, with peak incidence in the mid-20s to early-30s and another peak after age 60 (Vogel, Wilson, & Melvin, 2004).

NHL is much more prevalent, and incidence has doubled since the 1970s. Estimated new cases in 2005 are 56,390, and estimated deaths are 19,200 (American Cancer Society, 2005). The median age for diagnosis of NHL differs per subtype. For example, small lymphocytic lymphomas are seen in older adults; lymphoblastic lymphomas occur mostly in young adults; follicular lymphomas are seen at middle age; and Burkitt's lymphomas usually occur in children and young adults (Vogel et al., 2004). Both HD and NHL have a male predominance, with a lifetime risk of 1 in 48 for men and 1 in 57 for women (Vogel et al.).

Risk Factors and Prevention

The etiology of HD is unknown, and after many years of research, understanding of the risk factors for developing HD is minimal. Pathologically, HD has an inflammatory appearance suggestive of an infectious etiology (Cheson, 2001). Studies have determined the best candidate to be the Epstein-Barr virus, which is known to cause infectious mononucleosis (Cheson). People are three times more likely to develop HD if they have had infectious mononucleosis (Cheson). A suggested genetic predisposition to HD estimated that 4.5% of all cases have a familial component (Grossbard, 2002). No conclusive evidence suggests any environmental or chemical factors (e.g., woodworking, farming, industrial chemicals, herbicides) or behavioral components (e.g., smoking, alcohol consumption, diet, activity) as risk factors for developing HD (Grossbard). However, there appears to be an increased risk of HD in people with HIV or AIDS and patients post–solid organ or bone marrow transplantation (BMT) (Cheson; Grossbard).

Most cases of NHL have no known cause; however, the risk of developing NHL increases with age. Both immune deficiency (congenital or acquired) and autoimmune disorders have been found to increase the risk of NHL (Grossbard, 2002). This includes patients with HIV/AIDS, rheumatoid arthritis, or Sjögren's syndrome or those who are post–solid organ or marrow transplantation. Several viruses have been found to increase the risk of some lymphoma subtypes. Human herpes virus-8 has been linked to body cavity lymphoma; hepatitis C is linked to immunocytoma; human T-cell lymphotropic virus-1 is linked to T-cell lymphoma; and the virus *Helicobacter pylori* has been linked to gastric mucosa–associated lymphoid tissue (MALT) lymphomas (Cheson, 2001). Some research has shown that certain chemical agents, herbicides, pesticides, ionizing radiation, and dark hair dyes formulated before 1980 can increase the risk for NHL (Vogel et al., 2004). Limited evidence suggests that lifestyle factors such as smoking, alcohol consumption, and a high-fat diet can increase the risk for NHL (Hoffman et al., 2000).

There are no known preventive measures for HD or NHL. However, if the incidence of HIV/AIDS could be decreased, that may affect HD and NHL incidence. Avoidance of chemical agents, radiation, and hair dye also may slightly decrease the incidence.

Diagnosis

Lymphadenopathy is the most common presenting symptom of HD and NHL. To make a diagnosis, a lymph node biopsy must be performed. Excisional biopsy, incisional biopsy, or fine needle aspiration are the most commonly used biopsy techniques. Once the biopsy is obtained, specific testing needs to be done on the specimen to determine the lymphoma subtype, including immunophenotyping, cytogenetic studies, and molecular studies (Hoffman et al., 2000). Based on the results of the tests, the pathologist can make the diagnosis of HD or NHL and determine the lymphoma subtype.

The key to a pathologic diagnosis of HD is identification of the Reed-Sternberg cell. The diagnosis of NHL, however, is not based on one type of cell but on combined results of flow cytometry and cytogenetic and molecular testing (Cheson, 2001).

Many components are involved in the staging process for HD or NHL after a pathologic diagnosis is made. The first part should include a thorough history and physical examination, with close attention to any report of B symptoms. Other initial testing should include complete blood count with differential, chemistries including renal and liver function panels, chest radiograph or a computed tomography (CT) scan of the chest, CT scans of the abdomen and pelvis, and a bone marrow biopsy and aspirate (Hoffman et al., 2000). Additional lab results that are important for diagnostic and prognostic purposes include erythrocyte sedimentation rate (ESR), lactate dehydrogenase, and a beta-2 microglobulin level. Other testing that may be performed based on history, physical examination, and subtype of lymphoma include magnetic resonance imaging, ultrasonography, nuclear scans including gallium, positron emission tomography, bone scans, and lumbar puncture for cerebrospinal fluid analysis (Grossbard, 2002).

The Ann Arbor staging system was originally developed for HD, and now its use has extended to NHL as well. The Ann Arbor staging classification (see Table 13-1) has been used for more than 30 years as a universal system for a variety of lymphomas and is the best way to describe the extent of anatomic disease (American Joint Committee on Cancer [AJCC], 2002).

Numerous classification schemes have been proposed for lymphomas over the years, but they are confusing. In 1982, the Working Formulation was introduced and provided simple clinical groupings (AJCC, 2002). However, with increased knowledge of the immune system and understanding of the lymphomas, a new classification system was developed. In 1994, the International Lymphoma Study Group introduced the Revised European-American Classification of Lymphoid Neoplasms (REAL), which took into account morphology, immunophenotype, and genetic and clinical features (AJCC). In 1997, the European Association of Hematopathologists and the Society

Table 13-1. Ann Arbor Staging System

Stage	Characteristics
I	Involvement of single LN region (I) or localized involvement of a single extralymphatic site in absence of LN involvement (IE)
II	Involvement of two or more LN regions on the same side of the diaphragm (II) or localized involvement of a single extralymphatic site with regional LN involvement with or without involvement of LN regions on same side of the diaphragm (IIE)
III	Involvement of LN regions of both sides of the diaphragm (III), which also may include extralymphatic extension in association with adjacent LN involvement (IIIE)
IV	Diffuse involvement of one or more extralymphatic organs, with or without associated LN involvement; or isolated extralymphatic organ involvement in the absence of adjacent regional LN involvement but in conjunction with disease in distant sites

Substage	Characteristics
A	Asymptomatic
B	Fever, night sweats, or weight loss
D	Skin involvement
E	Extralymphatic disease
GI	Gastrointestinal involvement
H	Hepatic involvement
L	Lung involvement
M	Bone marrow involvement
O	Osseous (bone) involvement
Pcard	Pericardium involvement
P	Pleural involvement
S	Spleen involvement
Softis	Soft tissue involvement
Thy	Thyroid involvement
W	Waldeyer's ring (tonsil, naso-oropharynx lymphoid tissue) involvement

Note. From *AJCC Cancer Staging Manual* (6th ed., pp. 395–400), by the American Joint Committee on Cancer, 2002, New York: Springer-Verlag. Copyright 2002 by the American Joint Committee on Cancer. Adapted with permission.

for Hematopathology developed the broader World Health Organization classification of lymphoid malignancies to include myeloid and histiocytic neoplasms (see Figure 13-1) based on the principles of the REAL classification (Harris et al., 1999).

Figure 13-1. World Health Organization Classification of Lymphoid Neoplasms

B-Cell Neoplasms
- Precursor B-cell neoplasm
  - Precursor B lymphoblastic leukemia/lymphoma
- Mature B-cell neoplasms
  - Chronic lymphocytic leukemia/small lymphocytic lymphoma
  - B-cell prolymphocytic leukemia
  - Lymphoplasmacytic lymphoma
  - Splenic marginal zone lymphoma
  - Hairy cell leukemia
  - Plasma cell myeloma
  - Solitary plasmacytoma of bone
  - Extraosseous plasmacytoma
  - Extranodal marginal zone B-cell lymphoma of mucosa-associated lymphoid tissue (MALT lymphoma)
  - Nodal marginal zone B-cell lymphoma
  - Follicular lymphoma
  - Mantle cell lymphoma
  - Diffuse large B-cell lymphoma
  - Mediastinal (thymic) large B-cell lymphoma
  - Intravascular large B-cell lymphoma
  - Primary effusion lymphoma
  - Burkitt's lymphoma/leukemia

T-Cell and NK-Cell Neoplasms
- Precursor T-cell neoplasms
  - Precursor T-lymphoblastic leukemia/lymphoma
  - Blastic NK-cell lymphoma

Mature T-Cell and NK-Cell Neoplasms
- T-cell prolymphocytic leukemia
- T-cell large granular lymphocytic leukemia
- Aggressive NK-cell leukemia
- Adult T-cell leukemia/lymphoma
- Extranodal NK/T-cell lymphoma, nasal type
- Enteropathy-type T-cell lymphoma
- Hepatosplenic T-cell lymphoma
- Subcutaneous panniculitis-like T-cell lymphoma
- Mycosis fungoides/Sezary syndrome
- Primary cutaneous anaplastic large cell lymphoma
- Peripheral T-cell lymphoma, unspecified
- Angioimmunoblastic T-cell lymphoma
- Anaplastic large cell lymphoma

Hodgkin Lymphoma
- Nodular lymphocyte predominant Hodgkin lymphoma
- Classical Hodgkin lymphoma
  - Nodular sclerosis Hodgkin lymphoma
  - Lymphocyte-rich Hodgkin lymphoma
  - Mixed cellularity Hodgkin lymphoma
  - Lymphocyte-depleted Hodgkin lymphoma

Note. From *Pathology and Genetics of Tumours of Haematopoietic and Lymphoid Tissues*, by E.S. Jaffe, N.L. Harris, H. Stein, and J.W. Vardiman, 2001, Lyon, France: IARC Press. Copyright 2001 by IARC Press. Adapted with permission.

Treatment Modalities

Surgery

Most diagnoses of lymphoma do not involve surgical procedures either as treatment or during the staging process. The exceptions to this are those cell types that are localized, such as extranodal marginal zone B lymphoma of B-cell lymphoma or MALT type. Nutritional implications for surgery involve increased energy and protein needs postoperatively to ensure adequate wound healing. Multivitamin supplementation, especially with vitamin C and zinc, may be used to optimize wound healing. Many hospital protocols recommend supplementation with approximately 220 mg zinc once daily and 500 mg of vitamin C twice daily (Mayes & Gottschlich, 2003). This is especially important for the patient with cancer who may enter surgery already at nutritional risk. Nutritional risk can be determined preoperatively by nutrition screening or through the use of a nutritional risk index (see Appendix J). Most research has indicated that patients who have experienced significant weight loss and/or hypoalbuminemia will benefit from preoperative nutritional support (Yeatman, 2000).

Radiation Therapy

The use of ionizing radiation is standard treatment for certain diagnoses of lymphoma. These include localized extranodal marginal zone B lymphoma, localized mantle cell lymphoma, follicular lymphoma, diffuse large B-cell lymphoma, and localized HD. Radiation is the primary therapy for stages I and II of aggressive NHL. Long-term survival rates improve when radiation is combined with chemotherapy. Other types of lymphoma are primarily treated with combination chemotherapy, and radiation can be used to supplement the treatment protocol. Ionizing radiation targets cells in the radiation field and damages the DNA of the cell, which prevents the cells from replicating. Those normal cells in the radiation field are able to regenerate, whereas the malignant cells are destroyed. Nutrition problems arise when the radiation field involves areas of the gastrointestinal tract (see Appendix D). Depending on the radiation field, nutritional implications can include mucositis, esophagitis, xerostomia, nausea, vomiting, and diarrhea. Additionally, many patients experience significant fatigue that, in turn, affects their appetite and functional status.

Chemotherapy

Combination chemotherapy is the primary mode of therapy in most diagnoses of lymphoma. Additionally, other classes of biologic products, such as interleukin-2, interferon alpha, and rituximab (Rituxan®, Genentech, South San Francisco, CA), can be used to support or maximize the effect of the chemotherapy agents.

Chlorambucil (Leukeran®, GlaxoSmithKline, Research Triangle Park, NC) and fludarabine (Fludara®, Berlex, Richmond, CA) are used as single agent chemotherapy drugs to treat small lymphocytic lymphomas (Braunwald et al., 2004). Chlorambucil can cause mild nausea, anorexia, and immunosuppression. Fludarabine may result in anorexia, fatigue, bone and joint pain, fever, and immunosuppression.

The most common chemotherapy protocols for NHL include combinations of cyclophosphamide, vincristine, and prednisone (CVP) or with the addition of doxorubicin (CHOP). Other protocols for NHL include ESHAP (etoposide, cytarabine, cisplatin, and methylprednisolone) and ICE (ifosfamide, carboplatin, and etoposide). In HD, the most common regimens include ABVD (doxorubicin, bleomycin, vinblastine, and dacarbazine), MOPP (nitrogen mustard, vincristine, procarbazine, and prednisone), and the Stanford regimen (mechlorethamine, doxorubicin, vinblastine, prednisone, vincristine, bleomycin, and etoposide) (Braunwald et al., 2004). Primary side effects with nutritional implications from these specific medications are outlined in Table 13-2.

Bone Marrow Transplant

BMT is an additional treatment path for patients with lymphoma. It most often is used when current chemotherapy regimens have failed or because of a relapse. It is estimated that autologous BMT can provide cure for half of patients with HD who previously have failed effective chemotherapy regimens (Braunwald et al., 2004). The goal of BMT is to replace the malignant or defective cells in the bone marrow and restore normal hematopoiesis and immune function. This is achieved by infusing the patient's own bone marrow (autologous) or bone marrow from a donor (allogeneic) after receiving high-dose chemotherapy and/or radiation therapy.

Nutritional Implications

Weight Loss, Anorexia, and Cachexia

Most references estimate that more than 50% of all patients with cancer will experience some degree of weight loss, with approximately one-third losing more than 5% of their normal weight (Tisdale, 2002). Additionally, the existence of the wasting syndrome, commonly known as cachexia, is estimated to occur in approximately 50% of all patients with cancer and, ultimately, is responsible for approximately 20% of all cancer deaths (Brown, 2002; Inui, 2002; Mantovani, Maccio, Massa, & Madeddu, 2001). Malnutrition is a significant component for determination of prognosis (Aviles et al., 1995).

Much has been written about weight loss in patients with cancer. The mechanisms of this weight loss are different than in a situation produced solely from an energy deficit. In simple starvation, weight loss occurs primarily from fat stores. The body strives to preserve somatic and visceral protein compartments and generally reduces its metabolic requirement. In patients with cancer, weight loss may occur without noticeable changes in nutrient intake. In a study by Bosaeus, Daneryd, and Lundholm (2002), dietary intake was analyzed in 297 patients with cancer and was compared to measured energy expenditure and reported weight loss. This research documented no difference in caloric and protein intake for patients who maintained a stable weight from those who lost weight. The conclusion that other factors contributed to documented weight

Table 13-2. Nutritional Side Effects From Chemotherapeutic Agents Used in Treatment of Non-Hodgkin Lymphoma and Hodgkin Disease

Drug	Nausea	Vomiting	Diarrhea	Constipation	Anorexia	Dysgeusia	Fatigue	Immuno-suppression	Mucositis	Other
Bleomycin	~	~			✓	✓	✓		✓	
Carboplatin	✓	✓	~		✓	~		~	~	
Chlorambucil	✓	✓	~		✓	~		✓	~	
Cisplatin	✓	✓	~		~	~		~	~	
Cyclophos-phamide	✓	✓	~			~		✓	~	
Cytarabine (cytosine arabinoside)	✓	✓	✓		✓	✓	~	✓	✓	
Dacarbazine	✓	✓	~		✓		~	✓	~	
Doxorubicin	✓	✓	~			✓	~	✓	✓	
Etoposide	✓	✓						✓		
Fludarabine	~	~	~				✓	✓	~	
Ifosfamide	✓	✓			✓			✓		

(Continued on next page)

Table 13-2. Nutritional Side Effects From Chemotherapeutic Agents Used in Treatment of Non-Hodgkin Lymphoma and Hodgkin Disease *(Continued)*

Drug	Nausea	Vomiting	Diarrhea	Constipation	Anorexia	Dysgeusia	Fatigue	Immuno-suppression	Mucositis	Other
Nitrogen mustard (mechlorethamine)	√	√			√				√	
Prednisone								√		Hyper-glycemia
Procarbazine	√	√					√	√		No alcohol
Vincristine				√		~	~	~		

√ = Most common
~ = Less common
Note. Based on information from Chu & DeVita, 2004.

loss was consistent with much of the previous nutrition research in cancer. This weight loss and, specifically, the loss of skeletal muscle and the increased rate of lipolysis, are driven by cytokine activity and specific tumor catabolic products, such as the lipid mobilizing factor (LMF) and proteolysis inducing factor (PIF) (Belda-Iniesta et al., 2003; Tisdale, 2002). A literature review by Brown (2002) summarized the understanding that nutritional interventions that only attempt to increase caloric intake do not result in the regain of skeletal muscle and are inadequate to reverse the cachexia syndrome. Specific therapies targeting cytokines, LMF, and PIF have resulted in the preliminary evidence of improvement in all areas of nutritional status (Belda-Iniesta et al.; Tisdale). Successful interventions have included the use of thalidomide, eicosapentaenoic acid, melatonin, and omega-3 fatty acids (Tisdale).

As stated in the introduction, patients with lymphoma presenting with B symptoms are those at highest nutritional risk from the onset of diagnosis. Other patients with lymphoma or HD generally experience weight loss and anorexia as a side effect of treatment or in the progression of the disease. Therefore, prevention of weight loss is of primary importance. Addressing nutritional risk and importance of weight maintenance should happen in the initial interview and counseling session with the patient. Education should center on targeted calorie and protein requirements and strategies to accomplish these goals. Interventions can include increasing nutrient density, energy and protein sources, timing and frequency of meals, as well as prescribing specific agents to increase appetite. Appendix C provides detailed information regarding the management of nutrition impact symptoms.

Nausea and Vomiting

Most of the common chemotherapeutic regimens for lymphomas have potential to cause nausea and vomiting. Nutritional interventions can minimize symptoms, but the planned and consistent use of antiemetic regimens is crucial to treat side effects.

Clear liquids or rehydration solutions may be best tolerated during periods of acute nausea and vomiting. Odors often exacerbate nausea. Cold or room temperature foods have fewer odors. Foods such as yogurt, cottage cheese, fruit, or cold meat salads may help with these problems.

Dysgeusia

Taste changes have been noted to occur during times of tumor growth, as a result of chemotherapy agents, or during saliva changes with radiation therapy. Patients often express a strong bitter taste associated with meats, coffee, or tea, as well as intolerance to sweet flavors. Clinicians should acknowledge these changes and provide appropriate substitutions for these foods. For example, if the patient does not tolerate meats, then alternate sources of protein should be recommended.

Mucositis

Mucositis is an inflammation of the oral mucosa and can result in open mouth sores and increased potential for fungal infections. Nutritional interventions should focus on texture modification and avoidance of extremes in temperatures and highly acidic or spicy foods. The use of pain medications and aggressive oral hygiene will assist in minimizing these symptoms.

Immunosuppression

The chemotherapy regimens for lymphomas will result in immunosuppression. During periods of neutropenia, patients should be instructed on appropriate food safety measures to minimize food-borne illnesses. Different institutions approach nutrition recommendations for neutropenia with varying degrees of restriction. Minimally, patients should be discouraged from eating at buffets or salad bars and should ensure that meats and eggs are well cooked and fresh fruits and vegetables thoroughly washed. More detailed guidelines can be found in Appendix K.

Fatigue

Extreme fatigue affects appetite and functional status, both of which can impair nutritional intake. Suggestions to assist with dietary intake during periods of fatigue include use of liquid high-calorie, high-protein supplements, convenience foods, or other ready-to-eat food choices.

Assessment Guidelines

Patients with cancer are considered to be an at-risk population, and, thus, nutrition assessment data will center on those measures that confirm the diagnosis of malnutrition and identify potential risk factors that could lead to malnutrition. No one test measures nutritional status. That is why assessment draws from many indices to provide a complete picture of nutritional health. It is through experience that a clinician can weigh the results of multiple measures to critically evaluate the nutritional status of patients. This section will outline the most important parameters to use for patients with lymphoma.

Nutrition assessment is defined as "an evaluation of the nutritional status of individuals or populations through measurements of food and nutrient intake and evaluation of nutrition-related health indicators" (Lee & Nieman, 2003, p. 3). The determination of *nutritional status* involves evaluating indices that approximate the body's nutrient stores. Nutritional status is altered when stores of energy, protein, vitamins, or minerals fluctuate as a result of either increased need or increased utilization. These frequent alterations in nutritional status alert the practitioner of potential nutritional risk for all patients with cancer.

Nutritional risk attempts to project potential nutrition problems by using clinical judgment to assess the client's current problem(s). Certain factors increase or decrease a client's nutritional risk, especially for patients with cancer. It is important to remember that most nutrition problems seen in the hospitalized population are the result of the disease or its treatment. The patient will most likely have either an increased requirement for certain nutrients or an inability to consume enough nutrients or metabolize the ones that can be digested and absorbed. Therefore, knowing the pathophysiology, treatment, and clinical course of a disease or diagnosis allows one to assess an individual's nutritional risk.

Medical History and Physical

A thorough evaluation of the patient's medical history and physical examination is of top priority before initiating the first patient interview. Information that is gathered will identify previous medical history and comorbidities, such as diabetes mellitus, autoimmune disorders, or coronary heart disease, that may impact the nutrition care plan. Results from staging studies outline the basis for the therapeutic plan and can provide information about systemic problems that may impact ingestion, digestion, or metabolism of nutrients. The initial medical evaluation will generally include complete blood count, ESR, blood urea nitrogen, creatinine, electrolytes, liver function tests, and serum lipid evaluation, as well as CT scans and bone marrow biopsy (Braunwald et al., 2004). Other chemistries may include albumin and prealbumin, which can be used in the biochemical portion of the nutrition assessment. Physical examination can provide basic data that alert for potential nutrition problems, including an examination of the patient's dentition. Information on current medications should be obtained at this time and will allow for identification of potential drug-nutrient interactions.

Initial Patient Interview

The importance of a thorough initial interview cannot be minimized. This interview not only provides invaluable information for formulating the nutrition care plan but also establishes the initial rapport between the clinician and the patient. This rapport and development of trust will provide the foundation for success of all nutritional interventions.

Many social factors impact nutritional status. During the interview, it is important to identify these factors, as they will affect planning and execution of nutrition education and intervention. Interview questions that identify primary language, educational background, and support systems will impact how nutritional interventions are planned and conducted.

Another component of the initial interview is an evaluation of the patient's functional status. Functional status is the ability to perform self-care and activities of daily living and indirectly gives information about skeletal muscle function. One simple test is the handgrip dynamometry. Handgrip measure has long been a part of fitness assessment but is now more common in nutrition assessment. This type of test is especially useful for long-term follow-up in outpatient or rehabilitation settings. More comprehensive measures of functional status use either the Karnofsky performance score or the ECOG (Eastern Cooperative Oncology Group) performance scale (Barber & Rogers, 2003). Establishing a baseline measurement will allow the practitioner to monitor subsequent changes in functional status as the patient progresses through treatment.

Dietary Assessment

During the patient interview, information regarding appetite and digestion should be obtained. This includes evaluation of ability to chew, use and fit of dentures, problems swallowing, nausea, vomiting, constipation, diarrhea, heartburn, or any other symptoms that might interfere with the ability to maintain adequate nutritional intake. Patients with localized organ involvement may present with symptoms that interfere with adequate oral intake. For example, B-cell lymphoma of a MALT type may originate from *Helicobacter* gastritis. Symptoms of gastritis may include abdominal pain, indigestion, nausea, and/or vomiting.

Changes in appetite are common but can be unnoticed by the patient. It is crucial to ask probing questions that may identify those discrepancies when patients describe their dietary intake. One suggestion may be to have patients evaluate their appetite on a number scale from 0–10 (Barber & Rogers, 2003; Grant & Kravitz, 2000). The patient's family or significant others also may provide insight to any recent changes in appetite.

A thorough diet history would identify the patient's usual pattern of intake, food preferences (including ethnic, cultural, and religious influences), use of alcohol, and use of vitamin, mineral, herbal, or other type of supplements. Any previous nutrition education or medical nutrition therapy should be evaluated. Questions should address food allergies or other food intolerance. Be sure to note recent changes from their normal pattern of eating.

Many different tools can be used to gather dietary information. All methods have limitations for both reliability and validity (Lee & Nieman, 2003). In this population, a 24-hour recall is not adequate to provide a thorough picture of a patient's normal intake. Using a 24-hour recall combined with either a diet history or food frequency list provides a more accurate picture of the patient's intake. Patients can be requested to keep a food diary. This method allows patients to participate in their own care and provides ownership to a portion of their medical and nutrition care plans. During hospitalizations, nursing and nutrition staff can monitor actual intake using a calorie count. This method allows documentation of a patient's intake.

Analyzing the data gathered by these methods can be accomplished using a computerized nutrient analysis system or by using exchange lists to estimate approximate caloric and protein intake. In the clinical setting, the requirement for detailed calculations for analysis often is not necessary. Because of the limitations of assessment methods, the intake is an estimate. In general, the analysis method will be determined on how the information will be used. For example, to determine if the intervention to change the patient's food choices has improved the intake, a direct observation of food intake may be used and then assessed by counting the energy value and protein content of the food that was recorded.

Anthropometric Assessment

Anthropometric and body composition assessment allows the clinician to fully assess the body's compartments for energy storage. This will include assessment of fat stores and lean body mass. When disease or stress is present, the changes in the energy storage compartments are an important component of determining nutritional status and risk. The results of anthropometric assessment are used not only to identify goals for nutritional intervention but also to monitor changes that occur as a result of either those interventions or continued effects of disease and stress.

Keeping these issues at the forefront of the anthropometric assessment, detailed information about the patient's height, weight, highest adult weight, weight six months ago, and weight one month ago should be gathered. Calculations of percent of usual body weight and body mass index then should be calculated.

Weight does not distinguish body composition, but in an acute care situation, it often is not practical to gather body composition data. In an outpatient setting where patients are seen over time, measurement techniques, such as skin folds, bioelectrical impedance, and near-infrared interactance, can be easily accomplished. Having this baseline measurement allows the clinician to assess shifts in body compartments and document more accurately the sources of weight loss.

Skin fold measurement can be used to calculate upper arm muscle area and upper arm fat area. The comparison standards that are used to assess these results are based on NHANES (National Health and Nutrition Examination Survey) data with healthy individuals. This affects the validity in the cancer population, but from a practical standpoint, these baseline measurements can be used to compare the patient's own changes over time.

Biochemical Assessment

Biochemical assessment involves measuring nutritional markers and organ function, which are found in blood, urine, feces, and from samples of tissue. Interpretation for biochemical assessment must be made in the context of the diagnosis and medical treatment. Disease states, hydration status, and subsequent treatments can have considerable effects on the levels of the biochemical indices. Reference values may change and should be interpreted using values provided by the laboratory that conducted the tests.

Protein's unique function in supporting cellular growth and development elevates its significance in nutrition assessment. Unlike fat and carbohydrate, which can be stored, protein is not stored and, therefore, is affected in periods of stress and malnutrition. In the patient with cancer, assessment of protein status is most important. Historically, research in cancer and nutrition repeatedly has demonstrated loss of skeletal muscle and visceral proteins (Broder, Sandoval-Cros, & Berger, 1999; Inui, 2002). Furthermore, much of the more recent research has begun to clarify the role of proinflammatory cytokines and tumor-derived catabolic factors that drive these metabolic abnormalities (Mantovani, 2001; Tisdale, 2002).

Biochemical measures should include serum albumin, prealbumin, and, when possible, C-reactive protein and fibronectin. In patients with lymphoma, including those without bone marrow involvement, other measures of protein status may be skewed by changes in both hematologic and immune function. Transferrin, total iron-binding capacity, total lymphocyte count, or delayed cutaneous hypersensitivity testing would not be sound or practical to use in protein assessment.

Clinical Assessment

Clinical assessment will focus on examination for signs of muscle wasting, vitamin and mineral deficiency, and hydration status. Muscle wasting is most commonly noted in temporal muscle loss and in the bulk and size of skeletal muscles. Physical signs of vitamin and mineral deficiencies can be noted in the hair, skin, oral mucosa, teeth, and gums. These are difficult to distinguish in many cases but often are noted to be consistent with other measures of malnutrition. Hydration status is evaluated by both vital signs with increased pulse and orthostatic hypotension and from the physical examination by noting weight loss, lethargy, sunken eyes, absence of tears, dry mucous membranes, decreased capillary refill, and decreased skin turgor.

Establishing Nutrient Requirements

The final step for the nutrition assessment will involve calculation of nutrient and fluid requirements for the patient. Appendices F, G, H, and I provide guidelines for establishing nutritional requirements.

Energy Requirements

Not all patients with lymphoma are hypermetabolic, but patients presenting with B symptoms may have factors that contribute to hypermetabolism, including fever, night sweats, and weight loss. Therefore, energy requirements must be individualized for each patient. The use of indirect calorimetry allows the clinician to more accurately estimate energy needs, but in many situations, this is not feasible. Most clinicians use the Harris-Benedict equation to calculate basal energy expenditure, with additional activity and injury factors to allow for calculation of total energy requirements.

Protein Requirements

Protein needs, similar to energy requirements, are individualized for each patient. The clinician will consider visceral and somatic protein status as well as other conditions that may increase protein needs as factors that might influence protein requirements. Other factors include wound healing and the status of cancer treatment. Most patients with cancer will require a minimum of 1.0–1.5 g protein/kg unless there are extenuating circumstances, such as renal or hepatic insufficiency. If visceral and somatic protein stores are depleted, protein needs may have to increase from 1.5 to 2.0 g/kg of body weight. Some clinicians prefer to use calorie:nitrogen ratios to calculate energy needs. Most patients' protein needs will be met with a ratio of 150:1 (Martin, 2000).

Fluid Requirements

Baseline fluid requirements can be estimated using several different formulas. Many clinicians suggest using 1 ml of fluid per kilocalorie of energy. Other formulas use age, and others are based on body surface area. Fluid requirements will be increased beyond baseline for those patients with night sweats and fever. Some chemotherapy agents require that patients consume additional fluid to minimize organ toxicities. As discussed earlier, hydration status should be evaluated during the clinical assessment of the patient so that specific fluid interventions can be made if necessary.

Micronutrient Requirements

Baseline vitamin and mineral requirements should start with levels indicated by Recommended Dietary Allowances and Adequate Intakes. The recommendations are for healthy individuals, and no specific amounts have been developed for patients with cancer. It is general practice to suggest that all patients take a multivitamin meeting these baseline levels. It is important to note that certain chemotherapy agents interfere with utilization of some vitamins and minerals. In these situations, monitoring supplementation or recommending additional amounts may be warranted. The values for UL (tolerable upper intake levels) can guide the practitioner to ensure that the patient is not consuming excessive amounts of vitamins or minerals.

Summary

All patients diagnosed with HD or NHL should receive a complete nutrition assessment at the time of diagnosis and appropriate follow-up throughout treatment. The use of the Patient-Generated Subjective Global Assessment (Isenring, Bauer, & Capra, 2003; McCallum, 2000; Ottery, 1996) (see Appendix A) is an excellent tool for identifying at-risk patients throughout the treatment period.

A crucial component of the patient care plan is the development of measurable outcomes for medical nutrition therapy. Figure 13-2 summarizes outcomes of medical nutrition therapy for patients with NHL or HD.

Figure 13-2. Expected Outcomes for Medical Nutrition Therapy in Patients With Non-Hodgkin Lymphoma and Hodgkin Disease

- Weight and lean body mass are maintained within the established goal range through consumption of adequate energy and protein or with appropriate nutritional support.
- Hydration will be adequate as measured by clinical and physical assessment.
- The patient will consume adequate energy and protein to perform activities of daily living.
- The patient will consume appropriate foods to reduce treatment side effects.
- The patient will verbalize comprehension of neutropenic precautions.
- The patient will use appropriate and safe complementary nutrition therapies.

Note. Based on information from Luthringer & Kulakowski, 2000.

References

American Cancer Society. (2005). *Cancer facts and figures, 2005.* Atlanta, GA: Author.

American Joint Committee on Cancer. (2002). *AJCC cancer staging manual* (6th ed.). Chicago: Author.

Aviles, A., Yanez, J., Lopex, T., Garcia, E.L., Guzman, R., & Diaz-Maqueo, J.C. (1995). Malnutrition as an adverse prognostic factor in patients with diffuse large cell lymphoma. *Archives of Medical Research, 26,* 31–34.

Barber, M.D., & Rogers, B.B. (2003). *Advances in the management of tumor induced weight loss.* Retrieved March 15, 2004, from http://www.medscape.com/viewprogram/2008_pnt

Belda-Iniesta, C., de Castro Carpeno, J., Fresno Vara, J.A., Cejas Guerrero, P., Casado Saenz, E., Espinosa Arranz, E., et al. (2003). Eicosapentaenoic acid as a targeted therapy for cancer cachexia. *Journal of Clinical Oncology, 21,* 4657–4658.

Bosaeus, I., Daneryd, P., & Lundholm, K. (2002). Dietary intake, resting energy expenditure, weight loss and survival in cancer patients. *Journal of Nutrition, 132*(Suppl. 11), 3465S–3466S.

Braunwald, E., Fauci, A., Isselbacher, K.J., Kasper, D.L., Hauser, D.L., Longo, D.L., et al. (Eds.). (2004). *Harrison's principles of internal medicine* (15th ed.). Retrieved April 2004, from http://harrisons.accessmedicine.com

Broder, G., Sandoval-Cros, C., & Berger, A. (1999). Complications of cancer. *Cancer Control, 6,* 509–516.

Brown, J.K. (2002). A systematic review of the evidence on symptom management of cancer-related anorexia and cachexia. *Oncology Nursing Forum, 29,* 517–530.

Cheson, B.D. (2001). Hodgkin's disease and the non-Hodgkin's lymphomas. In R. Lenhard, Jr., R. Osteen, & T. Gansler (Eds.), *The American Cancer Society's clinical oncology* (pp. 497–516). Atlanta, GA: American Cancer Society.

Chu, E., & DeVita, V.T. (2004). *Physicians' cancer chemotherapy drug manual.* Sudbury, MA: Jones and Bartlett.

Grant, M., & Kravitz, K. (2000). Symptoms and their impact on nutrition. *Seminars in Oncology Nursing, 16,* 113–121.

Grossbard, M.L. (2002). *Malignant lymphomas.* Toronto, Ontario, Canada: BC Decker.

Gutaj, D. (2000). Lymphoma. *RN, 63*(8), 32–38.

Harris, N.L., Jaffe, E.S., Diebold, J., Flandrin, G., Muller-Hermelink, H.K., Vardiman, J., et al. (1999). World Health Organization classification of neoplastic diseases of the hematopoietic and lymphoid tissues: Report of the clinical advisory committee meeting—Airlie House, Virginia, November 1997. *Journal of Clinical Oncology, 17,* 3835–3849.

Hoffman, R., Benz, E.J., Shattil, S.J., Furie, B., Cohen, H.J., Silberstein, L.E., et al. (2000). *Hematology: Basic principles and practice* (3rd ed.). Philadelphia: Churchill Livingstone.

Inui, A. (2002). Cancer anorexia-cachexia syndrome: Current issues in research and management. *CA: A Cancer Journal for Clinicians, 52,* 72–91.

Isenring, E., Bauer, J., & Capra, S. (2003). The scored Patient-Generated Subjective Global Assessment (PG-SGA) and its association with quality of life in ambulatory patients receiving radiotherapy. *European Journal of Clinical Nutrition, 57,* 305–309.

Lee, R.D., & Nieman, D.C. (2003). *Nutritional assessment.* New York: McGraw-Hill.

Luthringer, S., & Kulakowski, K. (2000). Medical nutrition therapy protocols. In P.D. McCallum & C.G. Polisena (Eds.), *The clinical guide to oncology nutrition* (pp. 24–26). Chicago: American Dietetic Association.

Mantovani, G., Maccio, A., Massa, E., & Madeddu, C. (2001). Managing cancer-related anorexia, cachexia. *Drugs, 61,* 499–514.

Martin, C. (2000). Calorie, protein, fluid, and micronutrient requirements. In P.D. McCallum & C.G. Polisena (Eds.), *The clinical guide to oncology nutrition* (pp. 45–52). Chicago: American Dietetic Association.

Mayes, T., & Gottschlich, M.M. (2003). Burns and wound healing. In L.E. Matarase & M.M. Gottschlich (Eds.), *Contemporary nutrition support practice: A clinical guide* (2nd ed., pp. 595–615). Philadelphia: Saunders.

McCallum, P.D. (2000). Patient-Generated Subjective Global Assessment. In P.D. McCallum & C.G. Polisena (Eds.), *The clinical guide to oncology nutrition* (pp. 11–23). Chicago: American Dietetic Association.

National Cancer Institute. (2002). *What you need to know about non-Hodgkin's lymphoma.* Retrieved March 3, 2004, from http://www.cancer.gov/cancerinfo/wyntk/non-hodgkins-lymphoma

National Cancer Institute. (2003). *Adult non-Hodgkin's lymphoma.* Retrieved March 9, 2004, from http://www.cancer.gov/cancerinfo/pdq/treatment/adult-non-hodgkins/healthprofessional/

Ottery, F. (1996). Definition of standardized nutritional assessment and interventional pathways in oncology. *Journal of Nutrition, 12*(Suppl. 1), S15–S19.

Tisdale, M.J. (2001). Cachexia in cancer patients. *Nature Reviews, 2,* 862–870.

Vogel, W.H., Wilson, M.A., & Melvin, M.S. (2004). *Advanced practice oncology and palliative care guidelines.* Philadelphia: Lippincott Williams and Wilkins.

Yeatman, T.J. (2000). Nutritional support for the surgical oncology patient. *Cancer Control, 7,* 563–565.

CHAPTER 14

Multiple Myeloma, Melanoma, and Sarcoma

Tinrin Chew, RD
Bernadette Festa, MS, RD
Maryellen O'Leary, RN

Multiple Myeloma

Overview

Multiple myeloma is a malignant disease that has the potential to affect every system in the body. Although incurable, the disease extends over a prolonged period of time with varying degrees of symptoms that may significantly impact the patient's quality of life. Peak age at diagnosis is 50–70 years (Turgeon, 1998; Varricchio, Pierce, Walker, & Ades, 1997). Multiple myeloma is a cancer of plasma cells in the bone marrow. Normally, plasma cells produce antibodies and play a key role in immune function. Uncontrolled growth of these cells leads to bone pain and fractures, anemia, infections, and other complications.

Etiology

The cause of multiple myeloma is unknown. Exposure to radiation, benzene, herbicides, and insecticides may play a role. Genetic factors and viral infection also may influence the risk of developing multiple myeloma, as well as a history of chronic infections or repeated allergenic stimulation (Pazdur, Coia, Hoskins, & Wagman, 2001; Varricchio et al., 1997).

Clinical Features and Treatment

Clinical features result from (a) a direct effect of the malignant cell population within the marrow, causing bone marrow depression, (b) an increased osteoclastic activity, causing bone destruction, and (c) the accumulation of

219

immunoglobulins throughout the body. The severity of the symptoms depends on the number of tumor cells present or the tumor burden. The most common presentation of multiple myeloma is bone pain together with anemia. Bone pain results from either destructive bone lesions or bone tenderness caused by extensive bone marrow involvement. Pain usually involves the back or chest or, less commonly, the arms and legs. Skeletal lesions may result in pathologic fractures (the vertebra), spinal cord compression, and hypercalcemia (caused by the breakdown of bone). Hypercalcemia, in turn, causes nausea, vomiting, constipation, frequent urination, dehydration, increased thirst, weakness, and mental status changes. Bone marrow depression with anemia and/or leukopenia and thrombocytopenia signifies replacement of normal cells with tumor cells. Symptoms of anemia include weakness, fatigue, and loss of appetite. This places the patient at enormous risk for infection, which increases throughout the course of the disease as the patient is treated with cytotoxic and steroid therapy (Varricchio et al., 1997).

The current treatment options for multiple myeloma include watchful waiting (for early or smoldering multiple myeloma), chemotherapy, immune-modulating drugs, and stem cell transplantation. An oral melphalan-prednisone combination is recommended for individuals older than age 70 and younger individuals who will not be undergoing stem cell transplantation. Melphalan (Alkeran®, GlaxoSmithKline, Research Triangle Park, NC), in turn, causes bone marrow suppression and renal insufficiency. The side effects of prednisone are dyspepsia, hyperglycemia, fluid and sodium retention, steroid psychosis, and myopathy. This therapy is given for four days every four weeks. VAD (vincristine [Oncovin®, Lilly, Indianapolis, IN], doxorubicin [Adriamycin®, Pfizer, New York, NY], dexamethasone [Decadron®, Merck, West Point, PA]) chemotherapy has been successful with patients who have not responded to initial treatment or have relapsed. Most chemotherapy agents have emetogenic potential; doxorubicin and vincristine have a moderate to very low percentage (respectively) for emetogenesis. With the onset and duration being four to eight hours, all patients are pretreated with antiemetics to reduce this side effect. This treatment regimen is administered intravenously for 4 days every 28 days, and dexamethasone is given orally over 4 days on a weekly basis. Interferon has been used as maintenance therapy following response to induction chemotherapy. Interferon can cause anorexia, fatigue, flu-like syndrome, thrombocytopenia, hepatic toxicity, and mental status changes (Pazdur et al., 2001; Varricchio et al., 1997).

Thalidomide (Thalomid®, Celgene, Warren, NJ) is an immune-modulating drug that may slow the growth of plasma cells and reduce their numbers. Thalidomide is useful in patients with newly diagnosed, relapsed, and refractory multiple myeloma. It is used alone or with prednisone as initial treatment. Side effects associated with this drug include neuropathy, constipation, and somnolence. Its lack of myelosuppression makes it amenable to be combined with cytotoxic chemotherapy. Bortezomib (Velcade®, Millennium Pharmaceuticals, Cambridge, MA) is one of a new class of drugs (protease inhibitor) that has shown effectiveness in treating patients with refractory multiple myeloma (Multiple Myeloma Research Foundation, 2002).

In the absence of curative treatment for multiple myeloma, supportive care to prevent or ameliorate complications and optimize the patient's quality of life assumes primary importance. Pain management with narcotics and non-narcotic alternatives helps to maintain physical activity, promote bone strength, and may counter bone loss. Anemia, especially in older adults, causes significant fatigue and weakness. Patients and families may need instruction in regard to energy conservation and adequate nutritional support. Blood transfusions provide temporary improvement, and erythropoietin (Epogen®, Amgen, Thousand Oaks, CA) has been shown to raise hemoglobin levels.

Infection remains the most common cause of death. Patients and their families must be taught the importance of recognizing and reporting early signs of infection (Varricchio et al., 1997).

Nutritional Implications

Hypercalcemia is one manifestation of the disease with nutritional implications. It leads to loss of appetite, nausea, and thirst, possibly impacting overall nutritional status. Restriction of dietary calcium is not indicated for these patients. The elevation of calcium is secondary to myeloma cells, which form in the hard, outer part of bone, damaging and weakening bones, and, hence, releasing calcium into the blood (Eldridge, Rock, & McCallum, 2001; National Cancer Institute [NCI], 2002).

Hypercalcemia, a metabolic problem, cannot be corrected by diet. Although calcium is not restricted in the diet, care should be taken to assess if the patient is receiving any supplemental forms of calcium via mineral intake (e.g., antacids) or high doses of vitamin D via supplements. A multivitamin usually is not a concern, especially if the amounts are not more than 100% of the daily value. If the patient has a low appetite and oral intake, multivitamins may be indicated. Hypercalcemia is more likely to occur in patients who are relatively immobile and have a poor fluid intake, so attention to these issues is needed as well. Routinely evaluate the total daily fluid intake as part of the overall assessment. See Appendix I for recommendations for fluid needs.

Medications to inhibit bone resorption, such as pamidronate (Aredia®, Novartis, East Hanover, NJ) or zoledronate (Zometa®, Novartis), usually are administered as part of the overall treatment. A rise in clinical lab values of serum creatinine may be secondary to the multiple myeloma itself or medications versus a need for any nutritional changes.

Because multiple myeloma is a chronic disease, patients often are treated with many chemotherapy regimens. Thus, it is very important to perform a thorough nutrition assessment and regularly follow these patients. Unless the patients are losing a lot of weight, they usually do not raise a nutritional red flag. This chronic disorder affects an older population group faced with bone pain, possible immobility because of the pain, and loss of appetite, all of which can trap patients in a downward nutritional spiral. Attention to adequate nutrient-dense calories, protein, and fluid is a necessity.

Chemotherapy such as VAD, bortezomib, and thalidomide cause the expected decrease in cell counts, both white and red blood cells. Bortezomib is a proteasome inhibitor and is the first treatment in more than a decade to be approved for patients with myeloid myeloma. It has been approved for patients who have received at least two prior therapies and have disease progression on the last therapy. Bortezomib may be combined with other chemotherapy treatments or radiation for an additive effect. The Summit Trial (Multiple Myeloma Research Foundation, 2002) noted the most common side effects in patients: nausea 64%, diarrhea and fatigue, each, 49%, low platelet counts 44%, constipation 43%, peripheral neuropathy 35%, and loss of appetite 34%. Nausea is largely controlled via antiemetics. Generally, this group is treated with greater caloric- and nutrient-dense foods, with attention to adequate liquids as dehydration is a concern, and with an antidiarrhea and low-lactose diet, as needed, although constipation may be more of a problem. Provide calorie-dense liquids, such as shakes made with plain yogurt, protein powder, and fruit, per the patients' preference.

Neuropathy appears to be a common symptom affecting these patients because of the chemotherapy medications used. Nutritionally, glutamine and vitamin B_6 have been studied for their neurologic effects. Supplemental glutamine has been reported to improve nutritional status, decrease intestinal injury and bacterial translocation, reduce endotoxemia, and improve overall survival. Savarese, Boucher, and Corey (1998) reported the use of oral glutamine to prevent paclitaxel-induced myalgias and arthralgias. Ten grams of glutamine mixed in water, juice, or foods, such as as yogurt or applesauce, three times daily for five days after paclitaxel administration has been used. Consider using glutamine anecdotally to help with minimizing or preventing worsening neuropathy.

Nutrition is invaluable in addressing the bloating and excess gas production seen in patients receiving bortezomib. Educate the patient and/or family regarding minimizing gas-producing foods such as vegetables and vegetable juices. Keep in mind the universal acceptance of the importance of including phytochemical-rich foods in the daily diet.

The use of prednisone and other steroid medications such as dexamethasone (Decadron) temporarily may increase the appetite and blood glucose levels. Patient education on choosing foods with greater nutrient value and avoiding refined sugars and sweets is indicated.

Anemia is present in approximately two-thirds of patients at the time of diagnosis. However, during chemotherapy, there may be a further reduction in red blood cells, hemoglobin, and hematocrit. Attention to adequate building blocks of cells as protein, iron, and vitamin B_{12} is necessary, even though anemia is a clinical manifestation of multiple myeloma. Patient education should address building blocks. Basic guidelines for a low bacteria or neutropenic diet are found in Appendix K.

Assessment Guidelines

Because multiple myeloma usually is diagnosed in middle-aged or older populations, a complete nutrition assessment should be addressed, taking into account other comorbidities such as diabetes, heart disease, and osteoporosis. Lab values should be reviewed and monitored with the same frequency as those of patients with cancer; however, certain lab values should be looked at more closely.

Complete blood count—anemia is inherent in the disease; assess specifically for any nutrition-induced anemia, as in monitoring serum ferritin.

Chemistry panel—assess kidney function. Serum creatinine rises with myeloma activities, chemotherapy medications, and secondary to hypercalcemia. Ensure the patient is maintaining adequate hydration.

The patients' type of treatment may be one of the following (International Myeloma Foundation, 2003).

Stabilizing—countering the life-threatening disruptions to body chemistry. Limited nutritional intervention should be provided at this stage until the patient is stabilized.

Palliative—in advanced cancer, approximately 85% of patients experience anorexia and cachexia; the great majority suffer from intense fatigue, unrelieved by napping or resting. Support the patient by encouraging small, frequent meals and liquids of high-calorie density that are appealing to sight, taste, and smell. Encourage easy-to-consume foods that take a minimum amount of energy to eat (e.g., soft foods, puddings, shakes).

Remission inducing—use of chemotherapy or radiation therapy to kill malignant cells. The goal of preserving functional status is to ensure quality of life (activities of daily living, weight stability, and skeletal muscle mass preservation, as able). Focus on aggressive nutrition to preserve weight and lean body mass.

Curative—bone marrow transplants.

Nutritional Plan

To date, no specific diet has been developed for patients with multiple myeloma. Rather, these patients generally use the same recommendations suggested for other patients with cancer (see Appendix C). Attention to adequate hydration and appropriate protein and calcium intake, once the disease is controlled, is important. A complete assessment of the patient's use of any vitamin, mineral, or herbal supplements should be completed. Caution should be used with vitamin C supplements, as high doses (> 1,000 mg/day) may be counterproductive in myeloma and may further compromise kidney function.

Care Plan

A multidisciplinary approach should be a model used in all oncology settings and should include
- Nursing—assessment and support, initial and ongoing
- Pharmacy support—bisphosphonates (for myeloma bone disease), antidepressants, and pain management, as needed
- Nutrition education and support—initial and ongoing
- Psychosocial support—depression can be severe, especially because of the chronic nature of disease and the need for pain management.

Expected Outcomes of Therapy

Promising new therapies for multiple myeloma have increased the response rate from 30%–40% to 60%–70% (NCI, 2002). Early intervention can help to support the patient during treatment, which may be a long course. Attention to maintaining weight and preserving lean body mass during treatment is the goal. A secondary goal is preventing large amounts of weight gain if the patient is on steroids and preserving the functionality of patients in the older population.

Melanoma

Overview

This malignant cutaneous tumor originates from a melanocyte, which derives from the neural crest and migrates, most commonly, to the skin and less commonly to the eye, central nervous system, and respiratory, gastrointestinal, or genitourinary tract. Melanoma usually is curable in early stages. It is known to have long periods of remission before recurring. It is likely to spread to other parts of the body and be fatal. Because melanoma occurs primarily on the skin, public and professional education has resulted in this malignancy being detected at earlier, curable stages.

Incidence

The incidence of melanoma has been increasing. It now ranks as the fifth most common malignancy in the United States (Jemal et al., 2005; Rigel, Friedman, & Kopf, 1996). Among Whites, melanoma occurs most frequently in fair-skinned, light-haired individuals who sunburn easily and rarely or never tan. African Americans are at a lower risk than Whites. In men, melanoma often is found on the trunk (the area between the shoulders and the hips), head, or neck. In women, it often develops on the lower legs. Melanoma accounts for approximately 4% of skin cancer cases, but it causes about 79% of skin cancer deaths (American Cancer Society [ACS], 2005). The number of new cases of melanoma in the United States is on the rise. ACS estimated that in 2005, 59,580 new cases of melanoma will occur in the United States, and approximately 7,770 people will die from this disease (Jemal et al.).

Risk Factors and Prevention

Malignant melanoma risk is related to
- Excessive sun exposure—ultraviolet radiation
- Severe blistering sunburns, especially before age 17
- Family history of melanoma
- Personal history of melanoma or skin cancer
- More than 50 nevi (ordinary moles)
- Fair skin
- Weakened immune system
- Dysplastic nevi (changes in mole formation).

Medical professionals should be able to identify people at high risk for melanoma. The most important risk factors include persistently changing moles, older age, dysplastic moles with or without familial melanoma, and ethnicity (being white) (Helfand, Mahon, Eden, Frame, & Orleans, 2001). People who suffer severe, blistering sunburns, particularly in childhood or teenage years, are at increased risk for melanoma (Abraham & Allegra, 2001; ACS, 2004).

Treatment Modalities

Melanomas that have not spread beyond the site at which they developed are highly curable. However, there is a high incidence of relapse in high-risk patients. High-risk patients are defined as those with lesions greater than 4 mm thick, with lymph node involvement, or both. Surgical excision is the primary treatment of melanoma (Varricchio et al., 1997).

Nodal dissection is indicated when nodal involvement is present. Chemotherapy and radiation therapy are not alternatives to surgery, and they have not proven to be as effective as adjuvant therapies. Chemotherapy drugs used to treat melanoma include carmustine (BiCNU®, Bristol-Myers Squibb Oncology Division, Princeton, NJ), cisplatin, and vinblastine; DTIC® (dacarbazine) (Bayer, West Haven, CT), cisplatin, and vinblastine is another combination. Temozolomide (Temodar®, Schering, Kenilworth, NJ) is a new drug that works similarly to DTIC but can be taken orally. Recent studies suggest that combining several chemotherapy agents with one or more immunotherapy drugs may be more effective (Cascinelli et al., 2001). Radiation therapy is used as palliative treatment of metastatic melanoma and as postoperative treatment for cutaneous melanoma of the head and neck region. Immunotherapy, such as interferon, also is used. Interferon alpha-2b is the first and most active adjuvant therapy identified, showing relapse-free survival benefits in high-risk patients (Cascinelli et al.).

Nutritional Implications

High-dose interferon alpha can cause flu-like symptoms, including fever, chills, body aches, severe tiredness, loss of appetite, and depression. Patients may experience nausea, vomiting, and diarrhea. All of these side effects could cause a significant drop in a patient's appetite and intake and, thus, compromise nutritional status. Patients can lose weight rapidly during the initial month of treatment, as it is given five days a week for four weeks. Side effects and weight loss eventually will level off as drug doses decrease and patients adjust to the treatment. Nevertheless, early nutritional intervention is crucial in reducing the amount of weight lost and maintaining muscle mass. A weight loss of 20–30 pounds or more is common. Chemotherapies can cause nausea, vomiting, neutropenia, and fatigue and, thus, potential weight loss and compromised nutritional status.

Assessment Guidelines

Although most patients with melanoma appear healthy upon initial presentation, a nutrition assessment still should be performed, taking into account possible comorbidities, such as diabetes and heart disease, that require special nutritional considerations during the course of melanoma treatment. Review of the patient's medical history, medication, and lab values is a part of standard nutrition assessment.

The patient's diet history, eating and drinking habits, and usage of vitamins and dietary or herbal supplements should be discussed and assessed to see if there are any potential deficiencies, excesses, or interference that would impact treatment. Excessive alcohol intake should be noted and discussed with the patient, as alcohol may impact liver function and inhibit nutrient uptake, especially if the patient already shows signs of macrocytic anemia. The patient's diet history provides a tool for education. Based on fluid intake, the clinician could advise how much fluid to add. Through diet history, one can accentuate what is good and modify what could be better. It is not necessary to alter the patient's diet dramatically during this stressful time.

During the first month of high-dose interferon alpha therapy, fluid, calorie, and protein needs are greater because weight loss is a major side effect of treatment. Fluid needs are calculated based on the patient's body weight: 30 cc/kg plus an extra 500 ml for fever and insensible fluid loss. The Harris-Benedict formula is the most commonly used method to calculate basal energy expenditure (BEE) (see Appendix F). The estimated energy requirement is the BEE multiplied by a hypermetabolic factor of 1.4. If weight loss occurs after one week of therapy, an additional 500 calories per day may be needed for weight gain as well as weight maintenance. Protein needs are calculated as 1.2–1.5 g/kg. The patient should be instructed to monitor his or her weight three times per week. However, in the clinical setting, weight should be recorded at each visit, and a clinician or dietitian should evaluate the patient on a weekly basis. Weekly assessment includes weight, biochemical data, fluid and food intake, and treatment-related nausea, vomiting, malaise, and bowel irregularities. Proper nutritional interventions would be initiated per the clinician's assessment for symptomatic management.

Once the patient is on the maintenance dose of interferon alpha, fluids, calories, and protein may be readjusted per the patient's weight, biochemical data, and clinician's assessment and judgments.

As part of a thorough clinical and nutritional assessment, evaluating the patient's support system and functional mobility is important. By understanding the patient's support system and social function, the clinician can help the patient to strategize how to meet nutritional, emotional, physical, and social needs. If the patient has no support system or has limited financial resources, the clinician should involve a social worker or refer the patient to community- or hospital-based support groups for further assistance. Understanding the patient's level of mobility helps the clinician to guide the patient's daily activities and exercise regimen. The patient should be strongly encouraged to maintain daily activities and exercise as much as possible despite becoming fatigued.

Special Considerations

Besides taking antiemetics, patients should consume small, frequent meals consisting of bland, low-fat, low-acidic foods to mitigate nausea. Dry, starchy foods, such as saltines, pretzels, bagels, and baked potatoes, tend to ameliorate nausea. Antidiarrheal agents and a low-fiber, bland diet should manage diarrhea. Nausea, vomiting, and diarrhea may subside; however, poor appetite and fatigue may continue throughout the treatment.

Diet should be high in protein and calories and rich with omega-3 fatty acids. Many researchers believe that omega-3 fatty acids have a direct effect to counter some of the catabolic mediators involved in cancer and cachexia (Fearon et al., 2003; Ottery, 1995; Varricchio et al., 1997). Because patients exhibit strong catabolic response with high-dose interferon, it may be important to include these fatty acids in daily nutritional planning. The ideal intake of omega-3 fatty acids presently is unclear. However, the U.S. Food and Drug Administration has ruled that an intake of up to 3 g/day of marine omega-3 fatty acids generally is recognized as safe for diet inclusion (Kris-Etherton, Harris, & Appel, 2002).

Because of severe flu-like symptoms and fatigue, it would be ideal to have meals that require minimum preparation, are packed with the most nutrients, and take the least energy to consume. Patients should enrich food with protein powder and/or flaxseed oil (contains omega-3 fatty acids) whenever possible. These could be added to hot cereals, mashed potatoes, cream soups, casserole dishes, meatloaf, fruit smoothies, gravies, and sauces for extra protein, calories, and nutrients. Nutrient-dense beverages (e.g., yogurt shakes, fruit smoothies, juices, soups, commercial high-calorie, high-protein liquid nutritional supplements) are highly recommended instead of water alone. Fluid needs are greater than usual, especially when patients are dealing with fever and chills. Encourage patients to drink fluids before and after their interferon injection.

Although it is easy to instruct patients to rest when flu-like symptoms and fatigue occur, small increments of exercise, such as walking, swimming, and isometric/resistance exercise, should be encouraged. When patients are more adjusted to the treatment, levels of activity and exercise should increase. Exercise helps to boost energy. Numerous recent studies have shown the benefits of exercise during cancer treatment, including improved sleep at night, better muscle maintenance, improved performance status, and better quality of life (Ardies, 2002; Dimeo, Schwartz, & Fietz, 2003; Segal et al., 2003).

Having adequate protein and calories to prevent severe weight loss is crucial and important to impart during a patient and family education session. Incorporation of five servings of fruits and vegetables should be emphasized as well. Creamed vegetable soup or juices and fruit smoothies are good ways to incorporate phytonutrients' anticancer, antioxidant, and cell regulatory benefits (Wallace, 2002).

Even with high-protein, high-calorie, and omega-3-rich diet, with some forms of exercise, some patients continue to lose weight. Novel agents and/or specific amino acids, such as anabolic agents and specific amino acids, creatine, N-acetyl-cysteine, glutamine, and arginine, may prove to be beneficial (Baracos, 2004). However, at present, little is known about the optimal amino acid mixtures that could support anabolism and function in patients with cancer.

Care Plan

Ideally, a multidisciplinary approach should be used in all oncology settings and include
- Nursing assessment and support
- Pharmacy support—physician-prescribed appetite stimulants; anabolic agents may be needed if weight loss becomes severe. Initiation of an antidepressant prior to interferon therapy may be beneficial if the patient has a preexisting history of depression.
- Nutrition education and support and ongoing follow-up. Fluid, calorie, and protein needs must continue to be adjusted at each follow-up assessment.
- Psychosocial support—depression can be severe, and the patient may have suicidal ideations. Coping mechanisms, a support system, and resources in the community should be available to the patient.

Expected Outcomes of Therapy

Early nutritional intervention and support upon the initiation of melanoma treatment, especially high-dose interferon alpha, can reduce the severity of weight loss and possibly reduce the level of treatment-related toxicities. Although no data show that nutritional intervention would ensure completion of treatment, many incidences indicate discontinuation of treatment because of drug toxicities and/or severe weight loss. Proper nutrition and hydration would decrease severity of weight loss and hospitalization associated with treatment-related side effects such as dehydration, nausea, vomiting, or diarrhea. It is expected that with adequate protein intake, exercise, and novel agents (either omega-3 fatty acids or anabolic steroids), patients will be able to maintain muscle mass and, thus, have an improved sense of well-being and functionality. Ultimately, the expected outcome of nutrition therapy is to see patients complete their therapy and achieve long-term survival.

Sarcoma

Overview

Sarcoma is composed of cells derived from connective tissue such as bone and cartilage, muscle, blood vessel, or lymphoid tissue. These tumors develop rapidly and metastasize through the lymph node channels. Ewing's sarcoma is a malignant tumor of the bone that arises in the medullary tissue and occurs more often in cylindrical bones, with pain, fever, and leukocytosis as prominent symptoms. Fibrosarcoma arises from collagen-producing fibroblasts. Soft tissue sarcomas are more commonly found in the extremities, with the second most common site being the retroperitoneum. Kaposi's sarcoma is a malignant neoplastic vascular proliferation characterized by the development of bluish-red cutaneous nodules, usually on the lower extremities, which spread slowly, increase in size and number, and spread to more proximal sites. These tumors often remain confined to the skin and subcutaneous tissue, but widespread visceral involvement may occur. They are grouped separately because they do not share the same clinical and microscopic characteristics as the other sarcomas and are treated differently (Jemal et al., 2005).

Incidence

Soft tissue sarcomas are very rare tumors, accounting for approximately 1% of newly diagnosed cancers in the United States. Primary malignant bone tumors also are rare, comprising approximately 0.2% of all new cancers in the United States (Jemal et al., 2005).

More than 30 different histologic subtypes of soft tissue sarcoma have been identified, and these tumors can be found anywhere in the body where soft tissues are located (see Table 14-1). Soft tissues where sarcomas may arise include adipose tissue, muscle tissue, connective tissue, nerve tissue, fibrous tissue, synovial tissue, and blood and lymph vessels.

Grading

Sarcomas commonly are graded as low, intermediate, or high. Low-grade sarcomas rarely spread to distant sites, whereas high-grade sarcomas have an increased incidence of metastasis, with the most common site being the lung (Jemal et al., 2005).

Table 14-1. Common Bone Tumors

Tumor	Benign	Malignant
Bone	Osteoid osteoma	Osteosarcoma
	Osteoblastoma	
Cartilage	Osteochondroma	Chondrosarcoma
	Enchondroma	
	Chondroblastoma	
Fibrous	Nonossifying fibroma	Malignant fibrous histiocytoma
Miscellaneous	Giant cell tumor	Ewing's sarcoma
	Hemangioma	Chorodoma
	Langerhans cell histiocytosis	Adamantinoma
	Unicameral bone cyst	Lymphoma
	Aneurysmal bone cyst	Multiple myeloma

Etiology

The etiology of sarcomas is unknown, but there are some predisposing factors, such as family history and exposure to high-dose radiation and chemicals (e.g., henoxyacetic acid, herbicides, chlorphenols in wood preservative). People with certain inherited diseases such as neurofibromatosis have been shown to have a higher risk of developing a soft tissue sarcoma.

Treatment

Treatment varies depending on the stage of the sarcoma. The following are treatment modalities (NCI, 2003).

- For low-grade soft tissue sarcoma (stages IA, IB, and IIA), surgery is considered the primary therapy. If the tumor is unresectable, high-dose preoperative radiation therapy may be used, followed by surgical resection and postoperative radiation therapy. For tumors of the retroperitoneum, trunk, and head and neck, postoperative radiation therapy is administered to maximize local control if negative margins cannot be obtained.

- For high-grade soft tissue sarcoma with or without distant metastasis (stages IIB, IIC, and III), surgery still is considered. If the tumor is unresectable, high-dose radiation therapy may be used, but poor local control is likely to result. In some situations, radiation therapy or chemotherapy may be used prior to surgery to shrink the tumor and possibly preserve limbs. Postoperative radiation therapy may follow.

- With distant metastasis (stage IV), surgery with curative intent is possible for patients with limited pulmonary metastases and with complete resection of the primary tumor. Chemotherapy and radiation therapy often are used for palliation when the tumor is unresectable. The most commonly used chemotherapeutic drugs are ifosfamide (Ifex®, Bristol-Myers Squibb Oncology) and doxorubicin. Drugs such as dacarbazine and methotrexate, vincristine, cisplatin (Platinol®, Bristol-Myers Squibb Oncology), paclitaxel (Taxol®, Bristol-Myers Squibb Oncology), and others are added in combination. When several drugs are used together, the regimen is given a shortened name, such as MAID (combined mesna, doxorubicin, ifosfamide, and dacarbazine) or AIM (doxorubicin, ifosfamide, and mesna).

Nutritional Implications

Depending on the site of sarcoma and treatment modalities, nutrition can be significantly impacted. Proper nutrition would ensure surgical success with lower infection rate, quicker recovery, and the physical stamina to undergo postoperative radiation therapy or chemotherapy.

Radiation to the head and neck, gastrointestinal (gastrointestinal stoma tumor), and abdominal areas (uterine sarcoma) requires special nutritional attention (see Appendix D).

When radiation is given to the head and neck area, mucositis, xerostomia, ageusia, dysphagia, and esophagitis all are possible side effects that impact a patient's ability to obtain adequate hydration and nutrition. If radiation is given to the gastric, abdominal, or pelvic field, a patient's nutrition could be compromised because of nausea, vomiting, dyspepsia, and diarrhea. Chemotherapeutic agents such as ifosfamide and cisplatin are highly emetogenic and require antiemetic agents for early and late onset nausea and vomiting. Eating is problematic for most patients during the first week of chemotherapy. Small, frequent meals that are bland, low fat, low acid, and room temperature generally are better tolerated. Food should not have a strong odor. Antinausea medication can cause constipation to last for up to a week. Stool softeners and laxative agents need to be considered. Magnesium-based laxative agents may work the best, as cisplatin has a hypomagnesemia effect. Mucositis may be seen in some patients; therefore, the diet needs to be modified to decrease mucosal irritation. Aggressive hydration, frequent voiding, and administration of mesna can prevent hemorrhagic cystitis related to ifosfamide. Treatment for advanced sarcoma can be rigorous and difficult to tolerate; treatment-related side effects affect a patient's nutrition and sense of well-being. Appendix C provides detailed information regarding symptom management.

Assessment Guidelines

Nutrition assessment for sarcoma is similar to all other types of cancer; see previous guidelines for multiple myeloma or melanoma and Appendicies F, G, H, and I.

Special Considerations for Nutrition Care Planning

It is advisable to have patients maintain body weight throughout treatment, unless weight loss is experienced prior to diagnosis or postsurgery. Because a diet that is high in protein is needed for all treatment modalities, it is important to include protein with every meal and snack. Diet should be modified per symptoms as radiation treatments progress. Radiation to the head and neck area would mandate a soft or pureed/liquid diet that is low in acid but high in protein, calories, and nutrient density. Radiation to the pelvic field requires a low-fiber, low-lactose diet with probiotics and soluble fiber (e.g., Benefiber® [Novartis], Citrucel® [GlaxoSmithKline]). For specific and detailed nutritional considerations, please consult Chapter 6 on gynecologic cancer and Appendices C and D.

Amino acids such as glutamine have proven to be beneficial to the health of intestinal epithelium (Miller, 1999; Reeds & Burrin, 2001), as they are a major fuel for the enterocytes. Depletion of glutamine can result in atrophy, ulceration, and necrosis of the gut epithelium. Thus, glutamine should be considered as a part of the standard nutrition therapy during radiation to the head and neck (Skubitz & Anderson, 1996), gastrointestinal area, or abdominal and pelvic field. Chemotherapy side effects, such as nausea, vomiting, and neutropenia, are common. The nutritional considerations will not be further elaborated in this section, as they have been discussed in previous sections.

Expected Outcomes of Therapy

Proper nutrition ensures a faster recovery from surgery, postoperative radiation, or chemotherapy. Early nutritional intervention and education will decrease potential treatment-related side effects and severity of side effects and, ultimately, improve the patient's sense of well-being and quality of life. The patient is expected to know how much and what type of fluids to consume to maintain adequate hydration and electrolyte balance. The patient also should have a clear understanding of diet and nutrition to manage side effects and to ensure proper healing and recovery.

References

Abraham, J., & Allegra, C.J. (2001). Skin cancer and melanoma. In U. Hegde & B. Gause (Eds.), *Bethesda handbook of clinical oncology* (pp. 249–268). Philadelphia: Lippincott Williams & Wilkins.

American Cancer Society. (2004). *Overview: How is melanoma skin cancer treated?* Retrieved April 4, 2004, from http://www.cancer.org/docroot/cri/content/cri_2_2_4x_how_is _melanoma_skin.cancer_treated_50.asp

American Cancer Society. (2005). *Cancer facts and figures, 2005.* Atlanta, GA: Author.

Ardies, C.M. (2002). Exercise, cachexia, and cancer therapy: A molecular rationale. *Nutrition and Cancer, 42,* 143–157.

Baracos, V.E. (2004). New approaches in reversing cancer-related weight loss. *Oncology Issues, 19*(Suppl.), 6–10. Retrieved February 11, 2005, from http://www.accc-cancer. org/ONIS/suppl_nutri2.asp

Cascinelli, N., Belli, F., MacKie, R.M., Santinami, M., Bufalino, R., & Morabito, A. (2001). Effect of long-term adjuvant therapy with interferon alpha-2a in patients with regional node metastases from cutaneous melanoma: A randomized trial. *Lancet, 358,* 866–869.

Dimeo, F., Schwartz, S., & Fietz, T. (2003). Effects of endurance training on the physical performance of patients with hematological malignancies during chemotherapy. *Supportive Care in Cancer, 11,* 623–628.

Eldridge, B., Rock, C.L., & McCallum, P.D. (2001). Nutrition and the patient with cancer. In A.M. Coulston, C.L. Rock, & E.R. Monsen (Eds.), *Nutrition in the prevention and treatment of disease* (pp. 397–411). San Diego, CA: Academic Press.

Fearon, K.C., Von Neyenfeldt, M.F., Moses, A.G., VanGeenen, R., Roy, A., & Couma, D.J. (2003). Effects of protein and energy dense N-3 fatty acid enriched oral supplement on loss of weight and lean tissue in cancer cachexia: A randomized double blind trial. *Gut, 52,* 1391–1392.

Helfand, M., Mahon, S.M., Eden, K.B., Frame, P.S., & Orleans, C.T. (2001). Screening for skin cancer. *American Journal of Preventive Medicine, 20*(Suppl. 3), 47–58.

Jemal, A., Murray, T., Ward, E., Samuels, A., Tiwari, R.C., Ghafoor, A., et al. (2005). Cancer statistics, 2005. *CA: A Cancer Journal for Clinicians, 55,* 10–30.

Kris-Etherton, P.M., Harris, W.S., & Appel, L.J. (2002). Fish consumption, fish oil, omega-3 fatty acids, and cardiovascular disease. American Heart Association Scientific Statement. *Circulation, 106,* 2747–2757.

Miller, A.L. (1999). Therapeutic consideration of L-glutamine: A review of the literature. *Alternative Medicine Review, 4,* 239–248.

Multiple Myeloma Research Foundation. (2002). *Myeloma treatments, Velcade.* Retrieved March 26, 2004, from http://www.multiplemyeloma.org/treatments/3.05.asp

National Cancer Institute. (2002). *What you need to know about multiple myeloma.* Retrieved April 4, 2004, from http://www.cancer.gov/cancerinfo/wyntk/myeloma

National Cancer Institute. (2003, December 12). *Adult soft tissue sarcoma (PDQ): Treatment.* Retrieved April 5, 2004, from http://www.cancer.gov/cancerinfo/pdq/treatment/adult-soft-tissue-sarcoma/HealthProfessional

Ottery, F. (1995). Supportive nutrition to prevent cachexia and improve quality of life. *Seminars in Oncology, 22*(Suppl. 3), 98–111.

Pazdur, R., Coia, L., Hoskins, W., & Wagman, L. (2001). *Cancer management: A multidisciplinary approach. Medical, surgical and radiation oncology* (5th ed.). Philadelphia: F.A. Davis.

Reeds, P.J., & Burrin, D.G. (2001). Glutamine and the bowel. *Journal of Nutrition, 131*(Suppl. 9), 2505S–2508S.

Savarese, D., Boucher, J., & Corey, B. (1998). Glutamine treatment of paclitaxel-induced myalgias and arthralgias. *Journal of Clinical Oncology, 12,* 3918–3919.

Segal, R.J., Reid, R.D., Courneya, K.S., Malone, S.C., Parliament, M.B., Scott, C.B., et al. (2003). Resistance exercise in men receiving androgen deprivation therapy for prostate cancer. *Journal of Clinical Oncology, 21,* 1653–1659.

Skubitz, K.M., & Anderson, P.M. (1996). Oral glutamine to prevent chemotherapy induced stomatitis: A pilot study. *Journal of Laboratory and Clinical Medicine, 127*(2), 223–228.

Turgeon, M.L. (1999). *Clinical hematology: Theory and procedures* (3rd ed.). Chula Vista, CA: Scripps.

Varricchio, C., Pierce, M., Walker, C.L., & Ades, T.B. (1997). *A cancer source book for nurses* (7th ed.). Sudbury, MA: Jones and Bartlett.

Wallace, J.M. (2002). Nutritional and botanical modulation of the inflammatory cascade—eicosanoids, cyclooxygenases, and lipoxygenases—as an adjunct in cancer therapy. *Integrative Cancer Therapy, 1*(1), 7–37.

CHAPTER 15

Pediatric Cancers

Ria G. Hawks, RN, MS, CNS, CPNP
Elena J. Ladas, MS, RD

Incidence of Childhood Cancer

Each year, approximately 12,000 children and adolescents are diagnosed with cancer in the United States (Ries et al., 1999). The chance that a child will develop cancer is approximately 1 in 333 and is slightly more likely in males. The incidence of childhood cancer increased between 1975 and 1995, mainly because of an increased number of brain tumors diagnosed with the availability of magnetic resonance imaging (Smith, Freidlin, Ries, & Simon, 1998) and an increased number of lymphomas associated with HIV infection (Ries et al.). Cancer accounts for approximately 12% of childhood deaths, second only to accidents (Jemal et al., 2005).

Causes of Childhood Cancer

Children with cancer account for only 1% of all patients with cancer, and their cancers are distinct compared to adults. Pediatric tumors differ in diagnosis, clinical manifestations, and response to therapy and overall survival. Childhood cancer usually originates from blood-forming tissues or bones and muscles deep within, arising from ectodermal or mesodermal tissues. The endodermal layer gives rise to most adult malignancies, whereas environmental exposures have had the greatest influence over the decades (Baggott, Kelly, Fochtman, & Foley, 2002). Unlike cancer screening in adults, no effective screening is available for childhood cancer, and pediatric patients often present with disseminated disease. Yet, the cancer of childhood is very responsive to therapy, with an overall cure rate for all forms of childhood cancer of greater than 75% (Pizzo & Poplack, 2001). Unlike adults, the etiology of most childhood cancer remains unknown. Most cases of pediatric cancer occur in previously healthy children, and only a few are inherited or present at birth, most notably retinoblastoma. Some childhood cancers are attributable to ionizing radiation, such as brain tumors after cranial irradiation for acute lymphocytic leukemia (ALL) or thyroid cancer after neck and chest irradiation for Hodgkin lymphoma. They may develop as secondary malignancies as a result of chemotherapy, specifically alkylating agents. Other investigators have suggested that parental occupational exposure, maternal exposure, and environmental exposure may contribute to a child's risk of developing cancer; however, these hypotheses remain to be confirmed. Most childhood cancers seem to be caused by randomly occurring mutations in critical genes such as tumor suppressor genes, as has been demonstrated in Wilms' tumor (Kalapurakal et al., 2004).

Types of Cancer and Treatment Modalities

Acute leukemias, lymphomas, brain tumors, and "solid tumors" such as neuroblastoma and Wilms' tumor are the principal cancers observed in pediatric oncology. Incidence of a specific histology often correlates with age. Neuroblastoma is most common in infants and toddlers, ALL is seen most commonly in school-age children, and osteogenic sarcoma is primarily a disease of adolescents (Ries et al., 1999). Treatment modalities generally include surgery, chemotherapy, radiation therapy, and/or biologic therapies.

Acute Leukemias

Acute leukemias are the most common pediatric malignancy. Leukemias are subdivided according to the type of blood cell involved (lymphocytic, myeloid, monocytic). In contrast to adult leukemias, nearly all childhood leukemias are of acute onset, and the large majority (75%–80%) are ALL. Demographic features of ALL in childhood include a slight male preponderance, young age at diagnosis (three to five years), higher socioeconomic status, and increased frequency in Caucasians compared to African Americans (Colby-Graham & Chordas, 2003). Specific risk factors include *in utero* x-ray exposure and postnatal therapeutic irradiation. Children with Down syndrome, Bloom syndrome, ataxia-telangiectasia, Fanconi anemia, Wiskott-Aldrich syndrome, and related genetic disorders are at increased risk for the development of ALL (Pui, Relling, Campana, & Evans, 2002). Demographic features of acute myelogenous leukemia (AML) include an increased frequency in Hispanics and an increased risk associated with Down syndrome, *in utero* X-ray exposure or following treatment for another cancer.

Signs and symptoms of acute leukemias are fatigue, pallor, bleeding, fever, lymphadenopathy, bone pain, and occasionally headache, nausea, and vomiting. Diagnosis can be suspected by review of the peripheral blood smear and is confirmed by a bone marrow aspirate. Bone marrow studies typically include blast cell morphology, immunologic phenotype (markers of myeloid derivation or B or T lymphocyte lineage), and chromosome analysis. Risk stratification in ALL depends mainly on age and initial white blood cell (WBC) count, with an age of one to nine and a WBC count less than 50,000/mm³ considered favorable ("standard risk"). Adolescents and children with elevated WBC counts have inferior prognoses ("high risk"), as do children with certain cytogenetic findings, such as Philadelphia chromosome or t(9;22) translocation (Landier, 2001; Pui et al., 2002; Rubnitz & Pui, 2003; Smith et al., 1998). Infants (younger than 12 months) with ALL have a particularly poor prognosis and usually are treated on separate protocols (Pui et al.). Prognosis in AML depends more on disease subtype (promyelocytic being favorable), association with Down syndrome, and availability of an HLA-matched sibling donor for bone marrow transplant (Ebb & Weinstein, 1997). Outcome in all cases depends on response to initial treatment, with a poor outcome anticipated if the patient fails to attain remission.

ALL treatment comprises three distinct phases: (a) remission induction (usually corticosteroids, vincristine [Oncovin®, Lilly, Indianapolis, IN], and asparaginase [Elspar®, Merck, West Point, PA] with daunorubicin hydrochloride [Cerubidine®, Bedford Laboratories, Bedford, OH]), (b) consolidation (additional systemic therapy as well as central nervous system [CNS] prophylaxis with intrathecal methotrexate, adding additional drugs or cranial irradiation in high-risk patients and those with CNS involvement, (c) delayed induction (directed at eliminating residual disease), and (d) maintenance (prolonged therapy with vincristine, prednisone, methotrexate, and mercaptopurine [Purinethol®, Teva, North Wales, PA]) (Pui et al., 2002). Children with ALL are hospitalized initially but receive most treatment as outpatients. Overall cure rate is 80%, unlike adults, for whom the cure rate is 40%–50%. Infants, children with certain cytogenetic abnormalities, and patients failing to achieve remission have a significantly lower overall survival (Pui, 2000).

Treatment of AML is more intensive, requiring prolonged hospitalization. Therapy is based on infusions of cytarabine (Cytosar U®, Teva) and daunorubicin hydrochloride combined with other agents, resulting in marrow aplasia lasting for weeks. Children with matched sibling donors are referred for bone marrow transplant, whereas others receive additional chemotherapy. Overall, duration of AML treatment is shorter than that for ALL. Cure rates are approximately 60%–65% for patients receiving a matched-sibling transplant and 40%–50% for all others (Woods et al., 2001).

Lymphomas

The lymphomas most commonly observed in pediatric oncology are Hodgkin disease and non-Hodgkin lymphoma (NHL). Hodgkin disease is seen primarily in older children and adolescents and typically presents with lymph node enlargement in the neck and/or chest. An association with Epstein-Barr infection has long been suspected (Jarrett & MacKenzie, 1999). Patients with advanced-stage disease have additional involvement of the spleen and abdominal lymph nodes. "B symptoms" of weight loss, pruritus, and night sweats are less common than in adults. The most frequent histology is nodular sclerosis type. All patients receive chemotherapy, whereas radiation therapy is reserved for higher risk patients or those with delayed response to chemotherapy. Cure rates are in the range of 70%–95% (Pizzo & Poplack, 2001). Current treatment protocols emphasize risk-adapted strategies based on gender differences in susceptibility to late effects (Donaldson, Hancock, & Hoppe, 1999). For example, males have a greater risk of infertility following treatment with alkylating agents, whereas females are more susceptible to second malignant neoplasms following irradiation to the chest, and these late effects may be lessened by risk-adapted treatments that minimize exposure to specifically harmful modalities (Donaldson et al.).

Pediatric NHL is a group of disorders including Burkitt's, lymphoblastic, diffuse large cell, and other less common subtypes of lymphoma. The low-grade, indolent lymphomas of adults are not seen in children (Sandlund, Downing, & Crist, 1996). Demographic features include male preponderance and association with immunodeficiency syndromes, including HIV infection and postorgan transplant. Compared to Hodgkin disease, the age at presentation of NHL extends to toddlers, and in addition to lymphadenopathy, there may be visceral and bone marrow or CNS involvement. Treatment is similar to that for ALL, although generally of shorter duration. Cyclophosphamide (Cytoxan®, Bristol-Myers Squibb, New York, NY) is a key agent, and radiotherapy generally is not required. Rituximab (Rituxan®, Genentech, South San Francisco, CA), a monoclonal antibody targeting a B lymphocyte antigen expressed in diffuse large cell lymphomas, currently is under study (Plosker & Figgit, 2003). Cure rates for childhood NHL are in the range of 70%–95%, depending on extent of disease (localized versus disseminated) and presence of CNS disease.

Brain Tumors

Primary CNS tumors are a diverse group of disorders, which together represent the most common type of pediatric solid tumor. Pediatric brain tumors are the leading cause of both cancer-related morbidity and mortality (Packer et al., 2003). CNS tumors occur throughout childhood. The majority are infratentorial, presenting with signs of hydrocephalus (headache, vomiting, and lethargy) and cranial nerve dysfunction. The remainder are supratentorial, presenting with headache, weakness, endocrine disturbance, and seizures. Diagnostic evaluation includes detailed neurologic examination, magnetic resonance imaging, and, in some cases, lumbar puncture for cerebrospinal fluid cytology or tumor marker determination. Approximately half of all childhood CNS tumors are low-grade gliomas occurring in the optic chiasm, suprasellar region, midbrain, and cerebellum. They occur primarily in infants and young children. There is an increased risk of optic gliomas in children with neurofibromatosis type 1, justifying early screening (Rosser & Packer, 2002). Surgery for optic pathway, suprasellar, and diencephalic tumors may be limited to diagnostic biopsy or partial resection, whereas cerebellar astrocytomas usually can be completely resected. Depending on patient age, radiation therapy or chemotherapy may be indicated if residual tumor begins to grow or threatens adjacent vital structures. Overall survival rate exceeds 75%.

Primitive neuroectodermal tumors (PNETs), including cerebellar medulloblastoma, account for approximately one-fourth of pediatric brain tumors. They are characterized by rapid growth and propensity for dissemination throughout the neuraxis. Treatment includes management of hydrocephalus, aggressive resection, radiation therapy to brain and spine with tumor boost, and adjuvant chemotherapy. This approach is modified in very young children to defer or avoid radiation by use of intensive chemotherapy. Overall survival rates are approximately 75%, with localized medulloblastoma having the best outcome, less for disseminated medulloblastoma or supratentorial PNET, and less than 40% for infants with tumors that threaten adjacent vital structures (Pizzo & Poplack, 2001).

Ependymoma is the most common malignant brain tumor of infancy but also occurs throughout childhood and accounts for approximately 10% of childhood brain tumors (Pizzo & Poplack, 2001). Ependymomas are equally divided between supratentorial and infratentorial locations and between cellular ("benign") and anaplastic histologies. Most are localized, with dissemination at diagnosis in approximately 10% of cases (Pizzo & Poplack). Standard treatment includes surgery and involved field irradiation. Current protocols are evaluating the potential role of chemotherapy and second-look surgery in the treatment of ependymoma (Pollack, 1999).

High-grade astrocytomas occur mainly in the cerebral cortex or midbrain locations. They tend to be infiltrative, cause local mass effect, and may be multifocal, but rarely disseminate. Included in this group are anaplastic astrocytoma (grade III) and glioblastoma multiforme (grade IV), as well as gliosarcoma. Related intermediate grade tumors include giant cell astrocytoma, xanthoastrocytoma, and anaplastic oligodendroglioma. Surgical approaches range from biopsy to total excision, depending on location. Standard treatment includes radiation therapy and chemotherapy. Outcome varies with histology and extent of resection but generally is poor for incompletely resected high-grade astrocytomas (Packer, 1999). Diffuse intrinsic brain stem tumors usually are diagnosed radiologically and have a particularly poor outcome. Current protocols for high-grade astrocytomas are testing chemoradiotherapy and high-dose chemotherapy with autologous stem cell rescue. Advances in tumor biology and neuroscience hold promise for the future (Packer & Reddy, 2004).

Solid Tumors

Neuroblastoma is the most common malignancy of infants younger than age one and the most common extracranial solid tumor of childhood, accounting for 7% of childhood cancers. Nearly all cases are diagnosed by age five (Ries et al., 1999). Neuroblastoma arises from postsympathetic adrenergic ganglion cells (neuroblasts), and the primary tumor may originate in the neck, chest, abdomen, or pelvis. The disease is heterogenous both clinically and biologically (Castleberry, 1997). Infants present with localized tumors occasionally discovered on maternal ultrasound studies, although dissemination is the rule beyond age one. The primary tumor is most often located in the adrenal gland and may grow to a large size, crossing the midline. Bone metastases may cause a limp or refusal to bear weight and ecchymotic discoloration of the orbits ("raccoon eyes"). Paraspinous tumors may cause spinal cord compression with extremity weakness (Weinstein, Katzenstein, & Cohn, 2003). Neuroblastoma is metabolically active, and urine catecholamine metabolites are elevated at the time of diagnosis and relapse, making neuroblastoma one of the few childhood cancers with a distinct biologic marker by the ability to measure urinary catecholamines vanillylmandelic acid and homovanillic acid. However, screening in early infancy does not detect the life-threatening metastatic cases destined to present beyond age one (Spix et al., 2003).

Prognostic factors include age, stage, and pathologic features. Infants and children with localized tumors (low risk) are treated with surgery alone, which is curative in 90%–100% (Weinstein et al., 2003). Intermediate-risk patients (mainly infants with regionally extensive tumors) receive moderately intensive four-drug chemotherapy, with survival rates exceeding 80%. Patients with high-risk neuroblastoma (mostly children older than one with histologically aggressive tumors metastatic to bone, bone marrow, lymph nodes, and liver) generally undergo confirmatory biopsy, then receive dose-intensive induction chemotherapy, undergo attempted surgical resection of the tumor, and are further treated with radiation to sites of disease, high-dose chemotherapy with autologous stem cell rescue, and retinoic acid (a differentiation agent) (Weinstein et al.). In spite of this intensive approach, cure rates remain below 35% (Matthay et al., 1999). Newer approaches under evaluation include tandem autotransplants, targeted radio-immunoconjugate, and other cellular immune therapies.

Wilms' Tumor

Wilms' tumor, a cancer of the kidney, accounts for 6% of childhood cancers. The peak incidence is in children two to three years of age. The diagnosis is unusual beyond age 12, when primary renal tumors are more likely to be renal cell carcinomas. Wilms' tumor has interesting associations with syndromes of hemihypertrophy (including Beckwith-Weidemann syndrome), cryptorchidism, hypospadias, and aniridia. The tumor arises from nephrogenic rests (persistent embryonal remnants) and has characteristic chromosomal and molecular abnormalities of 11p13, 11p15, or LOH1p (Kalapurakal et al., 2004). Cases are classified pathologically as "favorable histology," with epithelial, blastemal, and stromal elements, and "unfavorable histology," which includes focal or diffuse anaplasia or clear cell sarcoma. Presenting signs and symptoms include asymptomatic or painful abdominal mass, painless hematuria, hypertension, and malaise. Occasionally, these patients may develop paraneoplastic syndromes, including erythrocytosis, hypercalcemia, Cushing's syndrome, or acquired Von Willebrand's coagulation defect. Treatment is based on staging after initial surgical exploration and attempted resection, determination of histology, and completion of metastatic evaluation. Therapy includes nephrectomy for all patients, dactinomycin (Cosmegen®, Merck) and vincristine therapy for patients with stage I or II disease, an addition of doxorubicin (Adriamycin®, Pfizer, New York, NY) and abdominal irradiation for stage III disease, and a combination of radiotherapy and multiagent chemotherapy for those with stage IV disease. Survival rates range from 96% for stage I to approximately 70% for patients with pulmonary metastases (D'Angio et al., 1989; Pizzo & Poplack, 2001).

Soft Tissue Sarcomas of Skeletal Muscular Origin

Rhabdomyosarcoma is the most common of the soft tissue sarcomas. There are two age peaks: two to four years and early to mid-adolescence. Although a small proportion can be associated with neurofibromatosis type 1 and Li-Fraumeni syndrome, most cases of rhabdomyosarcoma occur sporadically, with no known risk factor (McDowell, 2003).

There are two histologic variants, embryonal and alveolar, as well as several characteristic cytogenetic abnormalities (McDowell, 2003). Rhabdomyosarcoma generally presents as a painless lump with signs and symptoms varying by site: orbital—proptosis without erythema; parameningeal—dysphagia, "sinusitis" jaw pain, proptosis; extremity—painless lump; genitourinary—urinary frequency, obtrusive hematurias, scrotal mass (hernia), and grape-like protruding vaginal mass. Treatment requires a multimodality approach and is based on staging. Treatment includes surgery or lymph node dissection, with resection as a maximum nonmutilating, function-preserving operation, and chemotherapy with or without radiation. Prognosis is related to the site of origin, tumor burden, resectability, presence of metastases, and histopathology. Overall survival is approximately 70%. Patients with localized favorable sites have a greater than 85% survival rate, with the five-year survival for orbit tumors being greater than 95%. For those patients with localized, unfavorable sites, five-year survival is 55%–75%, and patients with metastatic disease at time of diagnosis have a poor outcome, less than 30% survival (Arndt & Crist, 1999).

Bone Tumors

Bone tumors account for 6% of childhood malignancies. They are most common in the second decade of life. The two common types of bone cancer are osteogenic sarcoma and Ewing's sarcoma. Osteogenic sarcoma is derived from a mesenchymal osseous progenitor (osteoblast), and the cause is unknown. A small proportion can be associated with Li-Fraumeni syndrome and hereditary retinoblastoma. Rarely, osteogenic sarcoma can develop as a secondary malignancy associated with radiation therapy for a previous primary malignancy. Osteogenic sarcoma most often occurs near the metaphyseal portion of the long bones: the distal femur, proximal tibia, and proximal humerus. Primary axial-skeletal tumors are rare (Arndt & Crist, 1999). Clinical symptoms are subtle but progress to swelling and pain of the affected area. The patient may present with a pathologic fracture of the affected bone. Patients often relate the onset of symptoms with a trauma to the involved bone, but this is incidental and not causal. Treatment consists of surgery (limb salvage or amputation) and chemotherapy. A biopsy is performed to establish the diagnosis, followed by neoadjuvant chemotherapy for usually 6–10 weeks and definitive surgery. Neoadjuvant therapy may render the primary tumor resectable as well as provide important prognostic pathologic information in response to chemotherapy (Kline & Sevier, 2003). The lungs and bones are the most common sites for metastatic disease. Unilateral or bilateral thoracotomies, dependent on factors such as number, time of occurrence, or previous therapy, may be performed with curative intent to remove pulmonary metastases. For patients with localized tumors, the chance of five-year survival is approximately 65%, and for patients with lung metastases at time of diagnosis, the five-year survival is 25%–35%. Resection of pulmonary metastases may be curative in up to 25% of patients with de novo recurrent metastases (Pizzo & Poplack, 2001).

Ewing's sarcoma of the bone is most common in the second decade of life and accounts for 4% of childhood and adolescent cancers. Ewing's tumor of bone belongs to a group of malignancies known as "small round blue cell tumor" arising from bone, which is of neural crest origin, not osseous origin (Weber & Sim, 2001). Caucasian children have a sixfold higher incidence over African American children. There are no other known risk factors, and sites of origin are equally distributed between axial and appendicular primary. The most common primary sites include the pelvis, proximal bones of the extremities, upper tibia, and ribs (Arndt & Crist, 1999). Common sites of metastases are the lung, bone, and bone marrow. Clinical symptoms at the time of presentation include pain, soft tissue swelling, and related symptoms because of the site of origin. Constitutional symptoms of low-grade fever and weight loss may occur in some patients. Treatment consists of biopsy, neoadjuvant chemotherapy (vincristine, doxorubicin, cyclophosphamide alternating with ifosfamide (Ifex®, Bristol-Myers Squibb Oncology, Princeton, NJ) and etoposide (VePesid®, Bristol-Myers Squibb Oncology), surgical resection, and/or local radiotherapy occurring after induction chemotherapy (Wexler et al., 1996). In contrast to osteogenic sarcoma, Ewing's tumor of bone is sensitive to radiotherapy, and mutilating surgery or amputation is not necessary. However, improved limb-salvage techniques and complete tumor removal have made surgical resection an option, eliminating the risk of radiation-induced sarcoma later in life (Weber & Sim). Overall five-year survival is 65%, with the probability of Ewing's tumor of bone in the pelvis, sacrum, or coccyx resulting in substantially poorer outcome.

Patterns of Care

Most pediatric cancer care is provided in hospital settings or associated outpatient clinics. Treatments generally are protocol-based (Alcoser & Rodgers, 2003). Appropriate supportive care measures are critical to ensure optimal outcomes. These include antiemetic agents, antibiotics, blood products, hematopoietic growth factors, and pain medications (Bryant, 2003).

All children must undergo evaluation of nutritional status, and their risk of nutritional deficiency is assessed in terms of their disease process and planned treatment. Children, like adults, manifest nutritional imbalance either at diagnosis or during treatment and require aggressive intervention and/or supplemental therapies. Although there is speculation that nausea and vomiting from cancer treatment may occur less often in younger children, it remains one of the most common causes of nutritional imbalance in children of all ages with cancer. Cisplatin, carboplatin, and high-dose cyclophosphamide are highly emetogenic chemotherapeutic regimens and often are used in combination to treat children with solid tumors or at the time of relapse for a variety of childhood cancers.

Vincristine, a common agent used in the treatment of childhood ALL, brain tumors, as well as other solid tumors, can cause severe constipation, leading to anorexia and possibly an ileus if not treated prophylactically. Dietitians can provide dietary guidance that will assist in preventing and treating this symptom. Patients with AML are especially susceptible to mouth sores, diarrhea, and anorexia. Patients undergoing myeloablative chemotherapy and stem cell transplant, such as a child with relapsed ALL or AML in first remission, will almost uniformly require supplemental feeding. Patients with brain tumors may have swallowing difficulties because of the cancer location or sequelae of surgery. They also may have nausea and vomiting. Patients with stage IV neuroblastoma are at significant risk for nutritional deficiencies because of their young age and aggressive therapy. Radiation to the abdomen, such as in Wilms' tumor, can cause nausea, vomiting, and diarrhea. Radiation to the head and neck in patients with rhabdomyosarcoma as well as various chemotherapy agents may cause mucositis and dysphagia. Although always considered in childhood, depression may contribute to anorexia, and attention is directed to maintaining caloric intake by oral supplementation, enteral feeding, or IV alimentation.

Nutritional Management of the Pediatric Patient With Cancer

The primary objective for nutritional intervention in children with cancer is to sustain growth both physically and mentally while undergoing anticancer therapy. In contrast to adults with cancer, children pose the challenge to clinicians of supporting growth while still enabling them to receive the recommended doses of anticancer therapy. Despite these objectives, malnutrition has been observed in the pediatric oncology population. Up to 50% of children present with overt malnutrition; however, this is largely contingent upon the diagnosis and stage of disease (Rickard et al., 1986). In children undergoing anticancer treatment, investigations have found the incidence of malnutrition to be 37.5%; however, this also is highly contingent upon treatment regimen (Van Eys, 1979).

A child's risk and degree of malnutrition depends on the diagnosis and selected treatment. Van Eys (1979) found that patients with advanced stage solid tumors, nonresponsive tumors, and recurrent disease have a high probability of becoming malnourished irrespective of their nutrition assessment at diagnosis. Other diagnoses that increase a child's risk of malnutrition are presented in Figure 15-1. Additional studies also have identified that children with ALL may present with undernutrition in contrast to overt malnutrition (Reilly et al., 1994), despite a number of publications reporting that in developed countries, children with ALL are not at high risk for overt malnutrition. Halton, Atkinson, and Barr (1998) found that height standard deviation scores significantly decreased in children undergoing treatment for ALL, despite adequate nutrient intake. The real magnitude of malnutrition in children with ALL, the most common childhood malignancy, is an increasing area of research initiatives. Significant controversy has evolved as to the gold standard for defining malnutrition. The most widely recommended criteria have been described elsewhere (Mauer et al., 1990; Waterlow, 1972) and are summarized in Figure 15-2.

Nutritional status has been correlated with treatment outcome, risk of infection, and decreased tolerance to chemotherapy; thus, increased attention

---

Figure 15-1. High-Risk Diagnoses

- Acute nonlymphocytic leukemia
- Ewing's sarcoma
- Medulloblastoma
- Nasopharyngeal cancers
- Neuroblastoma (stages III and IV)
- Rhabdomyosarcoma
- Wilms' tumor (stages III and IV)
- Advanced disease
- Relapsed disease
- Conditioning preparatory regimens— bone marrow transplant

Note. Based on information from Novy & Saavedra, 1997; Pizzo & Poplack, 2001.

Figure 15-2. Definitions of Malnutrition

- Five percent weight loss from preillness weight over a one month period or > 5% weight loss from weight for age greater than fifth percentile
- Height for age less than fifth percentile
- Weight and height less than fifth percentile
- Ideal body weight/height < 90%
- Triceps skin fold for age and gender less than the tenth percentile
- Body mass index for age and gender less than fifth percentile
- Serum albumin < 3.2 g/dl
- Oral intake < 80% of estimated needs

Note. Based on information from Kleinman, 2004; Sacks & Meek, 1997.

---

has emerged on providing proactive nutritional support. What has become progressively more apparent is that nutrition therapy should be initiated prior to the onset of malnutrition with the objective of preventing overt malnutrition from ensuing, rather than intervening once a child is clinically diagnosed with malnutrition. Thus, the clinician must give careful consideration to the intensity of upcoming therapy and expected incidence of nutritional complications.

Assessment Guidelines

The objective of nutrition screening is to identify children at risk for malnutrition and collect and date data that can serve as a baseline for future nutritional interventions (Kleinman, 2004). The American Academy of Pediatrics and the Children's Cancer Group have published criteria for routine nutrition screening. Upon identification of a patient at nutritional risk, the patient should be referred to a registered dietitian for a more in-depth nutrition assessment. A nutrition assessment has four primary components, which are commonly referred to as the ABCDs of nutrition assessment: anthropometric data, biochemical data, clinical presentation, and dietary intake.

Anthropometric Data

Anthropometric data use measurements of weight, height, head circumference (< 3 years of age), and muscle and fat stores. These measurements then are interpreted using different methods. Historically, the system developed by Waterlow (1972) has been used to determine different categories for nutritional status based on percentage of ideal body weight. An important feature of these measurements is that they should be followed and assessed serially to look at change over time (Kleinman, 2004).

The most accurate system for measuring anthropometric data is under debate. Investigators have recommended the use of body mass index (BMI), weight-for-height (WFH), and mid-upper arm circumference (MUAC) (Motil, 1998). The Centers for Disease Control and Prevention recommended the use of weight-for-length percentiles in children younger than two years of age and WFH percentiles or BMI in children older than two years of age (Kuczmarski et al., 2000). WFH and BMI for age percentiles are readily available and provide a quick assessment of nutritional status. These indices also have the benefit of not requiring trained technicians to perform tests. However, the formula used is contingent on the child's or adolescent's diagnosis. Brennan (1998) found that in patients with solid tumors, tricep skin fold thickness and MUAC were more sensitive in indicating nutritional status when compared to WFH. Because MUAC does not require a trained technician, its use is more applicable in children with solid tumors and neuroblastoma (Brennan).

Biochemical Data

The gold standard laboratory index for determining protein status is albumin; however, it is not without limitations. Studies have indicated that albumin is not sensitive enough to identify a patient at risk for malnutrition (Carter et al., 1983) and suggest that prealbumin is a more appropriate choice because of its shorter half-life. Others have suggested that transthyretin is a more sensitive marker, as it has been correlated with recent dietary intake and should rise within 10 days after initiating nutritional support (Motil, 1998). However, transthyretin also is an acute phase protein, which limits its usefulness in the clinical setting. Lymphocytes are not a good indicator for nutritional status because of the myelosuppression observed with most anticancer agents. Other indices such as liver function tests, renal profile, electrolytes, and glucose will provide the clinician with additional information on the status of organ function and are useful particularly in patients on enteral or parenteral feeding.

Clinical Presentation

Complications or side effects resulting from chemotherapy, radiation therapy, or surgery can hinder a child's oral intake. Nausea, vomiting, mucositis, and loss of appetite all may occur as a result of therapy and may require more aggressive nutritional intervention. Encouraging oral intake may help in the short term; however, recent studies have found that facilitating oral intake on its own does not mitigate these side effects. Nutritional interventions (i.e., oral supplements, appetite stimulants, tube feedings, total parenteral nutrition [TPN]) may be necessary to ensure that the patient meets his or her nutritional needs.

Dietary Intake

A three-day dietary recall is useful in identifying problems patients have in meeting the recommended intakes for carbohydrates, protein, and fat.

They are less informative of micronutrient intake. The recommended dietary allowances for infants, children, and adolescents are described in Table 15-1. Patients receiving less than 80% of the recommended nutritional needs through oral intake are at risk for becoming malnourished. The dietary recall can be useful in identifying weaknesses in the patient's dietary intake and can provide a base for recommendations. When completed at diagnosis, it can establish baseline data for comparison of intake throughout therapy. To assess micronutrient intake, a more detailed analysis is necessary. In most cases, a children's multivitamin/mineral supplement can be recommended to the patient to ensure adequate intake of vitamins and minerals. It should not provide more than 100% of the recommended daily allowance for any nutrient. Controversy exists over the safety of folate-containing supplements in patients treated with methotrexate-containing regimens. However, Schroder, Clausen, Ostergard, and Pressler (1986) found no significant differences in erythrocyte-methotrexate or frequencies of relapse. More recently, in a study of 79 children with ALL, multivitamin use was not associated with methotrexate toxicity or recurrence in patients supplementing with a low-dose multivitamin containing folate (Ladas, Kennedy, Huiling, & Kelly, 2003). Low-dose

Table 15-1. Dietary Reference Intakes

	Age	Kcal/Day	Protein (g/kg/day)
Infants			
Males	0–6 months	570	1.52*
	7–12 months	743	1.5
Females	0–6 months	520	1.52*
	7–12 months	676	1.5
Children			
Males	1–2 years	1,046	1.10
	3–8 years	1,742	0.95
	9–13 years	2,279	0.95
	14–18 years	3,152	0.85
Females	1–2 years	992	1.10
	3–8 years	1,642	0.95
	9–13 years	2,071	0.95
	14–18 years	2,368	0.85

*Represents adequate intake

Note. Based on information from the Food and Nutrition Board & the Institute of Medicine, 2000; Kleinman, 2004.

supplementation (within the dietary reference intakes) with folate likely is not deleterious in the context of cancer therapy; however, additional clinical trials are needed to confirm this hypothesis.

Nutritional Intervention

The goal of nutritional intervention is to maintain current weight and support optimal growth and development. Most patients will require nutritional intervention at some point during therapy. The clinician has four primary options for nutritional intervention: (a) dietary counseling to increase or modify intake from food sources, (b) oral supplements, (c) enteral tube feedings, or (d) TPN. Patients with diagnoses described in Figure 15-1 should be considered for proactive enteral nutrition at diagnosis to avoid severe malnutrition that has been commonly reported in children with these diagnoses. DeSwarte-Wallace, Firouzbakhsh, and Finklestein (2001) found that nasogastric or nasojejunal tube feedings were well-tolerated and cost-effective methods of nutritional intervention in children undergoing intensive anticancer regimens (DeSwarte-Wallace et al.). The authors did not observe any increase in complications or therapy-related side effects. Similar findings have been reported in the literature (Barron et al., 2000). Thus, enteral feedings are a safe and effective method of nutritional intervention in children undergoing intensive cycles of cancer therapy and are recommended as the preferred method of intervention.

Explicit algorithms have been published and serve as a useful guideline in choosing between enteral feedings and TPN (Sacks & Meek, 1997). Feeding by the enteral route is the preferred (oral or tube) route; however, in patients with disruptions to their gastrointestinal tract or patients who are unable to tolerate enteral feedings, TPN is a more appropriate choice.

Obesity

With the increase in the use of corticosteroids in the management and treatment of many childhood malignancies, new challenges in the nutritional management of pediatric patients with cancer have evolved. Obesity has increasingly become an area of concern in children undergoing therapy as well as survivors of childhood cancer (Oeffinger & Hudson, 2004). Children treated with corticosteroids now commonly increase two or four percentiles during their treatment. This is particularly true of children with certain types of brain tumors. These children should not be assessed as being well nourished based solely on weight. In many cases, these children are at risk for malnutrition. However, different nutritional intervention approaches may be more appropriately indicated for these patients. Ideally, intervention should include aspects of nutritional intake modification, behavior modification, nutritional education, as well as an appropriate exercise and activity plan. Cancer treatment should not be the cause of rapid weight loss during therapy in obese patients but should be addressed when cancer therapy is completed. Educating patients on improving the quality of the diet during the period of increases in appetite is an important component of nutrition therapy. Coordinating services with a registered dietitian for calorie counts and individualized nutrition counseling will assist patients and their families in making more appropriate choices in dietary intake.

Late Effects

The study of late effects of treatment is an increasing focus of pediatric oncology care. An estimated 1 out of every 900 young adults is a childhood cancer survivor (Bottomley & Kassner, 2003). A variety of medical complications of childhood cancer therapy have been encountered, including growth failure, learning disability, thyroid disorders, heart failure, and infertility. Survivors have a 2%–8% risk of second malignant neoplasms for 20 years from initial diagnosis (Bhatia & Sklar, 2002; Haddy, Mosher, Dinndorf, & Reaman, 2004). Conversely, some therapies have been found to be essentially free of late complications, such as the chemotherapy used for Wilms' tumor. It is recommended that all pediatric patients with cancer continue to be followed well beyond the period of immediate recurrence risk to monitor for late effects and long-term outcome (Harvey, Hobbie, Shaw, & Bottomley, 1999; Oeffinger & Hudson, 2004).

References

Alcoser, P.W., & Rodgers, C. (2003). Treatment strategies in childhood cancer. *Journal of Pediatric Nursing, 18*(2), 103–112.

Arndt, C.A., & Crist, W.M. (1999). Common musculoskeletal tumors of childhood and adolescence. *New England Journal of Medicine, 341,* 342–352.

Baggott, C.R., Kelly, K.P., Fochtman, D., & Foley, G.V. (2002). *Nursing care of children and adolescents with cancer* (3rd ed.). Philadelphia: Saunders.

Barron, M.A., Duncan, D.S., Green, G.J., Modrusan, D., Connolly, B., Chait, P., et al. (2000). Efficacy and safety of radiologically placed gastrostomy tubes in paediatric haematology/oncology patients. *Medical and Pediatric Oncology, 34*(3), 177–182.

Bhatia, S., & Sklar, C. (2002). Second cancers in survivors of childhood cancer. *National Reviews. Cancer, 2*(2), 124–132.

Bottomley, S.J., & Kassner, E. (2003). Late effects of childhood cancer therapy. *Journal of Pediatric Nursing, 18*(2), 126–133.

Brennan, B.M. (1998). Sensitive measures of the nutritional status of children with cancer in hospital and in the field. *International Journal of Cancer Supplement, 11,* 10–13.

Bryant, R. (2003). Managing side effects of childhood cancer treatment. *Journal of Pediatric Nursing, 18*(2), 113–125.

Carter, P., Carr, D., Van Eys, J., Ramirez, I., Coody, D., & Taylor, G. (1983). Energy and nutrient intake of children with cancer. *Journal of the American Dietetic Association, 82,* 610–615.

Castleberry, R.P. (1997). Biology and treatment of neuroblastoma. *Pediatric Clinics of North America, 44*, 919–937.

Colby-Graham, M.F., & Chordas, C. (2003). The childhood leukemias. *Journal of Pediatric Nursing, 18*(2), 87–95.

D'Angio, G.J., Breslow, N., Beckwith, J.B., Evans, A., Baum, H., deLorimier, A., et al. (1989). Treatment of Wilms' tumor. Results of the Third National Wilms' Tumor Study. *Cancer, 64*, 349–360.

DeSwarte-Wallace, J., Firouzbakhsh, S., & Finklestein, J.Z. (2001). Using research to change practice: Enteral feedings for pediatric oncology patients. *Journal of Pediatric Oncology Nursing, 18*(5), 217–223.

Donaldson, S.S., Hancock, S.L., & Hoppe, R.T. (1999). The Janeway lecture. Hodgkin's disease—Finding the balance between cure and late effects. *The Cancer Journal From Scientific American, 5*, 325–333.

Ebb, D.H., & Weinstein, H.J. (1997). Diagnosis and treatment of childhood acute myelogenous leukemia. *Pediatric Clinics of North America, 44*, 847–862.

Food and Nutrition Board & the Institute of Medicine. (2002). *Dietary reference intakes for energy, carbohydrate, fat, fatty acids, cholesterol, protein, and amino acids.* Washington, DC: National Academies Press.

Haddy, T.B., Mosher, R.B., Dinndorf, P.A., & Reaman, G.H. (2004). Second neoplasms in survivors of childhood and adolescent cancer are often treatable. *Journal of Adolescent Health, 34*, 324–329.

Halton, J.M., Atkinson, S.A., & Barr, R.D. (1998). Growth and body composition in response to chemotherapy in children with acute lymphoblastic leukemia. *International Journal of Cancer Supplement, 11*, 81–84.

Harvey, J., Hobbie, W.L., Shaw, S., & Bottomley, S. (1999). Providing quality care in childhood cancer survivorship: Learning from the past, looking to the future. *Journal of Pediatric Oncology Nursing, 16*(3), 117–125.

Jarrett, R.F., & MacKenzie, J. (1999). Epstein-Barr virus and other candidate viruses in the pathogenesis of Hodgkin's disease. *Seminars in Hematology, 36*, 260–269.

Jemal, A., Murray, T., Ward, E., Samuels, A., Tiwari, R.C., Ghafoor, A., et al. (2005). Cancer statistics, 2005. *CA: A Cancer Journal for Clinicians, 55*, 10–30.

Kalapurakal, J.A., Dome, J.S., Perlman, E.J., Malogolowkin, M., Haase, G.M., Grundy, P., et al. (2004). Management of Wilms' tumour: Current practice and future goals. *Lancet Oncology, 5*(1), 37–46.

Kleinman, R.E. (2004). Nutritional management of children with cancer. In R.E. Kleinman (Ed.), *Pediatric nutrition handbook* (pp. 709–717). Elk Grove Village, IL: American Academy of Pediatrics.

Kline, N.E., & Sevier, N. (2003). Solid tumors in children. *Journal of Pediatric Nursing, 18*(2), 96–102.

Kuczmarski, R.J., Ogden, C.L., Grummer-Strawn, L.M., Flegal, K.M., Guo, S.S., Wei, R., et al. (2000). CDC growth charts: United States. *Advance Data, 314*, 1–27.

Ladas, E.J., Kennedy, D.D., Huiling, L., & Kelly, K.M. (2003). Preliminary findings: Dietary folate and methotrexate (MTX) toxicity in children with acute lymphoblastic leukemia (ALL) [Abstract]. *American Society of Hematology, 102*, 11.

Landier, W. (2001). Childhood acute lymphoblastic leukemia: Current perspectives. *Oncology Nursing Forum, 28*, 823–833.

Matthay, K.K., Villablanca, J.G., Seeger, R.C., Stram, D.O., Harris, R.E., Ramsay, N.K., et al. (1999). Treatment of high-risk neuroblastoma with intensive chemotherapy, radiotherapy, autologous bone marrow transplantation, and 13-cis-retinoic acid. Children's Cancer Group. *New England Journal of Medicine, 341*, 1165–1173.

Mauer, A.M., Burgess, J.B., Donaldson, S.S., Rickard, K.A., Stallings, V.A., Van Eys, J., et al. (1990). Special nutritional needs of children with malignancies: A review. *JPEN Journal of Parenteral and Enteral Nutrition, 14*, 315–324.

McDowell, H.P. (2003). Update on childhood rhabdomyosarcoma. *Archives of Disease in Childhood, 88*, 354–357.

Motil, K.J. (1998). Sensitive measures of nutritional status in children in hospital and in the field [Review]. *International Journal of Cancer Supplement, 11,* 2–9.

Novy, M.A., & Saavedra, J.M. (1997). Nutrition therapy for the pediatric cancer patient [Abstract]. *Clinical Nutrition, 12*(4), 16–25.

Oeffinger, K.C., & Hudson, M.M. (2004). Long-term complications following childhood and adolescent cancer: Foundations for providing risk-based health care for survivors. *CA: A Cancer Journal for Clinicians, 54,* 208–236.

Packer, R.J. (1999). Primary central nervous system tumors in children. *Current Treatment Options in Neurology, 1,* 395–408.

Packer, R.J., Gurney, J.G., Punyko, J.A., Donaldson, S.S., Inskip, P.D., Stovall, M., et al. (2003). Long-term neurologic and neurosensory sequelae in adult survivors of a childhood brain tumor: Childhood cancer survivor study. *Journal of Clinical Oncology, 21,* 3255–3261.

Packer, R.J., & Reddy, A. (2004). New treatments in pediatric brain tumors. *Current Treatment Options in Neurology, 6,* 377–389.

Pizzo, P.A., & Poplack, D.G. (Eds.). (2001). *Principles and practice of pediatric oncology* (4th ed.). Philadelphia: Lippincott Williams & Wilkins.

Plosker, G.L., & Figgitt, D.P. (2003). Rituximab: A review of its use in non-Hodgkin's lymphoma and chronic lymphocytic leukemia. *Drugs, 63,* 803–843.

Pollack, I.F. (1999). Pediatric brain tumors. *Seminars in Surgical Oncology, 16*(2), 73–90.

Pui, C.H. (2000). Acute lymphoblastic leukemia in children. *Current Opinion in Oncology, 12*(1), 3–12.

Pui, C.H., Relling, M.V., Campana, D., & Evans, W.E. (2002). Childhood acute lymphoblastic leukemia. *Reviews in Clinical and Experimental Hematology, 6*(2), 161–180.

Reilly, J.J., Odame, I., McColl, J.H., McAllister, P.J., Gibson, B.E., & Wharton, B.A. (1994). Does weight for height have prognostic significance in children with acute lymphoblastic leukemia? *American Journal of Pediatric Hematology/Oncology, 16*(3), 225–230.

Rickard, K.A., Coates, T.D., Grosfeld, J.L., Weetman, R.M., & Baehner, R.L. (1986). The value of nutrition support in children with cancer. *Cancer, 58*(Suppl. 8), 1904–1910.

Ries, L.A.G., Smith, M.A., Gurney, J.G., Linet, M., Tamran, T., Yourng, J.L., et al. (1999). *Cancer incidence and survival among children and adolescents, United States SEER Program 1975–1995* [NIH Pub. No. 99–4649]. Bethesda, MD: National Cancer Institute.

Rosser, T., & Packer, R.J. (2002). Neurofibromas in children with neurofibromatosis 1. *Journal of Child Neurology, 17,* 585–591.

Rubnitz, J.E., & Pui, C.H. (2003). Recent advances in the treatment and understanding of childhood acute lymphoblastic leukaemia. *Cancer Treatment Reviews, 29*(1), 31–44.

Sacks, N., & Meek, R.S. (1997). Nutritional support. In A.R. Ablin (Ed.), *Supportive care of children with cancer: Current therapy and guidelines from the children's cancer group* (pp. 193–208). Baltimore: Johns Hopkins University Press.

Sandlund, J.T., Downing, J.R., & Crist, W.M. (1996). Non-Hodgkin's lymphoma in childhood. *New England Journal of Medicine, 334,* 1238–1248.

Schroder, H., Clausen, N., Ostergard, E., & Pressler, T. (1986). Folic acid supplements in vitamin tablets: A determinant of hematological drug tolerance in maintenance therapy of childhood acute lymphoblastic leukemia. *Pediatric Hematology Oncology, 3*(3), 241–247.

Smith, M.A., Freidlin, B., Ries, L.A., & Simon, R. (1998). Trends in reported incidence of primary malignant brain tumors in children in the United States. *Journal of the National Cancer Institute, 90,* 1269–1277.

Spix, C., Michaelis, J., Berthold, F., Erttmann, R., Sander, J., & Schilling, F.H. (2003). Lead-time and over diagnosis estimation in neuroblastoma screening. *Statistics in Medicine, 22,* 2877–2892.

Van Eys, J. (1979). Malnutrition in children with cancer: Incidence and consequence. *Cancer, 43*(Suppl. 5), 2030–2035.

Waterlow, J.C. (1972). Classification and definition of protein-calorie malnutrition. *BMJ, 3,* 566–569.

Weber, K.L., & Sim, F.H. (2001). Ewing's sarcoma: Presentation and management. *Journal of Orthopaedic Science, 6,* 366–371.

Weinstein, J.L., Katzenstein, H.M., & Cohn, S.L. (2003). Advances in the diagnosis and treatment of neuroblastoma. *Oncologist, 8,* 278–292.

Wexler, L.H., DeLaney, T.F., Tsokos, M., Avila, N., Steinberg, S.M., Weaver-McClure, L., et al. (1996). Ifosfamide and etoposide plus vincristine, doxorubicin, and cyclophosphamide for newly diagnosed Ewing's sarcoma family of tumors. *Cancer, 78,* 901–911.

Woods, W.G., Neudorf, S., Gold, S., Sanders, J., Buckley, J.D., Barnard, D.R., et al. (2001). A comparison of allogeneic bone marrow transplantation, autologous bone marrow transplantation, and aggressive chemotherapy in children with acute myeloid leukemia in remission. *Blood, 97,* 56–62.

CHAPTER 16

Hematopoietic Stem Cell Transplantation

Mary Reilly Burgunder, RN, BSN, MS, OCN®
Barbara J. Dickson, RD, MS, CD

Introduction

Hematopoietic stem cell transplantation (HSCT) has emerged as a recognized and effective treatment modality for various malignant and nonmalignant diseases. More than 40,000 HSCT procedures are performed annually worldwide (Ball, Lister, & Law, 2000). Nutrition is an important part of the management of patients who undergo HSCT. As a component of medical care, nutrition assessment, management, and monitoring can affect patient outcomes and may influence the risk of complications and overall cost of the procedure (Rock, 2000).

This chapter reviews the basic principles and process of HSCT, the complications of HSCT most commonly associated with nutritional deficits, and the nutritional management of patients undergoing HSCT.

Overview

The first successful bone marrow transplant (BMT) was performed in 1968 to treat acute leukemia. The original principle for BMT was related to dose response to chemotherapy. Many malignancies exhibit a dose-related response to chemotherapy or radiation therapy; increasing the dose raises the number of cells that are destroyed. However, the dose of chemo- or radiotherapy is limited by marrow toxicity (Wilke-Shapiro, 1998). With an alternate source of stem cells available from a donor (allograft) or the patient's own cells harvested prior to therapy (autograft), lethal doses of therapy may be given regardless of marrow toxicity.

Another rationale for HSCT is to replace diseased or malfunctioning hematopoietic stem cells (HSCs) with healthy stem cells. An example of this would be HSCT for the treatment of aplastic anemia.

The third rationale is that post-transplant changes in the immune system may provide immunotherapeutic effects against residual tumor cells. This has been emphasized by the results of studies of allogeneic HSCT and the correlation between graft-versus-host disease (GVHD) and a decreased incidence of relapse (Simpson & Keating, 2000). The use of reduced-intensity or nonmyeloablative stem cell transplantation (NSCT) is increasing. The rationale behind NSCT is to induce optimal graft-versus-leukemia effects for elimination of all malignant cells by donor stem cells. This may successfully replace standard high-dose myeloablative chemoradiotherapy by providing a safer, better-tolerated therapeutic option for patients (Or et al., 2003).

Types of Hematopoietic Stem Cell Transplantation

There are three types of HSCT. *Autologous* HSCT is performed using the patient's own stem cells. These are collected from the peripheral blood prior to the patient receiving the conditioning or preparative regimen with chemotherapy alone or in combination with radiotherapy. *Allogeneic* HSCT is performed with HSCs from a donor. The donor may be related (usually a sibling or a parent) or unrelated. An unrelated donor may be identified through a registry of volunteer donors (e.g., National Marrow Donor Program) or a cord blood bank. *Syngeneic* HSCT is performed with a donor who is an identical twin. This type of transplant has less morbidity and mortality than an allogeneic HSCT but also has a higher rate of relapse.

Human leukocyte antigen (HLA) typing helps to identify donors. Generally, the best donor would be one who matches the recipient at each of the two alleles at HLA-A, HLA-B, and HLA-DR. This is termed a six-antigen match. HLA haplotype is inherited from only one parent (Rosner, Martell, & Trucco, 2000). Therefore, if a patient and sibling inherit the same two haplotypes from each parent, they are considered a six-antigen match and would be the preferred donor match (Wilke-Shapiro, 1998).

Indications for Hematopoietic Stem Cell Transplantation

As HSCT has developed over the past three decades, the list of diseases treated with it has grown and includes both malignant and nonmalignant diseases. According to the International Bone Marrow Transplant Registry/Autologous Blood and Marrow Transplant Registry (IBMTR/ABMTR, 2003), approximately 30,000 autologous transplants and 15,000 allogeneic transplants were performed worldwide in 2000. In North America in 2000, 10,550 autologous and 7,200 allogeneic HSCTs were reported to IBMTR. The greatest numbers of transplants were performed for multiple myeloma and non-Hodgkin lymphoma, followed by acute myelogenous leukemia, Hodgkin disease, and acute lymphocytic leukemia. A noninclusive listing of current diseases treated with HSCT is provided in Figure 16-1.

Figure 16-1. Diseases Treated With Hematopoietic Stem Cell Transplant

Malignant diseases
- Acute and chronic leukemias
- Hodgkin and non-Hodgkin lymphoma
- Multiple myeloma
- Solid tumors
  - Neuroblastoma
  - Ewing sarcoma
  - Testicular cancer
  - Breast cancer

Hematologic disorders
- Myelodysplastic syndromes
- Sickle cell anemia
- Congenital neutropenias
- Severe aplastic anemia
- Fanconi anemia

Immunodeficiencies/genetic disorders
- Severe combined immunodeficiency
- Wiskott-Aldrich syndrome
- Leukodystrophies
- Miscellaneous metabolic disorders

Autoimmune diseases
- Rheumatoid arthritis
- Systemic sclerosis
- Multiple sclerosis

Process

The process of HSCT begins with the patient evaluation. This first phase of the transplant process involves a comprehensive clinical and psychosocial evaluation to determine the patient's eligibility for HSCT. The transplant team performs a comprehensive history and physical examination, including past therapies received, comorbid medical conditions, and a review of systems. A thorough psychosocial evaluation is performed and includes a review of prior coping mechanisms, available support systems, caregiver availability, and financial and community resources. Critical laboratory and diagnostic data are obtained. Hematologic, hepatic, renal, immune, and infectious disease markers are performed. Diagnostic tests measure organ function and disease status and may include bone marrow biopsy, computed tomography (CT) scans, electrocardiogram, cardiac ejection fraction, pulmonary function test, and chest x-ray (Wilke-Shapiro, 1998).

Once a patient has been deemed eligible for HSCT and a donor has been identified, the next phase of the transplant process is the preparative or conditioning regimen. This may be administered in an inpatient or outpatient setting and may include chemotherapy, with or without radiation therapy or immunotherapy. The specific combination of chemotherapy with or without radiation depends on the underlying disease, the type of transplant, and prior therapy received by the patient (Wilke-Shapiro, 1998). Depending on the regimen, the conditioning phase may last one or several days prior to transplant. After conditioning, the stem cells are collected from the donor (or have been previously collected and cryopreserved) and infused into the patient. The recovery phase lasts for several weeks following the stem cell infusion and is associated with many complications.

Toxicities

Common toxicities after HSCT include mucositis, infection, and the potential for bleeding. These toxicities are related to the degree of aplasia and side effects of the conditioning regimen. Direct mucosal toxicity can vary from mild to severe depending on the type of conditioning regimen. Synergistic effects of chemotherapy and radiation therapy can exacerbate the mucosal toxicity, and grade 3 to 4 mucositis is not uncommon after total body irradiation. Mucositis generally presents within several days after the conditioning regimen as xerostomia, oropharyngeal pain, or ulcerations. The duration of mucositis usually parallels the duration of absolute neutropenia (Vargas & Silverman, 2000). Nutritional support becomes an important management issue if mucositis is severe. Pain management frequently requires the institution of opiates.

Infection in the gastrointestinal (GI) tract may affect the esophagus, stomach, duodenum, and colon. The esophagus is susceptible to fungal infection, usually with the *Candida* species. Viral infections of the esophagus may be because of herpes simplex virus or cytomegalovirus (CMV). If oral intake is compromised, management with IV antifungal or antiviral therapy is indicated. CMV or herpes viral infections may present with nausea, vomiting, or hematemesis. Bacterial infections of the colon may be related to the use of broad-spectrum antibiotics. The use of antibiotics may predispose the patient to infection, such as *Clostridium difficile.* CMV may present as colitis with lower GI bleeding, cramping, and diarrhea (Vargas & Silverman, 2000).

In addition to the aforementioned toxicities, patients who receive allogeneic HSCT are at risk for developing GVHD. GVHD has both acute and chronic phases. The onset of acute GVHD generally occurs between 14 and 60 days post transplant but may occur as early as the first week post transplant or well after day 100 post-transplant. Acute GVHD also may occur after the use of donor lymphocyte infusions for the treatment of relapse (Przepiorka & Cleary, 2000).

The three major organ systems involved with acute GVHD are skin, liver, and GI, with the most common clinical manifestations being fever, rash, nausea, diarrhea, and abnormal liver function (Przepiorka & Cleary, 2000). Acute skin GVHD generally presents with erythema or a maculopapular rash that may manifest on the palms of the hands and soles of the feet, the shoulders and back, the trunk, the head, and the extremities. Acute GVHD of the liver is manifested by elevated serum bilirubin and alkaline phosphatase with lesser abnormalities of the serum transaminases. GVHD of the liver that is unresponsive to treatment may lead to liver failure (Przepiorka & Cleary). Approximately 13%–20% of patients undergoing HSCT present with symptoms of heartburn, nausea, crampy abdominal pain, and food intolerance, suggesting upper GI tract involvement with GVHD. Diarrhea, lower abdominal pain, and cramping would suggest colonic and distal small bowel involvement with GVHD (Vargas & Silverman, 2000). Several liters of secretory diarrhea may be produced daily requiring aggressive rehydration to maintain fluid and electrolyte balance. Nutritionally, the secretory diarrhea induces a protein-losing enteropathy with marked decreases in total protein and albumin. Total parenteral nutrition (TPN) frequently is used to maintain adequate nutritional status in these patients (Vargas & Silverman).

Chronic GVHD generally develops 80–100 days post-transplantation. The syndrome is characterized by fibrosis and mucosal changes similar to autoimmune connective tissue diseases such as scleroderma. Discoloration of the skin, sclerosis, and joint inflammation are classic signs of chronic GVHD. Esophageal strictures and dysmotility are the most significant abnormalities in the GI system. Patients may present with chronic severe retrosternal pain and/or dysphagia, odynophagia, or total esophageal obstruction (Vargas & Silverman, 2000). Chronic liver injury and cholestasis from GVHD are characterized by elevations in alkaline phosphatase and bilirubin (Vargas & Silverman).

Veno-occlusive disease (VOD) of the liver is a serious complication following cytoreductive therapy and can be a major cause of morbidity and mortality during the first 80–100 days following HSCT. It is characterized by painful hepatomegaly, hyperbilirubinemia, fluid retention, and weight gain. Various conditioning regimens have been implicated as well as the presence of infection, use of antimicrobial agents, and pretransplant liver disease (Vinayek, Demetris, & Rakela, 2000).

Assessment Guidelines

Nutrition assessment helps to identify nutrition-related problems in patients throughout the transplant course. A clinician's subjective assessment, as well as objective measurements, is critical.

History, gathered both from the patient as well as the medical record, provides a basis for interpreting current nutritional status and needs. Relevant information includes weight history, diet, food allergies, use of nutritional supplements, subjective symptoms that might interfere with nutrient intake or absorption, level of activity, medical comorbidities, and previous surgeries.

Anthropometry aids in the determination of nutritional needs. Accurate measurement of height (or supine length in pediatrics), weight, and upper arm anthropometry can be used in the estimation of an "ideal" or "desirable" weight. Patients with multiple myeloma may present with decreased stature because of vertebral compression, necessitating an accurate height measurement.

For patients with elevated weight because of fluid retention or fat deposition without lean tissue gain, weight adjustments may be necessary for the purpose of estimating nutrient requirements and determining medication dosages. Both extremes of weight, too high and too low, seem to place transplant recipients at increased risk for poor outcome. Underweight patients (< 95% ideal body weight) seem to have an increased risk of death in the early post-transplant period (Deeg, Seidel, Bruemmer, Pepe, & Applebaum, 1995). Subsequent studies have reported that extremely underweight (70%–79% age-adjusted body mass index [BMI]) as well as overweight (120%–139% age-adjusted BMI) patients are at an increased risk for nonrelapse mortality post-transplant (Dickson et al., 1999). Whether nutritional intervention before transplant, to improve weight status, can beneficially impact post-transplant outcome remains to be determined. Weight status post-transplant is an important nutritional indicator and should be closely monitored. Sodium and fluid retention, fat deposition, glucose intolerance, and change in activity level may influence weight status.

Laboratory assessment is another objective evaluation to provide input into the nutrition care plan. Serum albumin is of limited value as a nutrition index, except when hepatic function is normal and no evidence is available of recent or ongoing metabolic stress. It is important to consider when evaluating calcium status and its role as a drug transport molecule, however. Serum transthyretin (prealbumin) is a more sensitive protein marker, but similar to albumin, it is unreliable in the presence of inflammation or metabolic stress. C-reactive protein (CRP) is an acute-phase reactant that increases during metabolic stress and inflammation. It can be used to interpret low levels of negative acute-phase proteins (Mueller, 2004). CRP also may be useful to predict major transplant-related complications. It has been shown to increase along with other proinflammatory cytokines, and these increases correlate with complications, including veno-occlusive liver disease, greater than grade II acute GVHD, and idiopathic pneumonia syndrome (Schots et al., 2003). Pre-transplant lipid levels (total cholesterol, triglycerides, high-density lipoprotein, low-density lipoprotein) are used to screen for preexisting lipid disorders and can guide post-transplant nutrition recommendations. Abnormal lipid levels post-transplant often are related to immunosuppressive medication effects (Carreras et al., 1989; Lopez-Miranda et al., 1992). This is a health concern because of the increasingly common risk of cardiovascular disease post–organ transplantation (Baum, 2001).

Evaluation of iron status has a special importance in transplantation because of the possible liver and other end organ damage from iron overload because of transfusions. This is also a concern post-transplant (McKay et al., 1996). Depending on the disease, patients may have received multiple transfusions pretransplant. Each unit of red cells contains 200–250 mg iron and requires six months to be excreted, without bleeding. Pretransplant iron status may change recommendations for vitamin C supplementation because of vitamin C's ability to improve iron absorption and act as a prooxidant. Baseline pre-transplant evaluation of renal and hepatic function will guide nutritional support recommendations. Other laboratory measures should be guided by the medical indications of the individual patient. These may include quantitative or qualitative fecal fat, serum levels of vitamins, and hydrogen breath test.

Nutritional Support

Total Parenteral Nutrition (TPN)

Peri-transplant nutritional concerns focus on the use of TPN and issues of refeeding (transitioning from TPN to oral intake). Effects of high-dose chemotherapy with or without total body irradiation, the subsequent neutropenia, and increased metabolic stress demands often require the use of artificial nutritional support. TPN has been a supportive modality since the early years of transplantation and is recognized as the standard of care for adult and pediatric allogeneic HSCT recipients (A.S.P.E.N. Board of Directors & the Clinical Guidelines Task Force, 2002). Weisdorf et al. (1987) first provided evidence that allogeneic transplant recipients receiving prophylactic TPN had an improvement in long-term outcome.

If possible, enteral nutrition should be used but may be poorly tolerated (Hopman et al., 2003) and requires intensive multidisciplinary efforts (Langdana, Tully, Molloy, Bourke, & O'Meara, 2001). Provision of TPN often becomes necessary. Protein requirements are estimated to be twice the recommended dietary allowance based upon weight and age (Charuhas, 2002). Energy requirements are based upon the basal energy expenditure (BEE) equation and adjusted for stress factors (Charuhas); this is generally 1.5 x BEE. Glutamine supplementation is controversial but may be of benefit, especially with GI morbidity (Murray & Pindoria, 2002). Fluid provision is critical because of the use of multiple nephrotoxins, and requirements are based upon body surface area for adults ($1,500 \text{ cc/m}^2$) and weight for children (Charuhas). Substrate distribution, as well as provision of vitamins, minerals, and electrolytes, is similar to that seen in the patient who is acutely ill. Appendices F, G, H, and I provide fomulas for calculating nutritional requirements.

Post-transplant, patients are at risk for food infections because of their immunocompromised state. Food safety is a major concern to decrease the risk of acquiring a food-related infection. The extent of food restrictions for the neutropenic patient is variable among institutions because of the lack of data regarding the "best" diet. Restrictions can vary from avoiding raw fruits and vegetables to more numerous restrictions. In the absence of GI problems, such as with GVHD, as close to a "regular" diet as possible should be achieved. Food safety guidelines for neutropenic diets are located in Appendix K.

Side effects, some of which are unique to HSCT, having nutritional support implications include GVHD, VOD, also known as sinusoidal obstructive syndrome (SOS), and immunosuppressive medication effects, such as hyperglycemia, lipid disorders, and osteoporosis.

As mentioned previously, GVHD can be an acute or chronic problem primarily affecting the skin, liver, or GI tract. Skin manifestations may range from mild erythroderma to severe bullous formation and skin sloughing. These changes require appropriate increases in provision of energy, protein, electrolytes, and minerals as with any severe skin injury (e.g., adequate intake of zinc and vitamin C for healing). When the liver is involved, severe cholestasis may occur, and fat digestion and absorption are problematic. If TPN includes manganese and copper, these may need to be discontinued because they are excreted via the biliary system, and levels may increase. Intestinal GVHD may be characterized by a continuum of symptoms from anorexia and early satiety to nausea, vomiting, voluminous diarrhea, and severe abdominal cramping (Wu et al., 1998). Abnormal losses of nutrients (e.g., zinc) in diarrhea output will need to be replaced (Charuhas, 2002), and energy and protein requirements may be increased.

Oral refeeding of patients with GI GVHD should be initiated as soon as appropriate to prevent gut atrophy, but it presents a challenge. Initiation may be based upon a decrease in stool volume to < 4–5 ml/kg/day at an unfed state or < 8–10 ml/kg/day at a fed state (Charuhas, 2002). Generally, a diet progression works best starting with isotonic fluids in limited quantity and gradually introducing foods and fluids that are low in lactose, insoluble fiber, acidity, fat, and caffeine. Figure 16-2 includes suggestions of foods to try post-transplant (Charuhas). Monitoring GI symptoms, as evidenced by pain and diarrhea, will guide diet progression. GI symptoms from GVHD and/or conditioning chemoradiotherapy may remain prominent in the post-transplant period and negatively affect quality of life (Hacker & Ferrans, 2003). Weight monitoring is very important to detect nutrition problems. Intestinal malabsorption may be present, requiring the use of pancreatic enzyme replacement, and GI motility tests may be indicated to obtain the correct diagnosis. Xerostomia, as an element of the sicca syndrome, may be observed, along with dysphagia and achalasia. Periodic esophageal dilations may be required for patients to maintain adequate oral intake. In extreme cases, enteral nutrition may be necessary to maintain adequate nutritional status.

VOD often involves sodium and fluid retention, and ascites may progress to hepatic failure. Reduction of sodium and fluid in TPN, enteral feeding, and/or oral intake often is necessary.

Corticosteroid-induced diabetes may be precipitated by the use of immunosuppressive medications. Pancreatic insulin secretion is impaired, glucose production is stimulated, and glucose utilization is inhibited. These alterations require careful blood sugar monitoring and use of basal and prandial insulins for management. Education regarding carbohydrate intake and encouragement of exercise are important aspects of management. Corticosteroids decrease bone formation and increase bone resorption through a number of different mechanisms (Carson & Blair, 1999). Corticosteroid-induced osteoporosis can become evident with decreases in bone density 6–12 months after beginning glucocorticoid therapy (Stern et al., 1996). Adequate intakes of calcium (1,500 mg/day for adults) and vitamin D (800 IU/day for adults) and encouragement of exercise are important (Charuhas, 2002).

NSCT is opening the arena of transplantation to patients previously ineligible for conventional stem cell transplants because of increased age or comorbidities. Although the preparative regimen is less toxic, these patients may develop GVHD and side effects similar to those of patients receiving a more toxic conditioning regimen, perhaps at a later time post-transplant (Mielcarek et al., 2003).

Figure 16-2. Gastrointestinal Diet

Suggestions of Foods to Try First
- Beverages (1 cup)
  - Tea, weak decaffeinated or brewed herb, except peppermint
  - Gatorade®
  - Rice milk
  - Lactaid® 100 milk
  - ½ strength: apple juice, Kool-Aid®, Tang®, cranberry drinks
- Cereals (½ cup)
  - Hot (made with water): cream of rice, Cream of Wheat®, Farina®, grits, Malt-o-Meal®
  - Cold: puffed rice, Rice Krispies®, Cheerios®
- Starches (allowed with 1 tsp. margarine)
  - White bread, plain bagel, English muffin (1 slice)
  - Pasta: macaroni, egg noodles, plain spaghetti (½ cup)
  - Potato (no skin), baked, or mashed (½ medium or ½ cup)
  - Rice, white (½ cup)
  - Saltines (2)
  - Pretzels (1 oz)
  - White dinner roll (1 each)
- Fruits (½ cup)
  - Applesauce, plain
  - Banana (½)
  - Peaches, canned in juice or light syrup
  - Pears, canned in juice or light syrup
- Other
  - Lifesavers®
  - Lemon drops
  - Broth, beef or chicken (1 cup)
  - Popsicle®
- Miscellaneous
  - Sugar (1 packet or teaspoon)
  - Salt as desired

If Tolerated, Try
- Protein sources (allowed with 1 tsp. margarine or mayonnaise)
  - Well-cooked chicken or turkey breast (no skin), baked, broiled, or boiled (½ breast or 3 oz)
  - Ham, lean (3 oz)
  - Egg, well cooked only (1)
  - Fish, baked or poached (3 oz)
  - Tuna, water-packed (¼ cup)
  - Liquid lactose-free nutritional supplements (½ cup)
- Other
  - Chicken rice or chicken noodle soup (1 cup)
  - Sandwiches made with low-fat mayonnaise on white bread: egg salad, tuna salad, chicken, turkey, or lean ham (½ sandwich)
  - Vanilla wafers/graham crackers (2)
  - Animal crackers (4)
  - Angel food cake
  - Carrots, well cooked (½ cup)
  - Green beans, well cooked (½ cup)
  - Sweet potatoes (peeled, mashed) (½ cup)

Note. From *Hematopoietic Stem Cell Transplantation—Nutrition Care Criteria* (2nd ed., p. 207), by P.M. Charuhas, 2002, Seattle, WA: Seattle Cancer Care Alliance. Copyright 2002 by Seattle Cancer Care Alliance. Reprinted with permission.

References

A.S.P.E.N. Board of Directors & the Clinical Guidelines Task Force. (2002). Guidelines for the use of parenteral and enteral nutrition in adult and pediatric patients. *Journal of Parenteral and Enteral Nutrition, 26*(Suppl. 1), 83SA–85SA, 124SA–126SA.

Ball, E.D., Lister, J., & Law, P. (2000). *Hematopoietic stem cell therapy.* Philadelphia: Churchill Livingstone.

Baum, C.L. (2001). Weight gain and cardiovascular risk after organ transplantation. *Journal of Parenteral and Enteral Nutrition, 25*(3), 114–119.

Carreras, E., Villamor, N., Reverter, J.C., Sierra, J., Granena, A., & Rozman, C. (1989). Hypertriglyceridemia in bone marrow transplant recipients: Another side effect of cyclosporine A. *Bone Marrow Transplantation, 4,* 385–388.

Carson, D.S., & Blair, M.M. (1999). Corticosteroid-induced osteoporosis. *U.S. Pharmacist,* (Suppl.), 3–14.

Charuhas, P.M. (2002). *Hematopoietic stem cell transplantation—nutrition care criteria* (2nd ed.). Seattle, WA: Seattle Cancer Care Alliance.

Deeg, H.J., Seidel, K., Bruemmer, B., Pepe, M.S., & Appelbaum, F.R. (1995). Impact of patient weight on non-relapse mortality after marrow transplantation. *Bone Marrow Transplantation, 15,* 461–468.

Dickson, T.M., Kusnierz-Glaz, C.R., Blume, K.G., Negrin, R.S., Hu, W.W., Shizuru, J.A., et al. (1999). Impact of admission body weight and chemotherapy dose adjustment on the outcome of autologous bone marrow transplantation. *Biology of Blood and Marrow Transplantation, 5,* 299–305.

Hacker, E.D., & Ferrans, C.E. (2003). Quality of life immediately after peripheral blood stem cell transplantation. *Cancer Nursing, 26,* 312–322.

Hopman, G.D., Pena, E.G., le Cessie, S., van Weel, M.H., Vossen, J.M., & Mearin, M.L. (2003). Tube feeding and bone marrow transplantation. *Medical and Pediatric Oncology, 40,* 375–379.

International Bone Marrow Transplant Registry/Autologous Blood and Marrow Registry. (2003). *State of the art in clinical transplantation summary slides.* Milwaukee, WI: Medical College of Wisconsin.

Langdana, A., Tully, N., Molloy, E., Bourke, B., & O'Meara, A. (2001). Intensive enteral nutrition support in paediatric bone marrow transplantation. *Bone Marrow Transplantation, 27,* 741–746.

Lopez-Miranda, J., Perez-Jimenez, F., Torres, A., Espino-Montoro, A., Gomez, P., Hidalgo-Rojas, L., et al. (1992). Effect of cyclosporin on plasma lipoproteins in bone marrow transplantation patients. *Clinical Biochemistry, 25,* 379–386.

McKay, P.J., Murphy, J.A., Cameron, S., Burnett, A.K., Campbell, M., Tansey, P., et al. (1996). Iron overload and liver dysfunction after allogeneic or autologous bone marrow transplantation. *Bone Marrow Transplantation, 17,* 63–66.

Mielcarek, M., Martin, P.J., Leisenring, W., Flowers, M.E., Maloney, D.G., Sandmaier, B.M., et al. (2003). Graft-versus-host disease after nonmyeloablative versus conventional hematopoietic stem cell transplantation. *Blood, 102,* 756–762.

Mueller, C. (2004). True or false: Serum hepatic protein concentrations measure nutritional status. *Support Line, 26*(1), 8–16.

Murray, S.M., & Pindoria, S. (2002). *Nutrition support for bone marrow transplant patients.* Chichester, UK: John Wiley & Sons.

Or, R., Shapira, M.Y., Resnick, I., Amar, A., Ackerstein, A., Samuel, S., et al. (2003). Non-myeloablative allogeneic stem cell transplantation for the treatment of chronic myeloid leukemia in first chronic phase. *Blood, 101,* 441–445.

Przepiorka, D., & Cleary, K. (2000). Therapy of acute graft versus host disease. In E.D. Ball, J. Lister, & P. Law (Eds.), *Hematopoietic stem cell therapy* (pp. 531–540). Philadelphia: Churchill Livingstone.

Rock, C.L. (2000). Nutritional issues and management in hematopoietic stem cell transplantation. In E.D. Ball, J. Lister, & P. Law (Eds.), *Hematopoietic stem cell therapy* (pp. 503–507). Philadelphia: Churchill Livingstone.

Rosner, G., Martell, J., & Trucco, M. (2000). Histocompatibility. In E.D. Ball, J. Lister, & P. Law (Eds.), *Hematopoietic stem cell therapy* (pp. 233–251). Philadelphia: Churchill Livingstone.

Schots, R., Kaufman, L., Van Riet, I., Ben Othman, T., De Waele, M., Van Camp, B., et al. (2003). Proinflammatory cytokines and their role in the development of major transplant-related complications in the early phase after allogeneic bone marrow transplantation. *Leukemia, 17,* 1150–1156.

Simpson, D.R., & Keating, A. (2000). Acute myelogeneous leukemia. In E.D. Ball, J. Lister, & P. Law (Eds.), *Hematopoietic stem cell therapy* (pp. 14–30). Philadelphia: Churchill Livingstone.

Stern, J.M., Chesnut, C.H., III, Bruemmer, B., Sullivan, K.M., Lenssen, P.S., Aker, S.N., et al. (1996). Bone density loss during treatment of chronic GVHD. *Bone Marrow Transplantation, 17,* 395–400.

Vargas, H.G., & Silverman, W.B. (2000). Mucositis and other complications. In E.D. Ball, J. Lister, & P. Law (Eds.), *Hematopoietic stem cell therapy* (pp. 557–561). Philadelphia: Churchill Livingstone.

Vinayek, R., Demetris, J., & Rakela, J. (2000). Liver disease in hematopoietic stem cell transplant recipients. In E.D. Ball, J. Lister, & P. Law (Eds.), *Hematopoietic stem cell therapy* (pp. 541–556). Philadelphia: Churchill Livingstone.

Weisdorf, S.A., Lysne, J., Wind, D., Haake, R.J., Sharp, H.L., Goldman, A., et al. (1987). Positive effect of prophylactic total parenteral nutrition on long-term outcome of bone marrow transplantation. *Transplantation, 43,* 833–838.

Wilke-Shapiro, T. (1998). Nursing implications of bone marrow and stem cell transplantation. In J.K. Itano & K.N. Taoka (Eds.), *Core curriculum for oncology nursing* (3rd ed., pp. 662–677). Philadelphia: W.B. Saunders.

Wu, D., Hockenbery, D.M., Brentnall, T.A., Baehr, P.H., Ponec, R.J., Kuver, R., et al. (1998). Persistent nausea and anorexia after marrow transplantation. *Transplantation, 66,* 1319–1324.

CHAPTER 17

Complementary and Alternative Medicine in Cancer Care

Jill Place, MA, RD

Introduction

Much confusion exists regarding the definitions of complementary, alternative, and integrative medicine (Caspi et al., 2003). It generally is believed that complementary and alternative medicine (CAM) encompasses a diverse set of healthcare modalities that are considered unconventional and controversial mainly because of the scarcity of good scientific human double-blind, placebo-controlled evidence about them. In cancer nutrition, CAM encompasses diet regimens, nutritional supplements, and many types of esoteric herbal systems and preparations, such as traditional Chinese medicine.

Overview

In a recent New Zealand study (Chrystal, Allen, Forgeson, & Isaacs, 2003), 47% of subjects used CAMs to improve the quality of their lives, and 30% believed them to be a cancer cure. Seventy-one percent of these subjects believed that the therapies were helpful in cancer management, and 89% deemed them safe. Reasons for use of alternative remedies included the belief that alternative treatments were less harmful than conventional ones, dissatisfaction with conventional treatments, and poor relationships with healthcare providers (Shumay, Maskarinec, Kakai, & Gorley, 2001).

More than 80% of oncologists in a particular study considered CAMs to be ineffective, felt they could not promote their use, and generally had negative perceptions about them (Salmenpera, Suominen, & Vertio, 2003). However, up to 80% of patients with cancer use CAMs (Sparber et al., 2000; Wernecke et al., 2004).

Because of this dismissive view of CAM by traditional oncologists, the majority of patients with cancer using them do not report their use. In a study by Werknecke et al. (2004), only 46% of participants reported using CAM, and in Chrystal et al. (2003), approximately one-third told their doctors they were using CAM. Only 7% of participants used their oncologist for information about CAM use in another study, preferring instead to consult their friends and family (39%) or the Internet (19%) (Eng et al., 2003). The majority of patients with cancer depend upon faulty information from unscientific sources to make choices about CAM. This could explain why less than half of the subjects in the Wernecke et al. study had only a cursory understanding of the CAMs they were using and another third had little or no idea why they were taking certain supplements.

There are inherent dangers in patients not reporting CAM use to their oncologists, not having a clear understanding of the function of CAM, and believing that the majority of them are safe. In one study (Malik & Gopalan, 2003), 53% of patients with breast cancer delayed conventional treatment in lieu of CAM, resulting in significant worsening of their conditions to stage III or IV. The lack of communication between doctors and patients about adverse side effects and negative drug interactions between CAM and conventional treatments may potentially cause harm. In the Wernecke et al. (2004) study, 12% took supplements that interfered with their treatment, and 11% took more than the recommended dosage. According to Shumay et al. (2001), patients with cancer need to be educated about CAM treatments and the possible dangers of CAM-drug interactions. Nurses, dietitians, and other support staff should implement a multidisciplinary approach to cancer treatment that promotes better doctor-patient communication and more patient education about CAM.

Health Paradigms Shift

Oncology cannot ignore CAM use. Revenue from total visits to U.S. CAM practitioners nearly doubled from 1990 to 1997 to almost $12 billion, which was more revenue than total visits in 1997 to primary care physicians. Sales of dietary supplements have more than doubled since 1994 and topped $15 billion in 2000. Because of public pressure, government funding for CAM research has increased more than 50 times in 10 years, from $2 million to $114 million (Eisenberg et al., 1998; Rosenthal & Rosenthal, 2001).

Another paradigm shift is occurring in the way many practitioners view medicine, particularly CAM nutrition practitioners. There is a growing focus on functional medicine, a science-based, patient-centered paradigm of health care that centers on biochemical individuality and web-like interconnections of physiologic factors that lead to dysfunction (Institute for Functional Medicine, 2004). The goal of functional medicine is to intervene nutritionally with diet and nutritional supplements before this dysfunction can cause damage and disease. The case for functional medicine grows stronger every day with the increasing amount of government and private double-blind, peer-reviewed journal research on diet and supplements. When the Human Genome Project isolated the human genome, the idea of functional medicine became even more viable. Preliminary research shows that individual genes can be influenced to turn off disease and turn on health by individualized nutritional intervention, another new paradigm called "nutrigenomics." According to Fogg-Johnson and Kaput (2003), "the science of nutrigenomics is the study of how naturally occurring chemicals in foods alter molecular expression of genetic information in each individual" (p. 60).

Dietitians and nurses are jumping on the CAM bandwagon. A 2003 study (Dutta et al.) revealed that nearly half of nursing schools offered some type of CAM curriculum, and more and more dietitians are acquiring a Certified Clinical Nutritionist (CCN) certification, a specialty credential in functional medicine. In the near future, dietitians and nurses may provide nutrition and supplement education in integrated cancer practices that combine conventional and complementary medical modalities. Most physicians do not have the time, expertise, or counseling skills to provide diet and nutritional supplement advice to their patients. Conventional and complementary methods usually are not effectively coordinated (Spiegel et al., 2003).

Seven Modifiable Factors for Cancer Inhibition

Traditional cancer treatment is "downstream" medicine that focuses on fixing the problem without regard to its effect on other body tissues or systems. Invading tumors are removed by surgery, and metastatic invaders are killed with chemotherapy and radiation therapy. Traditional medicine attempts to fix the host of side effects, such as using growth factors to combat the anemia and low red blood cell count resulting from chemotherapy, caused by these toxic treatments.

A functional medicine approach, however, is based on "upstream medicine." Its goal is prevention—to identify tissue-selective upstream modulators of genomic and proteomic expression and normalize tissue function where functional change has taken place that might lead to disease with diet, supplements, and other lifestyle changes without affecting surrounding, normally functioning tissues and organs (Bland, 2004).

Boik (2001) hinted that upstream medicine using natural compounds may be the answer to cancer prevention. Boik explained that "cancer cells are the descendants of a normal cell in which something has gone wrong" (p. 1). Cancer then proliferates because of DNA damage, interrupted cellular communication, and the ability of cancer cells to grow uncontrollably and metastasize. Boik listed seven much-researched factors for cancer inhibition that may be influenced by natural compounds. He stated that natural compounds act on cancer cells in three ways: directly on the cell, indirectly through changing the body's environment, and by boosting immune response. Natural compounds that can actively participate in all of these ways are likely most effective. A combination of compounds that cover all or most of the following seven inhibitory factors also may be effective. According to Boik, natural compounds may inhibit cancer by

1. **Reducing oxidative stress.** Higher oxidative stress leads to greater gene instability, which may cause greater gene mutation and eventual cancer growth. Many natural compounds may serve directly or indirectly as antioxidants that may inhibit cancer growth.

2. **Normalizing gene transcription.** Transcription factors are proteins that modulate gene expression. Normalizing them may turn on genes that inhibit cancer growth and turn off genes that cause cancer.

3. **Normalizing signal transduction.** Intracellular communication depends upon proteins that are abnormal and excessive in cancer cells. Normalizing these signal proteins may reduce cancer growth.

4. **Normalizing intercellular communication.** Cells talk to each other by cellular adhesion molecules and by forming gap junctions between cells. Cancer cells stop talking with other cells so that they can grow uncontrollably. Natural compounds may be able to normalize these cellular adhesion molecules and gap junction functions and restore communication.

5. **Blocking angiogenesis.** Angiogenesis, the growth of new blood vessels, is a normal bodily process. But, like cancer cells, tumor angiogenesis can grow out of control. Cancer may be inhibited by blocking the chemicals that produce angiogenesis, called angiogenic factors, or by changing the environment in which angiogenesis takes place.

6. **Blocking metastasis.** Metastasis is the invasion of cancer cells into the surrounding tissues and, eventually, the lymph so that the cancer spreads throughout the body. Natural compounds may normalize enzymes that promote invasion or stop it altogether.

7. **Boosting immunity.** Some believe that a failure of the immune system causes cancer. So, boosting immune response may directly kill cancer cells. But cancer cells have ways to mask themselves to avoid immune attack. Natural compounds may be able to directly boost immunity as well as mark cancer cells for destruction by immune cells.

Supplements for Cancer Inhibition

The majority of CAM oncology nutrition entails the use of nutritional supplements and supplement systems, such as traditional Chinese medicine. Most CAM supplements have very little cancer-specific human research to merit their use, especially as individual supplements, but Boik (2001) speculated that an entire program can be formulated based upon extrapolations of current research. CAM supplements used in cancer treatment need much more study.

Because supplements are so widely used by patients with cancer, nurses and dietitians need some research-supported information about them to pass on to their patients, including their degree of effectiveness, their possible effect upon the seven modifiable factors for cancer inhibition, and, most importantly, precautions and drug-supplement interactions. Table 17-1 provides information about supplements most frequently used by patients with cancer.

Complementary and Alternative Medicine Diets

Diets as cancer therapy run the gamut from healthy alternatives to supposed cures. They may concentrate upon a single food component, such as the Grape Cure, or changing the body's environment to improve cancer resistance, such as the Acid/Alkaline Diet. Most focus on increasing intake of unprocessed fruits, vegetables, and whole grains, and minimizing consumption of refined foods, fat, and animal products. Some of the most popular CAM cancer diets are described.

Gerson

Max Gerson, MD, originally developed this program, which prescribes a high-potassium, calorie-restricted, salt-restricted, initially protein-restricted diet. The regimen generally entails hourly feedings of phytonutrient-rich raw fruit and vegetable juices and raw veal liver juice. Protein is reinstituted after six weeks with mostly nonfat dairy products. Additional treatments include coffee enemas, niacin, potassium salts, castor oil, and injectable crude liver extract with vitamin B_{12} (Gerson & Hildenbrand, 1990; Hildenbrand et al., 1996). A 1990s retrospective review (Hildenbrand, Hildenbrand, Bradford, & Calvin, 1995) showed that melanoma survival rates were exceptionally higher in patients treated with Gerson therapy. Unfortunately, the study entailed small sample sizes in each cancer stage group and was conducted by the Gerson Research Organization. Clearly, independent research needs to be done on this regimen before it can be considered a viable cancer alternative.

Kelley/Gonzalez

Dentist William Kelley began this program of diet, supplement, and enzyme therapy in the 1960s, and it consists of a five-step program that includes metabolic supplementation (mostly with proteolytic pancreatic enzymes), detoxification (with coffee enemas), an adequate, proper, well-balanced diet, neurologic stimulation (with manipulation), and a spiritual attitude. Kelley developed 10 different diets with 95 variations, from strict vegetarian to all meat, and individualized them to each patient as he did the supplement regimen, which entailed up to 150 pills a day. Dietary recommendations include unprocessed organic foods, liberal use of butter and cream, rotation of meats, and whole-grain and nut porridge (Science of Optimum Health, 2003a, 2003b).

Table 17-1. Supplements Commonly Used by Patients With Cancer

Supplement or Other Natural Compound	Use	Reduces Oxidative Stress	Normalizes Gene Transcription	Normalizes Signal Transduction	Normalizes Intercellular Comm.	Blocks Angiogenesis	Blocks Metastasis	Boosts Immunity	Effectiveness	Precautions
Astragalus	Strong immune booster; antioxidant; anticoagulant; often used in traditional Chinese medicine in combination formulas such as *Bu Zhong Yi Qi Tang* and *Fei Liu Ping* (Chu et al., 1988; Upton, 1999; Wang et al., 1993)		X		X		X		Few human studies; more studies perhaps in the Orient	Contraindicated with anticoagulant and immunosuppressive drugs; more than 28 g may be immunosuppressive; reduces immunosuppression with cyclosporine
Bromelain (proteolytic enzymes)	Regulates immune system; with other therapies prolonged survival time; reduced chemotherapy side effects; improved tumor boundaries (Gonzalez & Isaacs, 1999; Hale et al., 2002; Kelly, 1996)	X	X	X	X	X		X	Promising effectiveness; used for more than 100 years in Europe; some animal and human studies	Caution with antiplatelet/anticoagulant drugs and supplements, folic acid, Mg, Fe, and Zn; GI disturbances; caution with IgE-mediated allergic reactions
Cat's claw	Antioxidant, immunostimulant, antiestrogenic and antiviral; induces cell death and inhibits leukemia and lymphoma; not cytotoxic to normal cells (Santa Maria et al., 1997; Sheng et al., 1998)		X		X				Research very preliminary; mostly in vitro studies; mechanisms not clear	Caution with anti-HTNs, CYP3A4 substrates, and immunosuppressant drugs; may cause headache, dizziness, and vomiting

(Continued on next page)

Table 17-1. Supplements Commonly Used by Patients With Cancer (Continued)

Supplement	Actions/Uses	Evidence markers	Efficacy	Contraindications/Cautions
EPA and DHA (fish oils, omega-3 fatty acids)	Inhibits tumor growth through free-radical mediation; inhibits inflammation, angiogenesis, and invasion enzymes; increases effectiveness of chemotherapy; may inhibit cancer-induced cachexia, but conflicting results (Batist et al., 2002; Bruera et al., 2003; Ogilvie et al., 2000; Tavani et al., 2003)	X X X X X X X X	Possibly effective; one of most-researched natural compounds	Contraindicated with anticoagulant/antiplatelet and antihypertensive drugs and oral contraceptives; doses of more than 3 g may depress immune system and raise blood sugar; possible mercury contamination with poorly manufactured products
Essiac	Tea and other products made with burdock, sorrel, rhubarb, and slippery elm; possibly estrogenic, antioxidant, anti-inflammatory, antimicrobial, and anticarcinogenic (Kaegi, 1998a; Richardson et al., 2000; Rowinsky et al., 2000)	X	No clinical trials; three human studies showed no effect; perceived benefit in one	Toxicity reported, especially from herb contamination and burdock root; one report of chemotherapy toxicity
Evening primrose oil (also borage, GLA, omega-6)	Increases effectiveness of chemotherapy; boosts efficiency of tamoxifen; antioxidant; boosts immune system (Kenny et al., 2000; Menendez et al., 2001)	X X X	Inconclusive evidence; better effect with combinations of lipids	May cause mild GI effects; contraindicated with anticoagulant/antiplatelet herbs and drugs; prolongs bleeding time

(Continued on next page)

Table 17-1. Supplements Commonly Used by Patients With Cancer (Continued)

Supplement or Other Natural Compound	Use	Reduces Oxidative Stress	Normalizes Gene Transcription	Normalizes Signal Transduction	Normalizes Intercellular Comm.	Blocks Angiogenesis	Blocks Metastasis	Boosts Immunity	Effectiveness	Precautions
Garlic	Antimicrobial, antibacterial, antifungal, antiviral, anti-inflammatory, anti-tumor; stimulates immunity; most research done with the vegetable form	X	X	X	X	X	X	X	Possibly effective for colorectal, prostate, and gastric cancers; ineffective for breast and lung cancers	Caution with many drugs, including saquinavir, NNRTIs, oral contraceptives, and anticoagulant/antiplatelets; stop one to two weeks before surgery as prolongs bleeding time
		(Dorant et al., 1995, 1996; Durak et al., 2003; Fleischauer et al., 2000)								
Ginger	Antiemetic; might help prevent chemotherapy-induced nausea when given following administration of IV compazine								Possibly effective against nausea with powered root 2–4 g daily	Interaction with many drugs including antacids, anticoagulants/antiplatelets, anti-DMs, anti-HTNs, H2-blockers, PPIs, and barbiturates; consult professional if patient is using many drugs
		(Ernst & Pittler, 2000; Lumb, 1993)								

(Continued on next page)

Table 17-1. Supplements Commonly Used by Patients With Cancer (Continued)

Supplement	Description					Research	Cautions
Ginseng (Panax and Siberian)	Stimulates natural killer cells and other immune activity; inhibits cancer cell growth in stomach, lung, liver, ovarian, and skin cancers; antioxidant	X	X	X		Insufficient reliable information; few human studies	Caution with many drugs, including anticoagulants/antiplatelets, MAOIs, antidiabetics, antipsychotics, immunosuppressants, and Coumadin®; interactions with several conditions, including DM; consult professional
	(Davydov & Krikorian, 2000; Shin et al., 2000; Yun & Choi, 1995)						
Glutamine	Lowers glutathione in cancer cells and increases it in normal cells; reduces chemotherapy and radiotherapy side effects; increases immune response	X	X	X	X	Many human and animal studies; conflicting results from studies on reducing varied effects of treatment	Caution with anticonvulsants and lactulose; caution with hepatic encephalopathy, mania, seizure disorders, and MSG sensitivity
	(Anderson et al., 1998; Daniele et al., 2001; Savarese et al., 1998b)						
Green tea (EGCG)	Antioxidant; generally reduces risk of bladder, esophageal, pancreatic, gastric, and breast cancers, and cervical dysplasia; inhibits angiogenesis; enhances the effects of doxorubicin	X	X	X	X	Few human studies, but strong possibility of effectiveness in many animal studies	Caution with many drugs, especially anticoagulants/antiplatelets, Coumadin and MAOIs; caution with many conditions including DM, HTN, kidney disorders, and bleeding disorders; have patient consult a professional for more precautions and suggestions for supplementation
	(Garbisa et al., 1999b; Kaegi, 1998b; Sadzuka et al., 2000)						

(Continued on next page)

Table 17-1. Supplements Commonly Used by Patients With Cancer (Continued)

Supplement or Other Natural Compound	Use	Reduces Oxidative Stress	Normalizes Gene Transcription	Normalizes Signal Transduction	Normalizes Intercellular Comm.	Blocks Angiogenesis	Blocks Metastasis	Boosts Immunity	Effectiveness	Precautions
Hydrazine sulfate	Possibly reduces cachexia; mechanism unclear (Loprinzi, Goldberg, et al., 1994; Loprinzi, Kuross, et al., 1994)								Ineffective in colorectal and lung cancers; somewhat effective in neuroblastoma and Hodgkin disease	Adverse GI, neurologic, and glycemic effects; caution with anti-DM drugs, CNS depressants, and MAOIs; causes many abnormal drug tests
IP-6 (inositol hexophosphate)	Strong chelator; possibly involved in cell signaling and growth; antioxidant; enhances immune response (Shamsuddin & Vucenik, 1999; Shamsuddin et al., 1997; Vucenik et al., 1998)		X		X		X		Weak research; no studies in humans	Caution with pregnant women and lactating mothers; may reduce absorption of Ca, Fe, and Zn; mostly safe
Iscador (European mistletoe)	Biological response modifier; stimulates immune system; cytotoxic (Ernst et al., 2003; Grossarth-Matichek et al., 2001; Kaegi, 1998c)		X		X				Does not improve patient survival in any form of cancer	Caution with antihypertensive and immunosuppressive drugs; large amounts may cause toxicity

(Continued on next page)

Table 17-1. Supplements Commonly Used by Patients With Cancer (Continued)

Supplement	Description								References	Effectiveness	Cautions
Melatonin	Potent antioxidant; possibly controls oncogene expression; effective against breast, brain, lung, prostate, head and neck, and GI cancers; reduces solid tumors and chemotherapy toxicity; inhibits cachexia	X	X	X	X	X	X	X	(Lissoni et al., 1997; Lissoni, Barni, et al., 1999; Lissoni, Tancini, et al., 1999)	Possibly effective; many human studies; third most researched cancer-related supplement	Caution with many types of medications; caution with HTN, DM, and seizure disorders; have patients consult a supplement professional because of many interactions
MGN-3	Combination of rice bran and enzymes from mycelia of Shiitake, Kawaratake, and Suehirotake mushrooms; improves immunity							X	(Ghoneum, 1998; FDA, 1999)	Insufficient reliable information; most research is small studies and done by physician who invented product	None known; FDA is seeking permanent injunction for unapproved drug product promoted as treatment for cancer
Mushrooms (Beta-Glucans, Coriolus, Lentinan, Schizophyllan, Maitake [D fraction], Reishi, Shiitake, Kombucha, PSK, PSP)	Powerful immune stimulants; induce cell differentiation and cell death; inhibit cancer invasion; positive outcomes with breast, colorectal, lung, hepatic, nasopharyngeal, prostate, and gastric cancers; polysaccharides	X	X	X			X	X	(Borchers et al., 1999; deVere White et al., 2002; Ross et al., 1999)	Most researched of cancer-related supplements; used as cancer drug in Japan; possibly effective; research done with supplement, not food	Well-tolerated; caution with immunosuppressive antiplatelet/anticoagulant drugs; one episode of eosinophilia with large amount of powder (4 g); a tincture or decoction is form best used for supplementation, but studies have also used IVs, capsules, teas, tablets, and powders

(Continued on next page)

Table 17-1. Supplements Commonly Used by Patients With Cancer (Continued)

Supplement or Other Natural Compound	Use	Reduces Oxidative Stress	Normalizes Gene Transcription	Normalizes Signal Transduction	Normalizes Intercellular Comm.	Blocks Angiogenesis	Blocks Metastasis	Boosts Immunity	Effectiveness	Precautions
Resveratrol	Substance in grapes and wine; antioxidant; inhibits platelet aggregation, promotes apoptosis, and inhibits tumor growth	X	X	X	X	X		X	Preliminary, insufficient information for effectiveness	Has weak phytoestrogenic effect and may not be appropriate for those with breast cancer; few adverse reactions but may be contraindicated with anticoagulant/antiplatelet drugs and herbs; inhibits cytochrome P-450 enzymes so may also be contraindicated with CYP3A4 substrates
	(Carbo et al., 1999; Huang et al., 1999)									
Selenium	Antioxidant; easily participates in redox reactions; organic selenium works best; strongest association for cancer prevention in breast, prostate, and colorectal cancers; used in conjunction with other	X	X	X	X	X	X	X	Possibly effective for prostate cancer; conflicting evidence for colorectal and breast cancers; few human studies; prevention trials have shown	Reduces the effectiveness of HMG-CoA reductase inhibitors; decreases the effectiveness of the combination of niacin and simvastatin; toxicity can cause abnormal ECG reading similar to myocardial infarction; doses more than 400 mcg per day for adults may cause symptoms
	(Clark et al., 1996, 1998; Helzlsouer et al., 2000)									

(Continued on next page)

Table 17-1. Supplements Commonly Used by Patients With Cancer (Continued)

Supplement	Properties							Evidence	Side effects/comments
Selenium (cont.)	antioxidants like vitamin E in clinical trials							correlation between low selenium levels and increased cancer risk	including hair loss, white horizontal streaking on fingernails, fatigue, irritability, nausea, vomiting, garlic odor on breath, thrombocytopenia, and a metallic taste; avoid supplements during treatment
Shark cartilage (Neovastat [AE 941])	Antioxidant; has possible antimutagenic, anti-inflammatory, and analgesic effects; strong antiangiogenic properties; modulates apoptosis. (Batist et al., 2002; Neovastat clinical trial abstracts, 2001)	X	X			X		Very preliminary studies; effective against renal cell carcinoma; not effective against many advanced cancers but no other study types	Causes many side effects including nausea and vomiting, taste problems, constipation, hypotension, edema, hypercalcemia, and malaise; also causes acute hepatitis symptoms including elevated liver enzymes; acidic fruit juice can decrease potency; no known drug interactions
Soy (genistein and daidzein)	Most active isoflavones act as antioxidants, antimutagens, and antiproliferators for a wide variety of cancer cell lines; reduce menopausal symptoms; effective against prostate cancer; inhibit tumor growth through direct and indirect means. (Han et al., 2002; Horn-Ross et al., 2002; Lamartiniere, 2000)	X	X	X	X	X	X	Possible effectiveness against breast cancer, but evidence is conflicting and controversial; not enough evidence to merit use in most cancers except prostate cancer; many animal but few human studies	One to three servings of whole soy foods recommended instead of supplements for those with breast cancer because of phytoestrogenic effect; may increase risk of bladder cancer; caution with several types of drugs including estrogens, antibiotics, aromatase inhibitors, and Coumadin; may cause GI disturbances and allergic reactions; reduces iron absorption

(Continued on next page)

Table 17-1. Supplements Commonly Used by Patients With Cancer (Continued)

Supplement or Other Natural Compound	Use	Reduces Oxidative Stress	Normalizes Gene Transcription	Normalizes Signal Transduction	Normalizes Intercellular Comm.	Blocks Angiogenesis	Blocks Metastasis	Boosts Immunity	Effectiveness	Precautions
Traditional Chinese medicine	Polysaccharide blends with saponins such as Panax ginseng; stimulate immune system; biological response modifier; reduces chemotherapy toxicity; *Shi Quan Da Bu Tang* and *Bu Zhong Yi Qi Tang* most effective for cancer	X	X	X		X		X	Mostly animal studies so not enough evidence for effectiveness; possibly many more studies done in China	Mostly safe even when taken in conjunction with chemotherapy; see individual listings for astragalus, ginseng, and mushrooms for additional precautions; see herbalist or licensed acupuncturist for more information as these supplements are part of a much larger supplement system
	(Ebisuno et al., 1989; Ito & Shimura, 1985a, 1985b)									
Vitamin A	As ATRA (metabolite only available by prescription) and retinyl esters, effective against a variety of cancers; as beta-carotene, some	X	X	X	X	X	X	X	Possibly effective against breast cancer; many human studies with ATRA; ATRA approved for promyelocytic	High incidence of toxicity in doses > 15,000 IU; vitamin E increases absorption, enhances utilization, and prevents toxicity; toxicity symptoms include fatigue, irritability and other mood changes, anorexia, nausea and
	(The Alpha-Tocopherol, Beta-Carotene Cancer Prevention Study Group. 1994; Omenn et al., 1996)									

(Continued on next page)

Table 17-1. Supplements Commonly Used by Patients With Cancer (Continued)

									Effectiveness	Cautions/Side Effects
Vitamin A (cont.)	studies have shown causes cancer; antioxidant; enhances effect of chemotherapy; inhibits proliferation and increases differentiation								leukemia (80% remission in one study); inconsistent results; synthetic beta-carotene increased cancer risk, especially in smokers	vomiting, skin and nail changes, hair loss, anemia, leukopenia, leukocytosis, and thrombocytopenia; caution with many types of drugs including Coumadin, tetracyclines, and aminoglycosides; avoid supplements during treatment; consult professional for therapeutic doses
Vitamin C	Antioxidant; as prooxidant induces apoptosis; inhibits histamine; supports immunity; might decrease stomach, mouth, and esophageal cancers; conflicting evidence with breast cancer; mostly IV use for cancer trials (Labriola & Livingston, 1999; Prasad et al., 2002)	X	X	X	X	X	X		Possibly effective, but results inconclusive; not effective in patients with advanced cancer; possibly better results if used with other natural anticancer compounds	Doses greater than 2,000 mg may cause nausea, vomiting, esophagitis, heartburn, fatigue, flushing, headache, insomnia, diarrhea and other GI upsets; avoid supplements during treatment; may reduce effectiveness of chemotherapy; caution with many drugs including Coumadin, statins, and oral contraceptives; cancer cells uptake high doses but unknown if this is detrimental; high doses form oxalates and kidney stones; see professional for therapeutic doses

(Continued on next page)

Table 17-1. Supplements Commonly Used by Patients With Cancer (Continued)

Supplement or Other Natural Compound	Use	Reduces Oxidative Stress	Normalizes Gene Transcription	Normalizes Signal Transduction	Normalizes Intercellular Comm.	Blocks Angiogenesis	Blocks Metastasis	Boosts Immunity	Effectiveness	Precautions
Vitamin D	Deficiency linked to increased risk of breast, prostate, and colon cancers; as 1,25-D_3 (metabolite only available by prescription), has antitumor properties; may reduce expression of estrogen receptors; may increase half-life of ATRA	X	X	X	X	X	X		Not enough research to merit use in supplement form; usefulness hampered by toxicity; conversion of vitamin D supplements to 1,25-D_3 dependent upon body stores	Maximum daily tolerated dose of 1,25-D_3 1 to 2.5 mcg; may cause hypercalcemia; excess oral vitamin D more than 25 mcg (1,000 IU) may cause adverse effects such as osteoporosis, weight loss, anemia, pancreatitis, and seizures; interactions with many drugs including Tegretol®, Dilantin®, and thiazide diuretics; use therapeutic doses only under care of professional
	(Gross et al., 1998; Shokravi et al., 1995; Smith et al., 1999)									
Vitamin E	Antioxidant; most trials with a combination of other antioxidants; used topically on chemotherapy-induced skin	X	X	X	X	X	X	X	Possibly effective with cancers mentioned; best forms natural	Generally well-tolerated orally; avoid supplements during treatment; may reduce effectiveness of chemotherapy; interactions with several drugs including
	(Heinonen et al., 1998; Prasad et al., 2002; Virtamo et al., 2003)									

(Continued on next page)

Table 17-1. Supplements Commonly Used by Patients With Cancer (Continued)

Vitamin E (cont.)	ulcers (151); prevents recurrence of colorectal, prostate, breast, and gastric cancers		vitamin E succinate and alpha-tocopherol; human prevention trials but no human anticancer trials	Coumadin, anticoagulants/antiplatelets, and statins; interacts with several supplements/herbs such as lipid-based vitamins and other supplements and iron

ATRA—all-trans retinoic acid; Ca—calcium; CNS—central nervous system; DM—diabetes mellitus; ECG—electrocardiogram; FDA—U.S. Food and Drug Administration; Fe—iron; GI—gastrointestinal; HMG-CoA—3-hydroxy-3-methylglutaryl coenzyme A; HTN—hypertension; IgE—immunoglobulin E; IU—international units; MAOI—monoamine oxidase inhibitor; Mg—magnesium; NNRTI—non-nucleoside reverse transcriptase inhibitors; PPI—proton pump inhibitor; Zn—zinc

Note. © 2004, *Supplement Savvy, A Supplement Education System for Dietitians and Supplement Savvy Specialists: Cancer, Volume II.* Reprinted with permission of Jill Place, MA, RD, The Supplement Savvy RD.

Nicholas Gonzalez, MD, refined Kelley's program, dispensed with the spiritual and neurologic components, and added hair analysis to track progress. Initial studies have begun, but they are sparse and only have been conducted by Gonzalez and his colleagues. One recent study with mice (Saruc et al., 2004) indicated that the Gonzalez program might slow tumor growth and prolong pancreatic cancer survival. Another pilot study by Gonzalez showed an excellent survival rate among patients with adenocarcinoma (Gonzalez & Isaacs, 1999). Clearly, more independent study is needed.

Macrobiotics

George Ohsawa developed a diet-only approach to cancer and general health in the 1930s, and it was popularized in the United States by Michio Kushi, whose books on macrobiotics and cancer have made this regimen a CAM mainstay. Macrobiotics touts Oriental doctrines of rest, relaxation, and orderliness along with a return to the body's acid-alkaline balance by consuming mostly whole grains, vegetables, pickled foods, beans, sea vegetables, and, occasionally, fish (Kushi Institute, 2004). There is considerable anecdotal evidence and a few studies comparing those on the regimen with expected survival rates but no conclusive scientific research that macrobiotics is a viable cancer treatment (Kushi et al., 2001; Labriola, 2000).

Using Complementary and Alternative Medicine Knowledge With Patients

Some studies (Malik & Gopalan, 2003; Shumay et al., 2001; Wernecke et al., 2004) point to a reduced chance of recovery for those who shun conventional cancer treatment in favor of alternative cures. However, if patients are able to receive the full spectrum of alternative and conventional information about their condition at their first visit with an oncologist, they may be more equipped to make better treatment choices. All oncology professionals should

1. Gain more knowledge about CAM, especially about effectiveness and interactions with other treatments and drugs.
2. Gain more knowledge about effective ways to counsel this difficult patient population.
3. Focus mainly on "to do no harm." If patients are going to use CAM, practitioners have a responsibility to inform them of the potential hazards of the CAMs they are using.

Questions to Ask

To get a clear picture of what patients taking CAM are using, some example questions are listed. Include them as part of a patient questionnaire. It is helpful to have patients bring all of the supplements they are taking to their first consultation to determine supplement quality and toxic doses.

1. What types of CAM and nutritional supplements are you currently using (macrobiotics, acupuncture, vitamins, minerals, herbs)?
2. Who advised you to take them (health food store clerk, book on cancer, dietitian)?
3. Where did you get these supplements (health food store, dietitian, CAM practitioner)?
4. Why are you using these supplements? What do you think they will do for you?
5. Are you aware that some supplements may make the drugs you are taking less effective?

Advice to Patients

When giving advice to patients about supplements and other forms of CAM, it might be beneficial to cover the following points using short, easy-to-understand sentences to communicate your message. Negating the CAM experience most likely will not change behavior, but listening to, being accepting of, and educating patients with some solid information about CAMs might.

1. No current scientific research shows you can cure cancer by taking supplements or using CAMs.
2. Tell your doctor about the supplements and other CAMs you are using so that you can avoid supplement-drug interactions and other potential problems.
3. The best overall treatment for cancer might be an integrative approach of both conventional and alternative treatments. It is important to coordinate your cancer care with all of your practitioners.
4. The supplements you are taking (list them) may make the drugs you are taking (list them) less effective or have other effects (list them). Remember that all substances may cause harm if you take too much.
5. The U.S. Food and Drug Administration does not regulate supplements. Quality, safety, and effectiveness are questionable.
6. If you are interested in CAM for cancer care, it might be wise to consult a professional, such as an RN or dietitian, who specializes in alternative medicine. Recommendations from your friends, family, or the Internet may be inaccurate and possibly harmful.

Summary

A distinct dichotomy exists between CAM nutrition use by patients with cancer and CAM acceptance by oncologists. Up to 80% of patients with cancer are using CAM (Sparber et al., 2000; Wernecke et al., 2004), but more than 80% of oncologists do not approve of CAM usage (Salmenpera et al., 2003).

This dichotomy may lead to adverse side effects, drug-nutrient interactions, and overall reduced recovery from all types of cancer. CAM use is increasing, so oncologists and other cancer practitioners have a responsibility to learn more about CAM or refer their patients to nurses and dietitians who do to maximize their possibility of recovery.

References

The Alpha-Tocopherol, Beta-Carotene Cancer Prevention Study Group. (1994). The effect of vitamin E and beta-carotene on the incidence of lung cancer and other cancers in male smokers. *New England Journal of Medicine, 330,* 1029–1035.

Anderson, P.M., Ramsay, N.K., Shu, X.O., Rydholm, N., Rogosheske, J., Nicklow, R., et al. (1998). Effect of low-dose oral glutamine on painful stomatitis during bone marrow transplantation. *Bone Marrow Transplantation, 22,* 339–344.

Batist, G., Patenaude, F., Champagne, P., Croteau, D., Levinton, C., Hariton, C., et al. (2002). Neovastat (AE-941) in refractory renal cell carcinoma patients: Report of a phase II trial with two dose levels. *Annals of Oncology, 13,* 1259–1263.

Bland, J.S. (2004). *Nutrigenomic modulation of inflammatory disorders: Arthralgias, coronary heart disease, pms- and menopause-associated inflammation.* Gig Harbor, WA: Metagenics Educational Programs.

Boik, J. (2001). *Natural compounds in cancer therapy.* Princeton, MI: Oregon Medical Press.

Borchers, A.T., Stern, J.S., Hackman, R.M., Keen, C.L., & Gershwin, M.E. (1999). Mushrooms, tumors, and immunity. *Proceedings of the Society for Experimental Biology and Medicine, 221,* 281–293.

Bruera, E., Strasser, F., Palmer, J.L., Willey, J., Calder, K., Amyotte, G., et al. (2003). Effect of fish oil on appetite and other symptoms in patients with advanced cancer and anorexia/cachexia: A double-blind, placebo-controlled study. *Journal of Clinical Oncology, 2,* 129–134.

Carbo, N., Costelli, P., Baccino, F.M., Lopez-Soriano, F.J., & Argiles, J.M. (1999). Resveratrol, a natural product present in wine, decreases tumour growth in a rat tumour model. *Biochemical and Biophysical Research Communications, 254,* 739–743.

Caspi, O., Sechrest, L., Pitluk, H.C., Marshall, C.L., Bell, I.R., & Nichter, M. (2003). On the definition of complementary, alternative, and integrative medicine; societal megastereotypes vs. the patients' perspective. *Alternative Therapies in Health and Medicine, 9*(6), 58–62.

Chrystal, K., Allen, S., Forgeson, G., & Isaacs, R. (2003). The use of complementary/alternative medicine by cancer patients in a New Zealand regional cancer treatment centre. *New Zealand Medical Journal, 116*(1168), U296.

Chu, D.T., Wong, W.L., & Mavligit, G.M. (1988). Immunotherapy with Chinese medicinal herbs. II. Reversal of cyclophosphamide-induced immune suppression by administration of fractionated Astragalus membranaceus in vivo. *Journal of Clinincal and Laboratory Immunology, 25,* 125–129.

Clark, L.C., Combs, G.F., Turnbull, B.W., Slate, E.H., Chalker, D.K., Chow, J., et al. (1996). Effects of selenium supplementation for cancer prevention in patients with carcinoma of the skin. A randomized controlled trial. *JAMA, 276,* 1957–1963.

Clark, L.C., Dalkin, B., Krongrad, A., Combs, G.F., Jr., Turnbull, B.W., Slate, E.H., et al. (1998). Decreased incidence of prostate cancer with selenium supplementation: Results of a double-blind cancer prevention trial. *British Journal of Urology, 81,* 730–734.

Daniele, B., Perrone, F., Gallo, C., Pignata, S., De Martino, S., De Vivo, R., et al. (2001). Oral glutamine in the prevention of fluorouracil induced intestinal toxicity: A double blind, placebo controlled, randomized trial. *Gut, 48,* 28–33.

Davydov, M., & Krikorian, A.D. (2000). Eleutherococcus senticosus (Rupr. & Maxim.) Maxim. (Araliaceae) as an adaptogen: A closer look. *Journal of Ethnopharmacology, 72,* 345–393, 401–408.

deVere White, R.W., Hackman, R.M., Soares, S.E., Beckett, L.A., & Sun, B. (2002). Effects of a mushroom mycelium extract on the treatment of prostate cancer. *Urology, 60,* 640–644.

Dorant, E., van den Brandt, P.A., & Goldbohm, R.A. (1995). Allium vegetable consumption, garlic supplement intake, and female breast carcinoma incidence. *Breast Cancer Research and Treatment, 33,* 163–170.

Dorant, E., van den Brandt, P.A., & Goldbohm, R.A. (1996). A prospective cohort study on the relationship between onion and leek consumption, garlic supplement use and the risk of colorectal carcinoma in The Netherlands. *Carcinogenesis, 17,* 477–484.

Durak, I., Yilmaz, E., & Devrim, E. (2003). Consumption of aqueous garlic extract leads to significant improvement in patients with benign prostate hyperplasia and prostate cancer. *Nutrition Reviews, 23,* 199–204.

Dutta, A.P., Dutta, A.P., Bwayo, S., Xue, E., Akiyode, O., Ayuk-Egbe, P., et al. (2003). Complementary and alternative medicine instruction in nursing curricula. *Journal of the National Black Nurses Association, 14*(2), 30–33.

Ebisuno, S., Hirano, A., Kyoku, I., Ohkawa, T., Iijima, O., Fujii, Y., et al. (1989). Basal studies in combination with Chinese medicine in cancer chemotherapy. Protective effects on the toxic side effects of CDDP and antitumor effects with CDDP on murine bladder tumor (MBT-2). *Nippon Gan Chiryo Gakkai Shi, 24*(6), 1305–1312.

Eisenberg, D.M., Davis, R.B., Ettner, S.L., Appel, S., Wilkey, S., Van Rompay, M., et al. (1998). Trends in alternative medicine use in the United States, 1990–1997: Results of a follow-up national survey. *JAMA, 280,* 1569–1575.

Eng, J., Ramsum, D., Verhoef, M., Guns, E., Davison, J., & Gallagher, R. (2003). A population-based survey of complementary and alternative medicine use in men recently diagnosed with prostate cancer. *Integrated Cancer Therapy, 2*(3), 212–216.

Ernst, E., & Pittler, M.H. (2000). Efficacy of ginger for nausea and vomiting: A systematic review of randomized clinical trials. *British Journal of Anaesthesia, 84,* 367–371.

Ernst, E., Schmidt, K., & Steuer-Vogt, M.K. (2003). Mistletoe for cancer? A systematic review of randomized clinical trials. *International Journal of Cancer, 107,* 262–267.

Fleischauer, A.T., Poole, C., & Arab, L. (2000). Garlic consumption and cancer prevention: Meta-analyses of colorectal and stomach cancers. *American Journal of Clinical Nutrition, 72,* 1047–1052.

Fogg-Johnson, N., & Kaput, J. (2003). Nutrigenomics: An emerging scientific discipline. *Food Technology, 57*(4), 60–67.

Garbisa, S., Biggin, S., Cavallarin, N., Sartor, L., Benelli, R., & Albini, A. (1999). Tumor invasion: Molecular shears blunted by green tea. *Nature Medicine, 5,* 1216.

Gerson, M., & Hildenbrand, G.L. (Eds.). (1990). *A cancer therapy, results of fifty cases* (5th ed.). San Diego, CA: Gerson Institute.

Ghoneum, M. (1998). Enhancement of human natural killer cell activity by modified arabinoxylane from rice bran (MGN-3). *International Journal of Immunotherapy, 14,* 89–99.

Gonzalez, N. (2004). *Information on the treatment method.* Retrieved May 23, 2004, from http://www.dr-gonzalez.com/treatment_txt.htm

Gonzalez, N.J., & Isaacs, L.L. (1999). Evaluation of pancreatic proteolytic enzymes treatment of adenocarcinoma of the pancreas, with nutrition and detoxification support. *Nutrition and Cancer, 33*(2), 117–124.

Great Smokies Diagnostic Laboratories. (2003). *Genovations: Introducing breakthrough genetic assessment for customized intervention.* Retrieved April 23, 2004, from http://www.genovations.com/overview.html

Gross, C., Stanley, T., Hancock, S., & Feldman, D. (1998). Treatment of early recurrent prostate cancer with 1,24-dihydroxyvitamin D3. *Journal of Urology, 159,* 2035–2040.

Grossarth-Matichek, R., Kiene, H., Baumgartner, S.M., & Ziegler, R. (2001). Use of Iscador, an extract of European mistletoe (Viscum album), in cancer treatment: Prospective nonrandomized and randomized matched-pair studies nested within a cohort study. *Alternative Therapies in Health and Medicine, 7,* 57–78.

Hale, L.P., Greer, P.K., & Sempowski, G.D. (2002). Bromelain treatment alters leukocyte expression of cell surface molecules involved in cellular adhesion and activation. *Clinical Immunology, 104,* 83–90.

Han, K.K., Soares, J.M., Jr., Haidar, M.A., de Lima, G.R., & Baracat, E.C. (2002). Benefits of soy isoflavone therapeutic regimen on menopausal symptoms. *Obstetrics and Gynecology, 99,* 389–394.

Heinonen, O.P., Albanes, D., Virtamo, J., Taylor, P.R., Huttunen, J.K., Hartman, A.M., et al. (1998). Prostate cancer and supplementation with alpha-tocopherol and beta-carotene: Incidence and mortality in a controlled trial. *Journal of the National Cancer Institute, 90,* 440–446.

Helzlsouer, K.J., Huang, H.Y., Alberg, A.J., Hoffman, S., Burke, A., Norkus, E.P., et al. (2000). Association between alpha-tocopherol, gamma-tocopherol, selenium, and subsequent prostate cancer. *Journal of the National Cancer Institute, 92,* 2018–2023.

Hildenbrand, G.L., Hildenbrand, L.C., Bradford, K., & Calvin, S.W. (1995). Five-year survival rates of melanoma patients treated by diet therapy after the manner of Gerson: A retrospective review. *Alternative Therapies in Health and Medicine, 1*(4), 29–37.

Hildenbrand, G.L., Hildenbrand, L.C., Bradford, K., Rogers, D., Straus, C., & Calvin, S. (1996). The role of follow-up and retrospective data analysis in alternative cancer management: The Gerson experience. *Journal of Naturopathic Medicine, 6*(1), 49–56.

Horn-Ross, P.L., Hoggatt, K.J., & Lee, M.M. (2002). Phytoestrogens and thyroid cancer risk: The San Francisco Bay Area thyroid cancer study. *Cancer Epidemiology, Biomarkers and Prevention, 11,* 43–49.

Huang, C., Ma, W.Y., Goranson, A., & Dong, Z. (1999). Resveratrol suppresses cell transformation and induces apoptosis through a p53-dependent pathway. *Carcinogenesis, 20*(2), 237–242.

Institute for Functional Medicine. (2004). *What is functional medicine?* Retrieved May 29, 2004, from http://www.functionalmedicine.org/about/whatis.asp

Ito, H., & Shimura, K. (1985a). Studies on the antitumor activity of traditional chinese medicines. *Gan To Kagaku Ryoho, 12,* 2145–2148.

Ito, H., & Shimura, K. (1985a). Studies on the antitumor activity of traditional chinese medicines II. *Gan To Kagaku Ryoho, 12,* 2149–2154.

Kaegi, E. (1998a). Unconventional therapies for cancer: 1. Essiac. *Canadian Medical Association Journal, 158,* 897–902.

Kaegi, E. (1998b). Unconventional therapies for cancer: 2. Green tea. The Task Force on Alternative Therapies of the Canadian Breast Cancer Research Initiative. *Canadian Medical Association Journal, 158,* 1033–1035.

Kaegi E. (1998c). Unconventional therapies for cancer: 3. Iscador. *Canadian Medical Association Journal, 158,* 1157–1159.

Kelly, G.S. (1996). Bromelain: A literature review and discussion of its therapeutic applications. *Alternative Medicine Review, 1*(4), 243–257.

Kenny, F.S., Pinder, S.E., Ellis, I.O., Gee, J.M., Nicholson, R.I., Bryce, R.P., et al. (2000). Gamma linolenic acid with tamoxifen as primary therapy in breast cancer. *International Journal of Cancer, 85,* 643–648.

Kushi, L.H., Cunningham, J.E., Hebert, J.R., Lerman, R.H., Bandera, E.V., & Teas, J. (2001). The macrobiotic diet in cancer. *Journal of Nutrition, 131*(Suppl. 11), 3056S–3064S.

Kushi Institute. (2004). *What is macrobiotics?* Retrieved May 23, 2004, from http://www.kushiinstitute.org/whatismacro.html

Labriola, D. (2000). *Complementary cancer therapies.* Roseville, CA: Prima Publishing.

Labriola, D., & Livingston, R. (1999). Possible interactions between dietary antioxidants and chemotherapy. *Oncology, 13,* 1003–1008.

Lamartiniere, C.A. (2000). Protection against breast cancer with genistein: A component of soy. *American Journal of Clinical Nutrition, 71*(Suppl.), 1705S–1707S.

Lee, B.M., Lee, S.K., & Kim, H.S. (1998). Inhibition of oxidative DNA damage, 8-OHdG, and carbonyl contents in smokers treated with antioxidants (vitamin E, vitamin C, beta-carotene and red ginseng). *Cancer Letters, 132*, 219–227.

Lissoni, P., Barni, S., Mandala, M., Ardizzoia, A., Paolorossi, F., Vaghi, M., et al. (1999). Decreased toxicity and increased efficacy of cancer chemotherapy using the pineal hormone melatonin in metastatic solid tumor patients with poor clinical status. *European Journal of Cancer, 35*, 1688–1692.

Lissoni, P., Paolorossi, F., Ardizzoia, A., Barni, S., Chilelli, M., Mancuso, M., et al. (1997). A randomized study of chemotherapy with cisplatin plus etoposide versus chemoendocrine therapy with cisplatin, etoposide and the pineal hormone melatonin as a first-line treatment of advanced non-small cell lung cancer patients in a poor clinical state. *Journal of Pineal Research, 23*, 15–19.

Lissoni, P., Tancini, G., Paolorossi, F., Mandala, M., Ardizzoia, A., Malugani, F., et al. (1999). Chemoneuroendocrine therapy of metastatic breast cancer with persistent thrombocytopenia with weekly low-dose epirubicin plus melatonin: A phase II study. *Journal of Pineal Research, 26*(3), 169–173.

Loprinzi, C.L., Goldberg, R.M., Su, J.Q., Mailliard, J.A., Kuross, S.A., Maksymiuk, A.W., et al. (1994). Placebo-controlled trial of hydrazine sulfate in patients with newly diagnosed non-small-cell lung cancer. *Journal of Clinical Oncology, 12*, 1126–1129.

Loprinzi, C.L., Kuross, S.A., O'Fallon, J.R., Gesme, D.H., Jr., Gerstner, J.B., Rospond, R.M., et al. (1994). Randomized, placebo-controlled evaluation of hydrazine sulfate in patients with advanced colorectal cancer. *Journal of Clinical Oncology, 12*, 1121–1125.

Lumb, A.B. (1993). Mechanism of antiemetic effect of ginger. *Anaesthesia, 48*, 1118.

Malik, I.A., & Gopalan, S. (2003). Use of CAM results in delay in seeking medical advice for breast cancer. *European Journal of Epidemiology, 18*, 817–822.

Menendez, J.A., del Mar Barbacid, M., Montero, S., Sevilla, E., Escrich, E., Solanas, M., et al. (2001). Effects of gamma-linolenic acid and oleic acid on paclitaxel cytotoxicity in human breast cancer cells. *European Journal of Cancer, 37*, 402–413.

Neovastat clinical trial abstracts. (2001, March). Abstracts presented at the American Association for Cancer Research 92nd annual meeting, New Orleans, LA.

Ogilvie, G.K., Fettman, M.J., Mallinckrodt, C.H., Walton, J.A., Hansen, R.A., Davenport, D.J., et al. (2000). Effect of fish oil, arginine, and doxorubicin chemotherapy on remission and survival time for dogs with lymphoma: A double-blind, randomized, placebo-controlled study. *Cancer, 88*, 1916–1928.

Omenn, G.S., Goodman, G., Thornquist, M., Balmes, J., Cullen, M.R., Glass, A., et al. (1996). Risk factors for lung cancer and intervention effects in CARET, the beta-carotene and retinol efficiency trial. *Journal of the National Cancer Institute, 88*, 1560–1570.

Prasad, K.N., Cole, W.C., Kumar, B., & Che Prasad, K. (2002). Pros and cons of antioxidant use during radiation therapy. *Cancer Treatment Reviews, 28*, 79–91.

Richardson, M.A., Ramirez, T., Tamayo, C., Perez, C., & Palmer, J.L. (2000). Flor-Essence herbal tonic use in North America. *Herbalgram, 50*, 40–46.

Rizzi, R., Re, F., Bianchi, A., De Feo, V., de Simone, F., Bianchi, L., et al. (1993). Mutagenic and antimutagenic activities of Uncaria tomentosa and its extracts. *Journal of Ethnopharmacology, 38*(1), 63–77.

Rosenthal, R., & Rosenthal, R. (2001). *Exploring complementary and alternative medicine.* Washington, DC: National Academies Press.

Ross, G.D., Vetvicka, V., Yan, J., Xia, Y., & Vetvickova, J. (1999). Therapeutic intervention with complement and beta-glucan in cancer. *Immunopharmacology, 42*(1), 61–74.

Rowinsky, E.K., Johnson, T.R., Geyer, C.E., Jr., Hammond, L.A., Eckhardt, S.G., Drengler, R., et al. (2000). DX-8951f, a hexacyclic camptothecin analog, on a daily-times-five schedule: A phase I and pharmacokinetic study in patients with advanced solid malignancies. *Clinical Oncology, 18*, 3151–3163.

Sadzuka, Y., Sugiyama, T., & Sonobe, T. (2000). Efficacies of tea components on doxorubicin induced antitumor activity and reversal of multidrug resistance. *Toxicology Letters, 114,* 155–162.

Salmenpera, L., Suominen, T., & Vertio, H. (2003). Physicians' attitudes towards the use of complementary therapies (CTs) by cancer patients in Finland. *European Journal of Cancer Care, 12,* 358–364.

Santa Maria, A., Lopez, A., Diaz, M.M., Alban, J., Galan de Mera, A., Vicente Orellana, J.A., et al. (1997). Evaluation of the toxicity of Uncaria tomentosa by bioassays in vitro. *Journal of Ethnopharmacology, 57,* 183–187.

Saruc, M., Standop, S., Standop, J., Nozawa, F., Itami, A., Pandey, K.K., et al. (2004). Pancreatic enzyme extract improves survival in murine pancreatic cancer. *Pancreas, 28,* 401–412.

Savarese, D., Boucher, J., & Corey, B. (1998). Glutamine treatment of paclitaxel-induced myalgias and arthralgias [Letter]. *Journal of Clinical Oncology, 16,* 3918–3919.

Science of Optimum Health. (2003a). *Dietary recommendations.* Retrieved May 23, 2004, from http://www.drkelleycancerprogram.com/13.html

Science of Optimum Health. (2003b). *Dr. Kelley's cancer program.* Retrieved May 23, 2004, from http://www.drkelleycancerprogram.com/3.html

Shamsuddin, A.M., & Vucenik, I. (1999). Mammary tumor inhibition by IP6: A review. *Anticancer Research, 19,* 3671–3674.

Shamsuddin, A.M., Vucenik, I., & Cole, K.E. (1997). IP6: A novel anti-cancer agent. *Life Sciences, 61,* 343–354.

Sheng, Y., Pero, R.W., Amiri, A., & Bryngelsson, C. (1998). Induction of apoptosis and inhibition of proliferation in human tumor cells treated with extracts of Uncaria tomentosa. *Anticancer Research, 18,* 3363–3368.

Shin, H.R., Kim, J.Y., Yun, T.K., Morgan, G., & Vainio, H. (2000). The cancer-preventive potential of Panax ginseng: A review of human and experimental evidence. *Cancer Causes and Control, 11,* 565–576.

Shokravi, M.T., Marcus, D.M., Aljoy, J., Egan, K., Saornil, M.A., & Albert, D.M. (1995). Vitamin D inhibits angiogenesis in transgenic murine retinoblastoma. *Investigative Ophthalmology and Visual Science, 36*(1), 83–87.

Shumay, D.M., Maskarinec, G., Kakai, H., & Gorley, C.C. (2001). Why some cancer patients choose complementary and alternative medicine instead of conventional treatment. *Journal of Family Practice, 50,* 1067.

Smith, D.C., Johnson, C.S., Freeman, C.C., Muindi, J., Wilson, J.W., & Trump, D.L. (1999). A phase I trial of calcitriol (1,25-dihydroxycholecalciferol) in patients with advanced malignancy. *Clinical Cancer Research, 5,* 1339–1345.

Sparber, A., Bauer, L., Curt, G., Eisenberg, D., Levin, T., & Parks, S. (2000). Use of complementary medicine by adult patients participating in cancer clinical trials. *Oncology Nursing Forum, 27,* 623–630.

Spiegel, W., Zidek, T., Vutuc, C., Maier, M., Isak, K., & Micksche, M. (2003). Complementary therapies in cancer patients: Prevalence and patients' motives. *Wien Klin Wochenschr, 115,* 705–709.

Tavani, A., Pelucchi, C., Parpinel, M., Negri, E., Franceschi, S., Levi, F., et al. (2003). n-3 polyunsaturated fatty acid intake and cancer risk in Italy and Switzerland. *International Journal of Cancer, 105,* 113–116.

Upton, R. (Ed.). (1999). *Astragalus root: Analytical, quality control, and therapeutic monograph.* Santa Cruz, CA: American Herbal Pharmacopoeia.

U.S. Food and Drug Administration. (1999, December). *FDA takes action against firm marketing unapproved drugs.* Retrieved May 31, 2004, from http://www.fda.gov/bbs/topics/ANSWERS/ANS00988.html

Virtamo, J., Pietinen, P., Huttunen, J.K., Korhonen, P., Malila, N., Virtanen, M.J., et al. (2003). Incidence of cancer and mortality following alpha-tocopherol and beta-carotene supplementation: A postintervention follow-up. *JAMA, 290,* 476–485.

Vucenik, I., Zhang, Z.S., & Shamsuddin, A.M. (1998). IP6 in treatment of liver cancer. II. Intra-tumoral injection of IP6 regresses pre-existing human liver cancer xenotransplanted in nude mice. *Anticancer Research, 18,* 4091–4096.

Wang, S.R., Guo, Z.Q., & Liao, J.Z. (1993). Experimental study on the effects of 18 kinds of Chinese herbal medicines for the synthesis of thromboxane A2 and PGI2. *Chung Kuo Chung His I Chieh Ho Tsa Chih, 13*(3), 167–170.

Wernecke, U., Earl, J., Seydel, C., Horn, O., Crichton, P., & Fannon, D. (2004). Potential health risks of complementary alternative medicines in cancer patients. *British Journal of Cancer, 90,* 408–413.

Yun, T.K., & Choi, S.Y. (1995). Preventive effect of ginseng intake against various human cancers: A case control study on 1987 pairs. *Cancer Epidemiology, Biomarkers and Prevention, 4,* 401–408.

CHAPTER 18

Immunonutrition:
The Role of Specialized Nutritional Support for Patients With Cancer

Colleen A. Gill, MS, RD
Kathleen Murphy-Ende, RN, PhD, AOCNP

Overview

Evidence of the role of nutrition in the etiology and treatment of cancer evolved from epidemiologic studies done in the 1970s (Shils, 1994). Early research explored the connection between nutrition and the development of cancer and the aspects of diet that might be manipulated to decrease a population's cancer rates. The effect of nutritional support during cancer therapies or in minimizing the risk of recurrence in individuals with cancer has been a neglected area of investigation, as there are at least 10 times the number of etiologic studies as studies on nutrition and outcome. Nutrition as a critical component of the continuum of cancer care remains in its infancy.

Historically, nutritional interventions were begun late in the disease trajectory, if at all, because of concerns that nutritional support would "feed the tumor," eroding efforts to eradicate the tumor burden with chemotherapy and radiation. These concerns were exacerbated by data showing increased infection rates with total parenteral nutrition (TPN) (American College of Physicians, 1989). The detrimental impact of malnutrition was first quantified with the results from 12 Eastern Cooperative Oncology Group trials (DeWys et al., 1980) documenting the poor prognosis associated with weight loss in patients with cancer, an association that has been validated through subsequent research (Andreyev, Norman, Oates, & Cunningham, 1998; Bosaeus, Daneryd, & Lundholm, 2002).

The critical question has been whether weight loss is simply an irreversible early marker of a cancer resistant to treatment or if it independently reduces the ability of some patients to respond to therapies. Andreyev et al.'s (1998) research indicated that the reason patients with weight loss did poorly is that they received less treatment. These patients were far more prone to toxicities that resulted in dose reduction and shortened treatment courses. Where weight loss was reversed, survival improved significantly.

Oncologists and nurse practitioners may be ambivalent about offering aggressive nutritional support where research is equivocal and they feel unable to offer clear recommendations. In contrast, patients and families often actively explore nutritional interventions. Without direction from healthcare providers, patients and families are forced to rely on advice from friends, family, and purveyors of products. The emotional impact of anorexia and weight loss for patients with cancer includes altered body image, and for families, a loss of being able to nurture (Peteet, Medeiros, Slavin, & Walsh-Burke, 1981). Evaluating current research can ease the valid concerns of the healthcare provider while helping practitioners guide patients toward nutritional interventions that can improve their nutritional status and quality of life.

The intent of this chapter is to review research that demonstrates the potential benefit of specialized nutritional products to patients with cancer experiencing weight loss or anticipating surgery. Recently, research efforts in the area of nutritional factors impacting inflammation and immune function have led to specialized products designed for the patient with cancer. It is essential that the healthcare team (a) screen and identify at-risk patients, allowing early intervention, (b) continually reassess nutritional status to identify and treat new or confounding issues, and (c) offer appropriate and timely nutritional interventions. Planning effective therapies will require that the team differentiate between patients experiencing reversible weight loss and those with cachexia.

Weight Loss in the Patient With Cancer: Reversible Anorexia or Tumor-Induced Cachexia?

Regardless of cancer diagnosis, unintentional weight loss of more than 5% predicts a poor prognosis even after adjusting for performance status (DeWys et al., 1980). In a 1998 study, patients with weight loss received lower chemotherapy doses initially and developed more frequent and more severe dose-limiting toxicities, correlating with decreased response, shorter disease-free and overall survival, lower quality of life, and poorer performance status (Andreyev et al., 1998). Others have documented adverse outcomes associated with cancer cachexia, including deterioration in functional status, decreased quality of life (Inui, 2002), and increased healthcare costs (Tchekmedyian, 1998).

The term "cachexia" is derived from the Greek words *kakos*, meaning "bad," and *hexis*, meaning "condition." Primary cancer cachexia results from tumor-induced metabolic abnormalities, whereas secondary cachexia is caused by mechanical problems limiting intake. These physical barriers may include tumor-related obstruction and treatment-related gastrointestinal (GI) damage resulting in an impaired ability to ingest or absorb food. Because the development and severity of cachexia can vary considerably in patients with an apparently identical cancer and disease stage, variations in tumor phenotype and host response may be important contributory factors. Anorexia, a loss of appetite accompanied by early satiety, is present in up to 80% of patients with GI tumors and in 60% of those with lung cancer (Bruera, 1997), yet it occurs less frequently with breast or hematologic malignancies.

Adaptation to simple starvation leads to a significant decline in resting energy needs, but cancer cachexia often is associated with an increased metabolic rate, dependent on tumor type (Knox, 1983). The increased calorie needs seen in lung and pancreatic cancers are not matched by an increase in appetite and intake (Bosaeus et al., 2002). This lack of compensation is related to changes in the normal feedback mechanisms that usually trigger appetite when calories are lacking.

Although weight loss in patients with cachexia often has been attributed to anorexia, cachexia involves more than a simple calorie deficit and can occur in the absence of anorexia (Tisdale, 2002). The energy deficit, if any, does not account for the degree of weight loss and the profound disappearance of adipose tissue and lean body mass that is seen, often early in the course of disease. Losses in starvation are primarily fat, as the body adapts to conserve its muscle mass. In cachexia, skeletal muscle and fat are lost at almost equivalent rates, impacting strength and quality of life (see Figure 18-1). Only recently has research been able to identify the tumor-related metabolic factors that lead to the wasting that frequently precedes any decline in intake.

Figure 18-1. Differences in Cachexia and Starvation

Cancer Cachexia	Starvation
Similar loss of lean body mass and fat stores (related to tumor-induced lipid mobilizing factor, proteolysis-inducing factor)	Loss of fat stores > loss of lean body mass
Marked negative nitrogen balance	Mild negative nitrogen balance
Anaerobic metabolism of glucose by tumor	Aerobic metabolism of glucose
Depressed appetite and anorexia	Normal appetite and hunger
Refeeding leads to gains in water and fat (if at all)	Refeeding restores lean body mass, weight

Note. Based on information from Bruera, 1997; Cariuk et al., 1997; Eden et al., 1984; Khan & Tisdale, 1999; Tisdale, 2002.

Changes in Fat Metabolism in Cachexia

Fat stores are depleted in cachexia because degradation of fat is increased, and the fat storage process is inhibited. Patients with cancer secrete a lipid mobilizing factor (LMF) that acts directly on fat cells to stimulate breakdown (Khan & Tisdale, 1999). LMF increases an uncoupling protein in the mitochondria, allowing the disposal of excess free fatty acids while protecting these tissues from the oxidative damage that would normally result (Bing et al., 2002). A second LMF-induced uncoupling protein breaks the tie between respiration and energy production, increasing energy expenditure through thermogenesis (Bing et al., 2000). Energy is released as heat instead of generating adenosine triphosphate from the oxidation of free fatty acids. Because normal thermogenesis from digestion is part of the feedback mechanisms that control appetite, generation of heat from burning energy reserves in a way that simultaneously inhibits intake is consistent with the nonadaptive alterations in cancer cachexia.

Alterations in Protein Metabolism in Cachexia

The proinflammatory environment of cachexia creates a shift toward production of acute phase proteins and a sharp decline in production of serum proteins and proteins in skeletal muscle. The magnitude of this inflammatory acute phase response is typically measured by C-reactive protein (CRP) levels and predicted decreased survival (McMillan, Canna, & McArdle, 2003; McMillan et al., 2001). It is associated with an increased rate of weight loss in lung and GI cancers and with lower Karnofsky performance status and global quality-of-life scores (Scott et al., 2003). This pattern of altered protein production is a response that is usually short term but becomes a chronic condition in inflammation and chronic disease, called a "chronic phase response" (Bengmark, 2001).

The vicious cycle of elevated cytokine levels and inflammation in this acute and chronic phase response lowers the insulin sensitivity of muscle, limiting protein synthesis. However, the net loss of skeletal muscle is more a consequence of its increased breakdown than of any reduction in synthesis. A circulating skeletal muscle proteolysis-inducing factor (PIF) has been found in the urine of patients losing weight of varying cancer diagnoses, but not in patients with burns, sepsis, or major surgery, even if they were losing more weight than the patients with cancer (Cariuk et al., 1997). Weight loss was greater, with increased loss of muscle in patients with pancreatic cancer (Wigmore, Todorov, et al., 2000) who were excreting PIF in their urine. PIF was found to be expressed in GI cancer tumor cells from patients with significant weight loss but not in those whose weight was stable (Cabal-Manzano, Bhargava, Torres-Duarte, Marshall, & Wainer, 2001). PIF has been shown to mark protein for degradation and to induce proteasome expression through an intracellular signaling cascade that can be blocked by eicosapentaenoic acid (EPA) (Whitehouse & Tisdale, 2003). Muscle losses are exacerbated by the decline in physical activity that results from depletion of lean body mass. The accelerated proteolysis is an energy-dependent pathway seen in a variety of wasting conditions, adding to the elevated energy needs seen in cachexia (Lecker, Solomon, Mitch, & Goldberg, 1999). This proteolysis is not related to any deficit in protein consumed, thus explaining the failure of appetite stimulants and traditional nutritional supplementation to reverse muscle breakdown.

Glucose Metabolism in Cachexia

Carbohydrate intake normally results in the secretion of insulin in response to elevated blood glucose levels, promoting synthesis of both fat and protein. An anabolic hormone, insulin inhibits the release of amino acids from muscle, limiting the breakdown of the body's lean body reserves (Tisdale, 2001). Under ideal circumstances, this provides glucose for energy while conserving muscle mass.

Glucose metabolism in cancer is altered in several ways. The preference for an increased uptake of glucose by the tumor is well known and is the scientific basis of the positron emission tomography scan. Converted into lactate rather than CO_2 because the anaerobic environment within the tumor cell provides insufficient oxygen to allow normal Krebs cycle activity to operate, the lactate is (re)synthesized into glucose in the liver in an energy-consuming process. This net energy drain increases the patient's caloric needs as much as 260 calories a day (Eden, Edstrom, Bennegard, Schersten, & Lundholm, 1984).

Other substrates for glucose production in the individual with cachexia include glycerol released from the fat tissue because of LMF-induced lipolysis and amino acids released from skeletal muscle because of PIF-induced proteolysis. LMF also stimulates glucose production in the liver. Although the tumor induces increased glucose production, it simultaneously makes glucose less available to the host by creating peripheral insulin resistance (Tayek, Manglik, & Abemayor, 1997), ultimately making it more available to cancer cells. Although patients may be alarmed by the thought of "feeding the tumor" with carbohydrate intake, it must be emphasized that it is not advisable to severely restrict total carbohydrate intake because it will not eliminate the tumor's fuel sources and can significantly affect the patient's ability to take in adequate calories.

Neuroendocrine Changes in Cachexia

Cytokines promote anorexia and early satiety through central and peripheral mechanisms (Kotler, 2000). The central effect in the brain is on the hypothalamus, controlling appetite. Interleukin-1 (IL-1) increases corticotrophin-releasing hormone while suppressing the production of appetite-enhancing neuropeptide Y, effectively dampening the brain's perception of hunger. There also is enhanced tryptophan uptake in the brain, elevating serotonin levels that increase signaling in the brain, curbing appetite, and leading to early satiety. Several mediators affect GI function, impacting gastric emptying, decreasing intestinal blood flow, and altering GI motility (Kotler).

Summary

Weight loss in patients with cancer occurs through two different, although frequently overlapping, pathways. Starvation is a major element in reversible weight loss, and anorexia-associated weight loss can be treated with proper nutrition and the manipulation of caloric density and frequency. Cachexia, or tumor-induced weight loss, leads to protein-calorie malnutrition characterized by involuntary weight loss, tissue wasting, anorexia, lower performance status, and eventually death (Inui, 2002). Multiple cytokines in combination with other tumor-related factors are involved in the development of a generalized inflammatory state in tumor-induced weight loss. These mediators create derangements in protein, carbohydrate and lipid metabolism, and neuroendocrine function, decreasing appetite and impacting GI function (Kotler, 2000). Inflammatory processes result in damage to surrounding tissues, with the body mounting an acute phase response associated with decreased survival in patients with cancer (Scott et al., 2002). The ineffective utilization of nutrients and inability to adapt to the malnourished state require that interventions include strategies that block these metabolic changes because traditional nutritional intervention strategies relying solely on increased caloric intake have been unsuccessful (Nayel, el-Ghoneimy, & el-Haddad, 1992; Ovesen, Allingstrup, Hannibal, Mortensen, & Hansen, 1993). Manipulation of the inflammatory response offers an opportunity to influence the progress of cachexia.

Nutritional Interventions for Weight Loss in Cancer

Calories First, but Composition Counts

Because weight loss decreases survival time and performance status, therapies that stabilize weight may extend survival and improve quality of life for some. Cumulative side effects of chemotherapy and radiation can exacerbate eating problems, with detrimental results in malnourished patients.

The Patient-Generated Subjective Global Assessment (PG-SGA) is a field-tested, validated assessment of nutritional status (see Appendix A). Detsky et al. (1984) pioneered the concept of physical assessment to identify patients at risk for malnutrition. Dr. Faith Ottery, a surgical oncologist, adapted this for patients with cancer (McMahon, Decker, & Ottery, 1998), adding the patient-generated section and validating it in the oncology population. Investigators have found it highly accurate in classifying nutritional risk (Bauer, Capra, & Ferguson, 2002). Although not formally validated, time constraints have led some clinics to eliminate the physical assessment section, shortening the screening process.

Reversible Weight Loss

Weight loss can develop at any point during therapy, reinforcing the need to have baseline assessments followed by surveillance and aggressive interventions throughout the treatment course. Interventions to maximize caloric intake and maintain activity level are useful for patients with cancer experiencing problems with symptoms limiting intake. Establishing a schedule with small, frequent meals and snacks, maximizing caloric density where needed, and using fluids with calories usually are successful strategies.

The use of fluids with calories has several benefits for patients with cancer because fluids require less effort than is required in chewing solid foods, rarely stimulate the gag reflex, and may speed gastric emptying, resulting in fewer complaints of early satiety. Oral supplements useful in maintaining weight in these patients include many commercially available formulas and homemade milkshake recipes. Assisting the patient in finding supplements that he or she can tolerate and willingly consume is the key. Including a variety of options in oral supplements can prevent the "burnout" that can occur when patients rely on one option.

Tumor-Mediated Weight Loss

The main targets for anticachectic therapies have included PIF, LMF, and cytokines. Only EPA-containing oral supplements or the combination of B-hydroxy-B-methyl butyrate (HMB), arginine, and glutamine have been shown to block some of these mediators and increase skeletal muscle mass. Appetite stimulants have produced weight gain but were ineffective in increasing lean body mass.

Fish oils from fatty fish, rich in EPA and docosahexaenoic acid (DHA), have become a primary focus of research as the role of inflammatory cytokines in cachexia is elucidated. These highly unsaturated fats impact cachexia mediators through their effects on the synthesis of prostaglandins, the fluidity of cell membranes, receptor function, cell-signaling mechanisms, and regulation of gene expression.

Prostaglandins are locally active hormone-like compounds with biologic effects in cell proliferation, tissue repair, blood clotting, inflammation, and immune cell behavior. When cytokines stimulate cell membranes rich in omega-6 fat, metabolites of arachidonic acid (AA) stimulate the breakup of NFkB-IkB complex in the cytoplasm. Free NFkB then enters the nucleus, turning on the genes that produce more cytokines and acute phase proteins, creating an inflammatory environment. AA content in cell membranes also is a source of PIF-stimulated prostaglandins involved in tagging protein for breakdown in skeletal muscle and in increasing the proteosome machinery to do so. Blocking this proteolysis may limit tumor growth because tumor protein synthesis may be controlled by the rate of protein degradation (Istfan, Wan, & Bistrian, 1992).

EPA and DHA block the effects of omega-6 fats by replacing them in the membrane and providing a counterbalancing source of noninflammatory prostaglandins, the PGE3 series. EPA and DHA are rapidly incorporated into the cell membrane, with a dose response of up to three grams per day (Blonk et al., 1990). This same dose stabilized the acute phase protein response markers of inflammation: CRP, ceruloplasmin, and fibrinogen (Barber, Ross, Preston, Shenkin, & Fearon, 1999). Fish oil also has been found to markedly inhibit the synthesis of the cytokines, tumor necrosis factor (TNF)-alpha and IL-1 (Caughey, Mantzioris, Gibson, Cleland, & James, 1996; Endres & von Schacky, 1996). EPA and DHA are well-known inhibitors of cyclooxygenase and leukoxygenase enzymes that are otherwise involved in the final conversion of omega-6 precursors into inflammatory prostaglandins (PGE2 series) and leukotrienes (Daly, Weintraub, Shou, Rosato, & Lucia, 1995). Because most cancer lines overexpress PGE2 receptors, blocking this stimulation is theorized to be one reason fish oil supplementation has been found to inhibit proliferation and invasion, increase apoptosis, and induce differentiation in cancer cells (Rose, Connolly, & Coleman, 1996). A recent review by Wallace (2002) summarized the benefits of nutrition therapies in modulating inflammation in cancer.

Clinical studies have documented weight stabilization in patients with pancreatic cancers whose diet was supplemented with fish oil (Wigmore, Barber, Ross, Tisdale, & Fearon, 2000; Wigmore et al., 1996), perhaps because of the normalization of inflammatory processes. EPA was able to inhibit PIF-induced weight loss (Barber, Fearon, Tisdale, McMillan, & Ross, 2001; Smith, Lorite, & Tisdale, 1999) and also blocked the stimulation of lipolysis by LMF (Price & Tisdale, 1998; Tisdale & Beck, 1991). EPA limited host weight loss, preserving fat and muscle in patients with cancer (Barber et al., 2001).

Research by Barber, Ross, Voss, Tisdale, and Fearon (1999) found that the use of an experimental oral supplement rich in fish oil was effective in the cachectic patient with pancreatic cancer who was losing weight at a rate of 2.9 kg/month. The experimental product, containing 310 calories, 16 g protein, and 1 g EPA per can, was prescribed at a goal of two cans per day. Use of the product was associated with an overall total improvement in caloric intake of almost 400 calories/day and a weight gain of 1 kg/month. The increased calories accounted for only 1.55 kg of the 3.9 kg swing in body weight per month. The remaining improvement was attributed to reduced metabolic inefficiencies, with a documented decline in resting energy expenditure per kg of weight (Barber, McMillan, Preston, Ross, & Fearon, 2000). Later trials showed decreased production of IL-6 and excretion of

PIF and stabilization of acute phase proteins, all indications of a normaliza-tion of metabolic activity (Barber et al., 2001). With supportive care alone, these patients historically experienced progressive weight loss (Wigmore, Plester, Richardson, & Fearon, 1997). In fact, increasing caloric support with TPN (Nixon et al., 1981) or traditional oral supplements (Nayel et al., 1992; Ovesen et al., 1993) has previously been unable to improve weight status in cachectic patients with cancer.

At first glance, a recent trial comparing supplementation with fish oil to an isonitrogenous, isocaloric control contradicted the earlier studies when it failed to find a significant difference in weight change between the groups (Fearon et al., 2003). However, neither group was fully compliant with in-take, which was significant because earlier studies suggested there is a dose threshold effect requiring two grams of EPA a day to make an impact on mediators of cachexia and achieve weight stabilization (Bruera et al., 2003; Fearon et al., 2001). In the experimental group, there was a dose-response relationship between the amount of supplement consumed and increases in weight and lean body mass, an association not found in the control group. As in previous trials, plasma EPA levels were associated with weight and lean body mass gains, both of which were tied to quality of life. Importantly, those receiving the omega-3 supplement showed increases in total energy expenditure and physical activity level, which restored them to a normal sedentary level (Moses, Slater, Preston, Barber, & Fearon, 2004).

Juven® (Abbott Laboratories, Abbott Park, IL) is a powdered supplement being evaluated for its benefit in preventing loss of muscle mass. It contains three nutrients targeting the metabolic problems associated with wasting: 3 g of HMB to minimize muscle protein breakdown and 14 g each of gluta-mine and arginine to support muscle protein synthesis and immune func-tion. Providing an additional protein support of 45 g, it is not appropriate for those with impaired liver and/or kidney function, nor is it a complete nutritional product.

Hydroxymethylglutaryl coenzyme A (HMG-CoA) is a metabolite of the amino acid leucine, important in regulating body protein stores by slowing muscle protein breakdown and increasing its deposition. HMG is a precur-sor of HMG-CoA, and it is theorized that HMB protects stressed or dam-aged cells that may not be able to make enough HMB-CoA, thus supporting membrane function.

Glutamine is depleted from muscle in infection and disease because of the increased needs of the GI tract and immune system. Supplementation may limit this cause of muscle breakdown.

Arginine is a semi-essential amino acid that produces a key regulatory chemical, nitric oxide. Requirements for arginine are elevated during anabo-lism and/or stress. Supplementation of arginine can cause an increase in growth hormone secretion that may minimize muscle loss.

Originally studied in the AIDS population (Clark et al., 2000), Juven led to gains in lean body mass and improvement in immune status. Wound healing benefits were seen in older adults (Williams, Abumrad, & Barbul, 2002). Cancer-related wasting was limited in one study, with gain in weight and lean body mass, while consuming less calories than the control group (May, Barber, D'Olimpio, Hourihane, & Abumrad, 2002). Research regarding the use of arginine and glutamine in cancer is reviewed later in this chapter.

Alternatives When Voluntary Oral Intake Fails

Although concerning to the patient and family, slow weight loss is not a threat to the patient's nutritional status or tolerance of therapy. The indiscriminate use of enteral and parenteral nutrition is not indicated for patients with cancer where reasonable oral intake can be anticipated to return within a week (Nitenberg & Raynard, 2000). The benefit of these interventions is limited to a subset of patients experiencing a prolonged period of GI toxicity or in which major surgery is anticipated. Malnourished patients in these situations are certainly candidates for these aggressive interventions.

Lopez and Tehrani (2001) suggested that nutrition therapy be individualized and hierarchic, using interventions only when the simplest option is not applicable to the patient. Balancing this, they also noted that aggressive support should not be avoided out of fear that it will promote tumor growth. Although specialized nutritional support might not be appropriate for every patient, it never should be withheld where curative or palliative therapy exists.

Enteral nutrition with tube feedings can bypass barriers in the upper GI tract or be used to supplement patients that have such significant problems with appetite and early satiety that they are left unable to voluntarily consume adequate calories. A meta-analysis showed lower risk of infection associated with the use of the enteral versus parenteral feedings, possibly because of preservation of GI integrity (Braunschweig, Levy, Sheehan, & Wang, 2001). Tube feedings for cachectic patients with tumor-induced weight loss should contain two servings of a fish oil–containing formula previously described, along with a fiber-containing formula providing the balance of the required caloric support.

Parenteral support can be used when using the GI tract is contraindicated because of complications limiting adequate absorption. Reviews by Bistrian (2001) and Jeejeebhoy (2001) have contradicted the belief that TPN increases infection risks compared to enteral nutrition. High levels of blood sugars clearly occurred at greater frequency in TPN patients in the past, possibly because tube-fed patients often did not reach goal support and were relatively underfed in comparison. Where individualized TPN formulas are used and overfeeding is avoided, blood glucose levels are controlled, and no increase in sepsis is seen.

In most cancer settings, unfortunately, parenteral nutrition has not been shown to improve patient outcomes or survival (Klein & Koretz, 1994). The exception to this was seen in a malnourished patient with cancer who, despite being relatively overfed by current guidelines, benefited from perioperative support with TPN, with one-third less complications and decreased mortality (Bozzetti et al., 2000).

Enhancement of Immune Function in the Patient With Cancer

Although cancer cells develop from normal host cells that have lost the necessary checks and balances on growth, the body is able to recognize these cells as different and mount an immune response against them. Cancer cells carry unique histocompatibility complex antigens and may be missing some normal antigens, making the cells identifiable as "non-self" by the immune cells of the body. Activated macrophages identify tumor antigens and signal T cells that initiate the inflammatory response and release of TNF, IL-1, and IL-6, increasing the effectiveness of natural killer cells. Unfortunately, cancer cells can vary in their degree of antigenicity and, therefore, the strength of the immune response against the tumor. Once the cancer forms a mass, antibodies find it difficult to penetrate the inner cells.

Optimally, the immune system works best with a balance between the pro- and anti-inflammatory cytokines to maximize immune function and healing. Local inflammation helps the host by initiating healing, but excessive inflammation injures tissue. The excessive production of inflammatory cytokines associated with cancer can disrupt this critical balance. Unbridled activity of natural defense and repair mechanisms then work against the host rather than destroying the tumor.

Nutritional Status and the Immune System

Every component of the immune system consists of carbohydrates, protein, and fat, thus requiring adequate nutritional support to be able to function properly. The impact of malnutrition on immune function is seen in research in third world countries where the leading cause of death for children under the age of five is infectious disease related to their malnourished status (Chandra, 1991). Infection magnifies any nutritional deficiency a person may have, and in the patient who is chronically malnourished, this becomes a vicious circle with escalating malnutrition and slower recovery from subsequent illnesses.

The impact of marginal nutritional deficiencies is not as well understood, but evidence suggests that immune function can be altered with borderline deficiencies. Multiple vitamin use improved immune function, especially in older adults, because of the limited intakes and age-related decline in immune function (Chandra, 1992). Supplements with the potential to boost immune function include multiple vitamins as well as 200–400 IU of vitamin

E, 500–1,000 mg of vitamin C, 10–15 mg of zinc, and 1–2 g of EPA and DHA with chronic inflammation (e.g., cancer) (Kline, 2002). Supplementation with antioxidants (such as vitamins E and C) *during* some cancer therapies remains controversial. Obtaining adequate protein, balancing the omega-6 to omega-3 ratio in the diet, limiting excess calories, and eating more fruits, vegetables, and whole grains to provide vitamins, minerals, fiber, and phytochemicals can ensure optimal function.

Omega-3 Fat

The ratio of omega-6 to omega-3 fats in the diet is critical to a balanced immune response. Inflammation at low levels enhances immune response, but when excessive or prolonged, it suppresses immune function (Young, 1994). Perioperative supplementation with EPA was found to reduce immunosuppression caused by postoperative chemoradiation therapy in patients with esophageal cancer (Takagi, Yamamori, Furukawa, Miyazaki, & Tashiro, 2001). In malnourished patients, supplementation increased the ratio of T-helper to T-suppressor cells and prolonged survival (Gogos et al., 1998).

Tumor-induced production of PGE2 prostaglandins from omega-6 fats promotes macrophage and lymphocyte production of IL-10, an immunosuppressive cytokine, while suppressing IL-12 (Stolina et al., 2000). Limiting inflammation restores this balance and enhances natural killer cell function (Baxevanis et al., 1993). The role of EPA and DHA in balancing immune response is one way these "healthy fats" may decrease cancer risk and progression (Terry, Rohan, & Wolk, 2003).

Glutamine

Blood levels of glutamine, a neutral amino acid, are depleted in patients with cancer, with a negative impact on host tissues that are dependent upon glutamine for function, particularly lymphocytes and the intestinal epithelial cells (Shewchuk, Baracos, & Field, 1997). Glutamine supplementation offers protection for the cells of the gut as a precursor of glutathione (GSH), part of the antioxidant enzyme GSH peroxidase (Ziegler, Bazargan, Leader, & Martindale, 2000). Because GSH levels in the tumor are associated with resistance to radiation and chemotherapy (Arrick & Nathan, 1984), the use of glutamine therapy initially was rejected, fearing it would protect the tumor (Chance, Cao, Kim, Nelson, & Fischer, 1988). In fact, because of differences in the tumor intracellular environment, glutamine supplementation appears to *decrease* GSH levels, which may *increase* tumor sensitivity to treatment (Rouse, Nwokedi, Woodliff, Epstein, & Klimberg, 1995). Many studies have shown decreased tumor growth with glutamine (Fahr, Kornbluth, Blossom, Schaeffer, & Klimberg, 1994; Klimberg et al., 1996).

More current evidence (Savarese, Savy, Vahdat, Wischmeyer, & Corey, 2003) suggested that glutamine supplementation may decrease the severity of chemotherapy- (Anderson, Schroeder, & Skubitz, 1998) and radiation-induced (Huang et al., 2000) mucositis, irinotecan-induced diarrhea (Savarese, Al-Zoubi, & Boucher, 2000), paclitaxel-induced neuropathy (Vahdat et al., 2001), hepatic venoocclusive disease in stem cell transplantation (Brown et al., 1998), and the cardiotoxicity that accompanies anthracycline use (Cao, Kennedy, & Klimberg, 1999). Glutamine is similarly metabolized when given IV or orally (Panigrahi, Gewolb, Bamford, & Horvath, 1997), but enteral administration provides more gut protection through topical contact (Kouznetsova, Bijlsma, van Leeuwen, Groot, & Houdijk, 1999). It decreases gut permeability (Bjarnason, MacPherson, & Hollander, 1995) and induces heat shock proteins, a natural defense mechanism enhancing cell survival (Wischmeyer, 2002). The efficacy apparently varies with the type of chemotherapy because it seems to offer no significant benefit for patients receiving 5-fluorouracil (Okuno et al., 1999). The degree of protection offered by glutamine may depend on the dose and frequency of adminis- tration. A recent review of the clinical evidence for the use of glutamine found it to be well tolerated and recommended 20–30 g/day, initiated early with maintenance for five days or longer (Garcia-de-Lorenzo et al., 2003). Optimal dosing may prove to be 0.5 g/kg, divided into three doses a day to improve topical contact. Supplementation may prevent GI, neurologic, and possibly cardiac complications of cancer therapy, reducing delays in therapy. It also may improve the therapeutic index of both chemotherapy and radiation therapy, increasing tumor kill while simultaneously protecting the host from toxicity.

Apart from the benefits to GI integrity, glutamine also supports immune function directly as a substrate for the cells of the immune system (Calder & Yaqoob, 1999). Glutamine has been shown to increase phagocytic activity of cells, a key mechanism of bacterial killing, and to increase lymphocyte activation and proliferation (Yaqoob & Calder, 1997), preventing the de- crease in lymphocyte counts in patients with esophageal cancer (Yoshida et al., 1998). The role of glutamine in supporting immune cells is one of several mechanisms through which it may be beneficial in critical illness and surgery.

Arginine

Arginine can become a conditionally essential amino acid during stress because of its ability to stimulate the immune system (Evoy, Lieberman, Fahey, & Daly, 1998). With four nitrogen atoms per molecule, arginine is the most abundant carrier of nitrogen in humans. Used in the synthesis of proteins, urea, nitric oxide, polyamines, glutamate, creatine, and proline, it has many physiologic functions. Arginine can increase T lymphocytes as well as enhance the effect of T-helper cells and the response of immune cells to antigens (Barbul, 1990). It is a building block of both the nucleic acids and proteins needed to make immune cells and also may stimulate immunity by increasing the production of growth hormone, prolactin, and insulin. Arginine's ability to upregulate immune parameters has been demonstrated in several studies of patients with cancer (Daly et al., 1988), although another study found no improvement in lymphocyte proliferation and monocyte function (McCarter, Gentilini, Gomez, & Daly, 1998).

The use of arginine in patients with cancer is controversial because arginine can suppress or enhance tumor growth depending on the relative activities of several metabolic pathways, which may vary with the stage of carcinogenesis (Mills, Shearer, Evans, & Caldwell, 1992). This may explain the contradictory results in the literature finding that arginine can stimulate (Dodd et al., 2000; Edwards et al., 1997; Park et al., 1992), inhibit (Ma, Hoper, Anderson, & Rowlands, 1996), or have no effect (Robinson et al., 1999) on the growth of tumors. In animals, arginine supplementation decreased colorectal tumor production during the initiation phase of carcinogenesis but stimulated growth during the promotion stage (Ma, Williamson, O'Rourke, & Rowlands, 1999). Ultimately, the benefit of arginine may depend on the relative immunogenicity of the tumor, as weakly immunogenic tumors may not be recognized by the immune system. Research with neuroblastomas appears to support this hypothesis, as weakly immunogenic tumors were stimulated by arginine, whereas it retarded the growth of immunogenic (C1300) tumors and prolonged host survival (Yeatman, Risley, & Brunson, 1991).

Arginine may fuel growth through increased synthesis of IGF-1, growth hormone, prolactin, insulin, and glucagons—all anabolic hormones that enhance immunity and wound healing but undeniably stimulate growth. In patients with breast cancer, supplemental arginine was found to increase breast cancer growth (Park et al., 1992). This stimulation of proliferation may prove beneficial if it sensitizes the tumor to therapy or host defenses. In fact, arginine was shown to improve the response of women to chemotherapy, increase host defenses, and limit immunosuppression (Brittenden et al., 1994). In contrast, arginine *deprivation* therapy has been investigated as a potential treatment for some cancers, particularly melanoma and hepatocellular and prostate carcinomas (Dillon et al., 2004). These tumors frequently are deficient in argininosuccinate synthetase, making them unable to synthesize arginine and, thus, making it an essential amino acid for the growth of these tumors.

The positive or negative impact of arginine on cancer growth seems to be dependent on the immunogenicity of the particular tumor and on the requirement for arginine by that tumor as a growth substrate. Clearly, more research regarding arginine metabolism in tumor tissues is key before reasonable recommendations can be made.

The Role of the Gastrointestinal Tract in Immune Function

The physical barrier of the GI tract prevents trillions of microorganisms and foreign proteins from entering the body. More than a quarter of the GI tract is immunologically active tissue, known as gut associated lymphoid tissues (GALT), responding to foreign antigens by activating the immune response and producing antibodies, mostly sIgA. Malnutrition affects the gut's ability to maintain its varied functions. As the gut atrophies, junctions between the cells are loosened, and pathogens can enter the bloodstream through the gaps. The phenomenon of bacterial translocation occurs with localized or systemic injury, both common events for the patient with cancer undergoing chemotherapy, radiation therapy, or major surgery. Exacerbating this, malnutrition also affects the immune system's ability to recognize antigens and to mount a response. Finally, adaptations made by bacteria to a declining food supply result in their stimulation of cytokines in an inflammatory response, leading to increased bacterial translocation.

Both IV and oral forms of glutamine are protective in helping the gut to meet its needs for energy and repair. Glutamine also has a direct effect on the gut-associated immune cells that are a critical component of gut barrier function, significantly increasing intestinal T-cell counts (Gismondo et al., 1998).

The "friendly" bacteria in probiotics produce antimicrobial agents that are toxic to pathogenic flora, reducing the risk of host infection. Using dietary fiber as their food, they provide nutrients to the gut and detoxify carcinogens in the GI tract. Poor diet and stress disrupt the balance between good and bad bacteria (Bengmark, 2001). Trials using probiotics in enteral formulas found a significant decrease in infection and length of stay (Beniwal et al., 2003).

Nutritional Interventions in the Surgical Patient With Cancer

The Perioperative Period

When surgery is superimposed on the debilitating side effects of cancer and its treatment, it is not surprising that malnutrition is a comorbid factor for most patients with cancer admitted to an intensive care unit (Jolliet et al., 1999). Where feasible, support with enteral nutrition is preferable to TPN (Braunschweig et al., 2001) with improved outcomes, especially where immune-enhancing diets (IEDs) are used (Braga, Gianotti, Balzano, et al., 1999; Gianotti et al., 1997). Although a combination of standard, fiber-containing formulas with two cans per day of an EPA-/DHA-containing formula is appropriate for many patients with cancer requiring tube feeding; the specialized IED formulas appear to be warranted for malnourished surgical patients with cancer. Heslin and Brennan (2000) suggested that patients who are malnourished benefit the most from *perioperative* nutritional support, stating that this must be considered for surgical patients who have experienced more than a 10% weight loss and/or who have a serum albumin level < 3.5 awaiting major surgery. The delayed gastric emptying that can lead to intolerance of tube feedings (Heyland, Tougas, King, & Cook, 1996) can be circumvented with jejunal feedings if needed.

In this perioperative environment, formulas designed to modulate immune response often are appropriate. These products include nutrients such as arginine, glutamine, omega-3 fatty acids, and polyribonucleotides shown to alter immune parameters in some studies (Braga, Gianotti, Vignali, & Di Carlo, 1998; Nitenberg & Raynard, 2000). These formulations are designed to stimulate immune surveillance (T-helper cells, phagocytosis, and lymphocytes) while limiting the extreme response seen in sepsis (C-reactive protein, IL-2, and IL-6). Several methodologic problems were seen in early studies with these products (McCowen & Bistrian, 2003), including failure to deliver close to goal feedings, control groups with lower protein support (Daly et al., 1992), and the inclusion of mixed diagnoses and nutritional risk. Although several studies have described a decrease in infectious complications, length of stay, and costs with using these formulas (Braga, Gianotti, Radaelli, et al., 1999; Heys, Walker, Smith, & Eremin, 1999), no statistically significant improvement in survival has been observed(Heslin & Brennan, 2000; Heyland et al., 2001).

The conflicting data generated by the initial research may be the result of a lack of stratification of patients, failing to segregate and treat those who were malnourished and most likely to benefit from these interventions. In a 2003 review, McCowen and Bistrian concluded that the use of immunonutrition in moderate illness is likely to be helpful, whereas severe sepsis is beyond the reach of any nutritional intervention, and mild illness is likely to improve regardless of feeding. IED use in malnourished patients with cancer showed significant clinical advantages (Riso et al., 2000). For well-nourished patients, more recent studies showed a benefit of *preoperative* IED but a significant increase in GI side effects and no additional benefit postoperatively (Gianotti et al., 2002).

Appropriate timing of nutritional intervention is critical, as several days of immunonutrition are required to improve immune parameters and achieve clinical efficacy in the reduction of infectious complications (Senkal et al., 1999). Preoperative immune modulation with omega-3 and arginine may control the inflammatory response, offsetting some of the typical immune depression seen after surgical insult. Given the limited volumes that often result from feeding intolerance following surgery, preoperative feedings allow the patient to reach the critical volumes needed to improve immune parameters (Braga et al., 1998). The patients who were malnourished benefited most, with the risk of infection dropping 14%, compared to 39% in the control-fed group. Well-nourished patients were helped as well, with infectious complications reducing from 27% to 10%, and preoperative support alone was beneficial and possibly adequate (Gianotti et al., 2002). In contrast, patients who were malnourished did best with *perioperative* support (Braga, Gianotti, Nespoli, Radaelli, & Di Carlo, 2002), and its use was cost effective (Gianotti, Braga, Frei, Greiner, & Di Carlo, 2000). For malnourished patients, optimal intervention should be proactive, initiated in advance of surgery to further improve outcome (Sacks, Genton, & Kudsk, 2003). Based on this research, many oncology surgeons have implemented programs that include a presurgical nutrition clinic where patients are evaluated and educated to consume an IED supplement preoperatively to improve surgical outcomes.

The research involving IEDs typically includes one or more of the following elements, many of which have been reviewed in greater detail earlier in this chapter.

Glutamine

Glutamine is protective during critical illness through preservation of the gut barrier, with less systemic bacteremia (Salvalaggio & Campos, 2002; Salvalaggio et al., 2002). Glutamine's enhancement of heat shock protein expression, limiting proinflammatory cytokine release (Wischmeyer et al., 2001), may be critical in preventing the escalation of infection to multiorgan failure (Deitch, 2002). Recent meta-analyses concluded that glutamine use led to a lower rate of infectious complications and a shorter length of stay, especially among surgical patients.

Omega-3s

The role of omega-3 fat in an IED may be its ability to modulate the severity of the host immune response. Omega-3 fat was associated with a reduction in the production of prostaglandins associated with the catabolic aspects of the immune response (Swails et al., 1997).

Arginine

Arginine's inclusion in IED formulas may be of benefit in patients undergoing surgery because of its effect on wound healing and nitrogen balance (Daly et al., 1995). As a substrate for nitric oxide, a simple compound with profound metabolic effects, arginine is felt to be potentially either immune enhancing or immunosuppressive, depending on the quantity involved. The amount of arginine in IED solutions may be critical, as studies using lower concentrations at 6 g/l generally led to negative results, whereas those using solutions with > 12 g/l typically were positive (McCowen & Bistrian, 2003). Arginine supplementation alone was not beneficial in one medical intensive care unit study (Caparros, Lopez, & Grau, 2001). A meta-analysis by Heyland et al. (2003) concluded that arginine-containing formulas reduced length of stay and infectious complications in elective surgical patients.

In contrast, some investigators have suggested that negative effects may occur with the use of arginine-containing formulas in critically ill patients with sepsis, systemic inflammatory response syndrome, or organ failure.

They hypothesize that this may be because of the enhancement of an already escalated inflammatory response. Heyland et al. (2003) suggested that therapies effective in critical illness *decrease* rather than *stimulate* the inflammatory process, concluding that immunonutrition in critically ill patients with sepsis therefore might be harmful. This position remains controversial, as one study showed decreased mortality with IED use, although the effect was only evident in the least sick group of patients with sepsis who had baseline Apache II scores of 10–15 (Galban et al., 2000). A recent review of research investigating the role of arginine as a mediator or modulator of sepsis (Zaloga, Siddiqui, Terry, & Marik, 2004) concluded that arginine-containing IED formulas are safe and effective in patients with sepsis. Future trials using IEDs with adequate arginine content should clarify the current controversy.

Arginine alone was evaluated in one study of patients with head and neck cancers who were randomized to an arginine-supplemented or a control formula. Researchers found no difference in outcome indices, although there was a trend toward increased survival in the arginine group (van Bokhorst-De Van Der Schueren et al., 2001). Unfortunately, this pilot study was statistically underpowered, and a larger sample size may have resulted in significant differences between the groups. Most studies have included arginine, nucleotides, and omega-3 fats in a single IED formulation and have shown significant benefit in malnourished surgical patients with cancer. Despite the possible risk of stimulating tumor growth, the use of an IED is beneficial in the perioperative environment for the surgical patient with cancer, especially if he or she is malnourished. In this setting, the benefits in wound healing and immune enhancement override theoretical concerns.

Nucleotides

Although nucleotides are plentiful in breast milk and may be immunomodulatory in infants, no human studies show that the addition of nucleotides might be beneficial in IED. Animal studies showed an enhanced immune response to fungal challenge (Fanslow, Kulkarni, Van Buren, & Rudolph, 1988), and supplemental nucleotides helped to maintain cellular immune function during stress (Van Buren & Rudolph, 1997).

Consensus Recommendations on Immune-Enhancing Diets

Expert panel recommendations (Sacks et al., 2003) advised the early initiation of an IED for the patient who is malnourished, offering preoperative treatment for five to seven days to improve clinical outcome. Unless limited by renal or hepatic dysfunction, at least one liter should be provided daily, advancing as tolerated to this volume or until at least 50%–60% of nutrient needs are met.

The panel recommended that patients who are in the following categories be considered candidates for IED therapy.

1. Patients who are moderately or severely malnourished, albumin < 3.5, undergoing elective esophageal, gastric, pancreatic, or hepatobiliary surgery. The patient who is more severely malnourished would be expected to benefit the most.
2. Patients who are severely malnourished with an albumin < 2.8, undergoing colon or rectal surgery
3. Patients with preexisting malnutrition undergoing major head and neck surgery

Patients with cancer who should **not** be considered candidates for IED therapy include

1. Patients with sepsis with Apache scores > 15
2. Patients expected to resume an oral diet in five days
3. Patients with bowel obstruction distal to the access for feeding.

Practical strategies (McCowen & Bistrian, 2003) to reach IED objectives include

1. Arginine content is > 12g/l, ~ 4% of energy, with 1 g omega-3/1,000 calories.
2. Duration should be > 3 days, preferably 5–10 days (optimally initiated prior to surgery).
3. Nasogastric feeding should be used aggressively, with nursing protocols to advance feeding every four to six hours, and gastric residuals of 200 ml should be accepted.
4. Feeding goals should approach 25 kcal/kg, with > 800 ml/day delivered.

Summary

Current research suggests benefits of nutritional support to prevent or minimize weight loss in patients with cancer. The impact of nutritional intake and status on immune function and the inflammatory process has sparked interest in the development of specialized nutritional products for the person living with cancer (see Figure 18-2). Nurses and dietitians need to identify patients at risk for weight loss and offer nutritional supplements and education based on current research findings.

The use of immune-enhancing formulas for surgical patients with cancer is appropriate, especially when patients are malnourished. Because these formulas are most effective when used perioperatively, the implementation of presurgical nutrition clinics can improve outcomes for patients with cancer.

Figure 18-2. Algorithm for Nutritional Intervention Using Specialized Immunonutrition

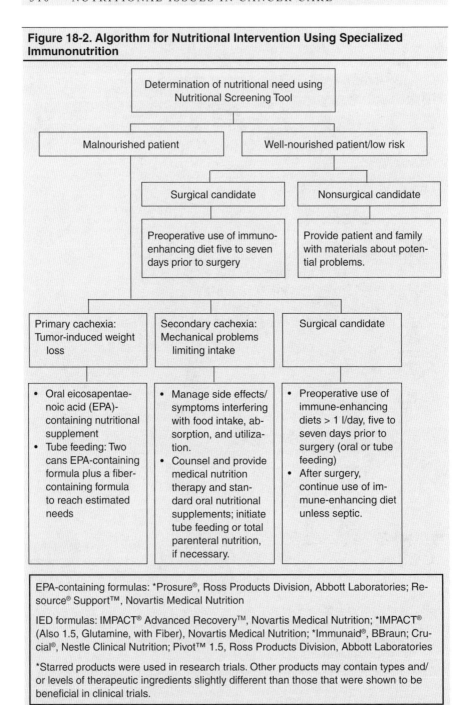

EPA-containing formulas: *Prosure®, Ross Products Division, Abbott Laboratories; Resource® Support™, Novartis Medical Nutrition

IED formulas: IMPACT® Advanced Recovery™, Novartis Medical Nutrition; *IMPACT® (Also 1.5, Glutamine, with Fiber), Novartis Medical Nutrition; *Immunaid®, BBraun; Crucial®, Nestle Clinical Nutrition; Pivot™ 1.5, Ross Products Division, Abbott Laboratories

*Starred products were used in research trials. Other products may contain types and/ or levels of therapeutic ingredients slightly different than those that were shown to be beneficial in clinical trials.

Note. Based on information from Barber et al., 2000; McCowen & Bistrian, 2003; Ovesen et al., 1993; Sacks et al., 2003.

References

American College of Physicians. (1989). Parenteral nutrition in patients receiving cancer chemotherapy. *Annals of Internal Medicine, 110,* 734–736.

Anderson, P.M., Schroeder, G., & Skubitz, K.M. (1998). Oral glutamine reduces the duration and severity of stomatitis after cytotoxic cancer chemotherapy. *Cancer, 83,* 1433–1439.

Andreyev, H.J., Norman, A.R., Oates, J., & Cunningham, D. (1998). Why do patients with weight loss have a worse outcome when undergoing chemotherapy for GI malignancies? *European Journal of Cancer, 34,* 503–509.

Arrick, B.A., & Nathan, C.F. (1984). Glutathione metabolism as a determinant of therapeutic efficacy: A review. *Cancer Research, 44,* 4224–4232.

Barber, M.D., Fearon, K.C., Tisdale, M.J., McMillan, D.C., & Ross, J.A. (2001). Effect of a fish oil-enriched nutritional supplement on metabolic mediators in patients with pancreatic cancer cachexia. *Nutrition and Cancer, 40*(2), 118–124.

Barber, M.D., McMillan, D.C., Preston, T., Ross, J.A., & Fearon, K.C. (2000). Metabolic response to feeding in weight-losing pancreatic cancer patients and its modulation by a fish-oil-enriched nutritional supplement. *Clinical Science (London), 98,* 389–399.

Barber, M.D., Ross, J.A., Preston, T., Shenkin, A., & Fearon, K.C. (1999). Fish oil-enriched nutritional supplement attenuates progression of the acute-phase response in weight-losing patients with advanced pancreatic cancer. *Journal of Nutrition, 129,* 1120–1125.

Barber, M.D., Ross, J.A., Voss, A.C., Tisdale, M.J., & Fearon, K.C. (1999). The effect of an oral nutritional supplement enriched with fish oil on weight-loss in patients with pancreatic cancer. *British Journal of Cancer, 81*(1), 80–86.

Barbul, A. (1990). Arginine and immune function. *Nutrition, 6*(1), 53–58; discussion 59–62.

Bauer, J., Capra, S., & Ferguson, M. (2002). Use of the scored patient-generated subjective global assessment (PG-SGA) as a nutrition assessment tool in patients with cancer. *European Journal of Clinical Nutrition, 56,* 779–785.

Baxevanis, C.N., Reclos, G.J., Gritzapis, A.D., Dedousis, G.V., Missitzis, I., & Papamichail, M. (1993). Elevated prostaglandin E2 production by monocytes is responsible for the depressed levels of natural killer and lymphokine-activated killer cell function in patients with breast cancer. *Cancer, 72,* 491–501.

Bengmark, S. (2001). Nutritional modulation of acute and chronic phase responses. *Nutrition, 17,* 489–485.

Beniwal, R.S., Arena, V.C., Thomas, L., Narla, S., Imperiale, T.F., Chaudhry, R.A., et al. (2003). A randomized trial of yogurt for prevention of antibiotic-associated diarrhea. *Digestive Diseases and Sciences, 48,* 2077–2082.

Bing, C., Brown, M., King, P., Collins, P., Tisdale, M.J., & Williams, G. (2000). Increased gene expression of brown fat uncoupling protein (UCP)1 and skeletal muscle UCP2 and UCP3 in MAC16-induced cancer cachexia. *Cancer Research, 60,* 2405–2410.

Bing, C., Russell, S.T., Beckett, E.E., Collins, P., Taylor, S., Barraclough, R., et al. (2002). Expression of uncoupling proteins-1, -2 and -3 mRNA is induced by an adenocarcinoma-derived lipid-mobilizing factor. *British Journal of Cancer, 86,* 612–618.

Bistrian, B.R. (2001). Update on total parenteral nutrition. *American Journal of Clinical Nutrition, 74*(2), 153–154.

Bjarnason, I., MacPherson, A., & Hollander, D. (1995). Intestinal permeability: An overview. *Gastroenterology, 108,* 1566–1581.

Blonk, M.C., Bilo, H.J., Nauta, J.J., Popp-Snijders, C., Mulder, C., & Donker, A.J. (1990). Dose-response effects of fish-oil supplementation in healthy volunteers. *American Journal of Clinical Nutrition, 52*(1), 120–127.

Bosaeus, I., Daneryd, P., & Lundholm, K. (2002). Dietary intake, resting energy expenditure, weight loss and survival in cancer patients. *Journal of Nutrition, 132*(Suppl. 11), 3465S–3466S.

Bozzetti, F., Gavazzi, C., Miceli, R., Rossi, N., Mariani, L., Cozzaglio, L., et al. (2000). Perioperative total parenteral nutrition in malnourished, gastrointestinal cancer patients: A randomized, clinical trial. *Journal of Parenteral and Enteral Nutrition, 24*(1), 7–14.

Braga, M., Gianotti, L., Balzano, G., Vignali, A., Gentilini, O., Zerbi, A., et al. (1999). Artificial nutrition after major pancreatic resection. Results of a prospective randomized clinical trial [Abstract]. *Journal of Parenteral and Enteral Nutrition, 23*(1), S2.

Braga, M., Gianotti, L., Nespoli, L., Radaelli, G., & Di Carlo, V. (2002). Nutritional approach in malnourished surgical patients: A prospective randomized study. *Archives of Surgery, 137*(2), 174–180.

Braga, M., Gianotti, L., Radaelli, G., Vignali, A., Mari, G., Gentilini, O., et al. (1999). Perioperative immunonutrition in patients undergoing cancer surgery: Results of a randomized double-blind phase 3 trial. *Archives of Surgery, 134*, 428–433.

Braga, M., Gianotti, L., Vignali, A., & Di Carlo, V. (1998). Immunonutrition in gastric cancer surgical patients. *Nutrition, 14*, 831–835.

Braunschweig, C.L., Levy, P., Sheean, P.M., & Wang, X. (2001). Enteral compared with parenteral nutrition: A meta-analysis. *American Journal of Clinical Nutrition, 74*, 534–542.

Brittenden, J., Park, K.G., Heys, S.D., Ross, C., Ashby, J., Ah-See, A., et al. (1994). L-arginine stimulates host defenses in patients with breast cancer. *Surgery, 115*(2), 205–212.

Brown, S.A., Goringe, A., Fegan, C., Davies, S.V., Giddings, J., Whittaker, J.A., et al. (1998). Parenteral glutamine protects hepatic function during bone marrow transplantation. *Bone Marrow Transplantation, 22*, 281–284.

Bruera, E. (1997). ABC of palliative care. Anorexia, cachexia, and nutrition. *BMJ, 315*, 1219–1222.

Bruera, E., Strasser, F., Palmer, J.L., Willey, J., Calder, K., Amyotte, G., et al. (2003). Effect of fish oil on appetite and other symptoms in patients with advanced cancer and anorexia/cachexia: A double-blind, placebo-controlled study. *Journal of Clinical Oncology, 21*(1), 129–134.

Cabal-Manzano, R., Bhargava, P., Torres-Duarte, A., Marshall, J., & Wainer, I.W. (2001). Proteolysis-inducing factor is expressed in tumours of patients with GI cancers and correlates with weight loss. *British Journal of Cancer, 84*, 1599–1601.

Calder, P.C., & Yaqoob, P. (1999). Glutamine and the immune system. *Amino Acids, 17*(3), 227–241.

Cao, Y., Kennedy, R., & Klimberg, V.S. (1999). Glutamine protects against doxorubicin-induced cardiotoxicity. *Journal of Surgical Research, 85*(1), 178–182.

Caparros, T., Lopez, J., & Grau, T. (2001). Early enteral nutrition in critically ill patients with a high-protein diet enriched with arginine, fiber, and antioxidants compared with a standard high-protein diet. The effect on nosocomial infections and outcome. *Journal of Parenteral and Enteral Nutrition, 25*, 299–308.

Cariuk, P., Lorite, M.J., Todorov, P.T., Field, W.N., Wigmore, S.J., & Tisdale, M.J. (1997). Induction of cachexia in mice by a product isolated from the urine of cachectic patients with cancer. *British Journal of Cancer, 76*, 606–613.

Caughey, G.E., Mantzioris, E., Gibson, R.A., Cleland, L.G., & James, M.J. (1996). The effect on human tumor necrosis factor alpha and interleukin 1 beta production of diets enriched in n-3 fatty acids from vegetable oil or fish oil. *American Journal of Clinical Nutrition, 63*(1), 116–122.

Chance, W.T., Cao, L., Kim, M.W., Nelson, J.L., & Fischer, J.E. (1988). Reduction of tumor growth following treatment with a glutamine antimetabolite. *Life Sciences, 42*(1), 87–94.

Chandra, R.K. (1991). 1990 McCollum Award lecture. Nutrition and immunity: Lessons from the past and new insights into the future. *American Journal of Clinical Nutrition, 53*, 1087–1101.

Chandra, R.K. (1992). Effect of vitamin and trace-element supplementation on immune responses and infection in elderly subjects. *Lancet, 340*, 1124–1127.

Clark, R.H., Feleke, G., Din, M., Yasmin, T., Singh, G., Khan, F.A., et al. (2000). Nutritional treatment for acquired immunodeficiency virus-associated wasting using beta-hydroxy beta-methylbutyrate, glutamine, and arginine: A randomized, double-blind, placebo-controlled study. *Journal of Parenteral and Enteral Nutrition, 24,* 133–139.

Daly, J.M., Lieberman, M.D., Goldfine, J., Shou, J., Weintraub, F., Rosato, E.F., et al. (1992). Enteral nutrition with supplemental arginine, RNA, and omega-3 fatty acids in patients after operation: Immunologic, metabolic, and clinical outcome. *Surgery, 112*(1), 56–67.

Daly, J.M., Reynolds, J., Thom, A., Kinsley, L., Dietrick-Gallagher, M., Shou, J., et al. (1988). Immune and metabolic effects of arginine in the surgical patient. *Annals of Surgery, 208,* 512–523.

Daly, J.M., Weintraub, F.N., Shou, J., Rosato, E.F., & Lucia, M. (1995). Enteral nutrition during multimodality therapy in upper gastrointestinal cancer patients. *Annals of Surgery, 221,* 327–338.

Deitch, E.A. (2002). Bacterial translocation or lymphatic drainage of toxic products from the gut: What is important in human beings? *Surgery, 131*(3), 241–244.

Detsky, A.S., Baker, J.P., Mendelson, R.A., Wolman, S.L., Wesson, D.E., & Jeejeebhoy, K.N. (1984). Evaluating the accuracy of nutritional assessment techniques applied to hospitalized patients: Methodology and comparisons. *Journal of Parenteral and Enteral Nutrition, 8,* 153–159.

DeWys, W.D., Begg, C., Lavin, P.T., Band, P.R., Bennett, J.M., Bertino, J.R., et al. (1980). Prognostic effect of weight loss prior to chemotherapy in cancer patients. Eastern Cooperative Oncology Group. *American Journal of Medicine, 69,* 491–497.

Dillon, B.J., Prieto, V.G., Curley, S.A., Ensor, C.M., Holtsberg, F.W., Bomalaski, J.S., et al. (2004). Incidence and distribution of argininosuccinate synthetase deficiency in human cancers: A method for identifying cancers sensitive to arginine deprivation. *Cancer, 100,* 826–833.

Dodd, F., Limoges, M., Boudreau, R.T., Rowden, G., Murphy, P.R., & Too, C.K. (2000). L-arginine inhibits apoptosis via a NO-dependent mechanism in Nb2 lymphoma cells. *Journal of Cellular Biochemistry, 77,* 624–634.

Eden, E., Edstrom, S., Bennegard, K., Schersten, T., & Lundholm, K. (1984). Glucose flux in relation to energy expenditure in malnourished patients with and without cancer during periods of fasting and feeding. *Cancer Research, 44,* 1718–1724.

Edwards, P.D., Topping, D., Kontaridis, M.I., Moldawer, L.L., Copeland, E.M., 3rd, & Lind, D. S. (1997). Arginine-enhanced enteral nutrition augments the growth of a nitric oxide-producing tumor. *Journal of Parenteral and Enteral Nutrition, 21,* 215–219.

Endres, S., & von Schacky, C. (1996). n-3 polyunsaturated fatty acids and human cytokine synthesis. *Current Opinion in Lipidology, 7*(1), 48–52.

Evoy, D., Lieberman, M.D., Fahey, T.J., 3rd, & Daly, J.M. (1998). Immunonutrition: The role of arginine. *Nutrition, 14,* 611–617.

Fahr, M.J., Kornbluth, J., Blossom, S., Schaeffer, R., & Klimberg, V.S. (1994). Glutamine enhances immunoregulation of tumor growth. *Journal of Parenteral and Enteral Nutrition, 18,* 471–476.

Fanslow, W.C., Kulkarni, A.D., Van Buren, C.T., & Rudolph, F.B. (1988). Effect of nucleotide restriction and supplementation on resistance to experimental murine candidiasis. *Journal of Parenteral and Enteral Nutrition, 12,* 49–52.

Fearon, K.C., von Meyenfeldt, M.F., Moses, A.G., Van Geenen, R., Roy, A., Gouma, D.J., et al. (2003). Effect of a protein and energy dense N-3 fatty acid enriched oral supplement on loss of weight and lean tissue in cancer cachexia: A randomised double blind trial. *Gut, 52,* 1479–1486.

Fearon, K.C.H., von Meyenfeldt, M., Moses, A.G.W., van Geenen, R., Roy, A., Gouma, D., et al. (2001). An energy and protein dense, high n-3 fatty acid oral supplement promotes weight gain in cancer cachexia. *European Journal of Cancer, 37*(Suppl. 6), S27–S28.

Galban, C., Montejo, J.C., Mesejo, A., Marco, P., Celaya, S., Sanchez-Segura, J.M., et al. (2000). An immune-enhancing enteral diet reduces mortality rate and episodes of bacteremia in septic intensive care unit patients. *Critical Care Medicine, 28,* 643–648.

Garcia-de-Lorenzo, A., Zarazaga, A., Garcia-Luna, P.P., Gonzalez-Huix, F., Lopez-Martinez, J., Mijan, A., et al. (2003). Clinical evidence for enteral nutritional support with glutamine: A systematic review. *Nutrition, 19*, 805–811.

Gianotti, L., Braga, M., Frei, A., Greiner, R., & Di Carlo, V. (2000). Health care resources consumed to treat postoperative infections: Cost saving by perioperative immunonutrition. *Shock, 14*, 325–330.

Gianotti, L., Braga, M., Nespoli, L., Radaelli, G., Beneduce, A., & Di Carlo, V. (2002). A randomized controlled trial of preoperative oral supplementation with a specialized diet in patients with GI cancer. *Gastroenterology, 122*, 1763–1770.

Gianotti, L., Braga, M., Vignali, A., Balzano, G., Zerbi, A., Bisagni, P., et al. (1997). Effect of route of delivery and formulation of postoperative nutritional support in patients undergoing major operations for malignant neoplasms. *Archives of Surgery, 132*, 1222–1229; discussion 1229–1230.

Gismondo, M.R., Drago, L., Fassina, M.C., Vaghi, I., Abbiati, R., & Grossi, E. (1998). Immunostimulating effect of oral glutamine. *Digestive Diseases and Sciences, 43*, 1752–1754.

Gogos, C.A., Ginopoulos, P., Salsa, B., Apostolidou, E., Zoumbos, N.C., & Kalfarentzos, F. (1998). Dietary omega-3 polyunsaturated fatty acids plus vitamin E restore immunodeficiency and prolong survival for severely ill patients with generalized malignancy: A randomized control trial. *Cancer, 82*, 395–402.

Heslin, M.J., & Brennan, M.F. (2000). Advances in perioperative nutrition: Cancer. *World Journal of Surgery, 24*, 1477–1485.

Heyland, D.K., Novak, F., Drover, J.W., Jain, M., Su, X., & Suchner, U. (2001). Should immunonutrition become routine in critically ill patients? A systematic review of the evidence. *JAMA, 286*, 944–953.

Heyland, D.K., Schroter-Nappe, D., Drover, J.W., Jain, M., Keefe, L., Dhaliwal, R., et al. (2003). Nutritional support in the critical care setting: Current practice in Canadian ICUs—Opportunities for improvement. *Journal of Parenteral and Enteral Nutrition, 27*, 74–83.

Heyland, D.K., Tougas, G., King, D., & Cook, D.J. (1996). Impaired gastric emptying in mechanically ventilated, critically ill patients. *Intensive Care Medicine, 22*, 1339–1344.

Heys, S.D., Walker, L.G., Smith, I., & Eremin, O. (1999). Enteral nutritional supplementation with key nutrients in patients with critical illness and cancer: A meta-analysis of randomized controlled clinical trials. *Annals of Surgery, 229*, 467–477.

Huang, E.Y., Leung, S.W., Wang, C.J., Chen, H.C., Sun, L.M., Fang, F.M., et al. (2000). Oral glutamine to alleviate radiation-induced oral mucositis: A pilot randomized trial. *International Journal of Radiation Oncology, Biology, Physics, 46*, 535–539.

Inui, A. (2002). Cancer anorexia-cachexia syndrome: Current issues in research and management. *CA: A Cancer Journal for Clinicians, 52*(2), 72–91.

Istfan, N.W., Wan, J.M., & Bistrian, B.R. (1992). Nutrition and tumor promotion: In vivo methods for measurement of cellular proliferation and protein metabolism. *Journal of Parenteral and Enteral Nutrition, 16*(6 Suppl.), 76S–82S.

Jeejeebhoy, K.N. (2001). Total parenteral nutrition: Potion or poison? *American Journal of Clinical Nutrition, 74*(2), 160–163.

Jolliet, P., Pichard, C., Biolo, G., Chiolero, R., Grimble, G., Leverve, X., et al. (1999). Enteral nutrition in intensive care patients: A practical approach. *Clinical Nutrition, 18*(1), 47–56.

Khan, S., & Tisdale, M.J. (1999). Catabolism of adipose tissue by a tumour-produced lipid-mobilising factor. *International Journal of Cancer, 80*, 444–447.

Klein, S., & Koretz, R.L. (1994). Nutrition support in patients with cancer: What do the data really show? *Nutrition in Clinical Practice, 9*(3), 91–100.

Klimberg, V.S., Kornbluth, J., Cao, Y., Dang, A., Blossom, S., & Schaeffer, R.F. (1996). Glutamine suppresses PGE2 synthesis and breast cancer growth. *Journal of Surgical Research, 63*, 293–297.

Kline, D.G. (2002). *Nutrition and immunity*. Ashland, NC: Nutrition Dimension.

Knox, L.S. (1983). Nutrition and cancer. *Nursing Clinics of North America, 18*(1), 97–109.

Kotler, D.P. (2000). Cachexia. *Annals of Internal Medicine, 133,* 622–634.

Kouznetsova, L., Bijlsma, P.B., van Leeuwen, P.A., Groot, J.A., & Houdijk, A.P. (1999). Glutamine reduces phorbol-12,13-dibutyrate-induced macromolecular hyperpermeability in HT-29Cl.19A intestinal cells. *Journal of Parenteral and Enteral Nutrition, 23,* 136–139.

Lecker, S.H., Solomon, V., Mitch, W.E., & Goldberg, A.L. (1999). Muscle protein breakdown and the critical role of the ubiquitin-proteasome pathway in normal and disease states. *Journal of Nutrition, 129*(1 Suppl.), 227S–237S.

Lopez, M.J., & Tehrani, H.Y. (2001). Nutrition and the patient with cancer. In R.E. Lenhard, R.T. Osteen, & T. Gansler (Eds.), *Clinical oncology* (pp. 811–822). Atlanta, GA: American Cancer Society.

Ma, Q., Hoper, M., Anderson, N., & Rowlands, B.J. (1996). Effect of supplemental L-arginine in a chemical-induced model of colorectal cancer. *World Journal of Surgery, 20,* 1087–1091.

Ma, Q., Williamson, K.E., O'Rourke, D., & Rowlands, B.J. (1999). The effects of l-arginine on crypt cell hyperproliferation in colorectal cancer. *Journal of Surgical Research, 81*(2), 181–188.

May, P.E., Barber, A., D'Olimpio, J.T., Hourihane, A., & Abumrad, N.N. (2002). Reversal of cancer-related wasting using oral supplementation with a combination of beta-hydroxy-beta-methylbutyrate, arginine, and glutamine. *American Journal of Surgery, 183,* 471–479.

McCarter, M.D., Gentilini, O.D., Gomez, M.E., & Daly, J.M. (1998). Preoperative oral supplement with immunonutrients in cancer patients. *Journal of Parenteral and Enteral Nutrition, 22,* 206–211.

McCowen, K.C., & Bistrian, B.R. (2003). Immunonutrition: Problematic or problem solving? *American Journal of Clinical Nutrition, 77,* 764–770.

McMahon, K., Decker, G., & Ottery, F.D. (1998). Integrating proactive nutritional assessment in clinical practices to prevent complications and cost. *Seminars in Oncology, 25*(2 Suppl. 6), 20–27.

McMillan, D.C., Canna, K., & McArdle, C.S. (2003). Systemic inflammatory response predicts survival following curative resection of colorectal cancer. *British Journal of Surgery, 90*(2), 215–219.

McMillan, D.C., Elahi, M.M., Sattar, N., Angerson, W.J., Johnstone, J., & McArdle, C.S. (2001). Measurement of the systemic inflammatory response predicts cancer-specific and non-cancer survival in patients with cancer. *Nutrition and Cancer, 41*(1–2), 64–69.

Mills, C.D., Shearer, J., Evans, R., & Caldwell, M.D. (1992). Macrophage arginine metabolism and the inhibition or stimulation of cancer. *Journal of Immunology, 149,* 2709–2714.

Moses, A.W.G., Slater, C., Preston, T., Barber, M.D., & Fearon, K.C.H. (2004). Reduced total energy expenditure and physical activity in cachectic patients with pancreatic cancer can be modulated by an energy and protein dense oral supplement enriched with n-3 fatty acids. *British Journal of Cancer, 90,* 996–1002.

Nayel, H., el-Ghoneimy, E., & el-Haddad, S. (1992). Impact of nutritional supplementation on treatment delay and morbidity in patients with head and neck tumors treated with irradiation. *Nutrition, 8*(1), 13–18.

Nitenberg, G., & Raynard, B. (2000). Nutritional support of the patient with cancer: Issues and dilemmas. *Critical Reviews in Oncology/Hematology, 34*(3), 137–168.

Nixon, D.W., Moffitt, S., Lawson, D.H., Ansley, J., Lynn, M.J., Kutner, M.H., et al. (1981). Total parenteral nutrition as an adjunct to chemotherapy of metastatic colorectal cancer. *Cancer Treatment Report, 65*(Suppl. 5), 121–128.

Okuno, S.H., Woodhouse, C.O., Loprinzi, C.L., Sloan, J.A., LaVasseur, B.I., Clemens-Schutjer, D., et al. (1999). Phase III controlled evaluation of glutamine for decreasing stomatitis in patients receiving fluorouracil (5-FU)-based chemotherapy. *American Journal of Clinical Oncology, 22,* 258–261.

Ovesen, L., Allingstrup, L., Hannibal, J., Mortensen, E.L., & Hansen, O.P. (1993). Effect of dietary counseling on food intake, body weight, response rate, survival, and quality of life in cancer patients undergoing chemotherapy: A prospective, randomized study. *Journal of Clinical Oncology, 11,* 2043–2049.

Panigrahi, P., Gewolb, I.H., Bamford, P., & Horvath, K. (1997). Role of glutamine in bacterial transcytosis and epithelial cell injury. *Journal of Parenteral and Enteral Nutrition, 21,* 75–80.

Park, K.G., Heys, S.D., Blessing, K., Kelly, P., McNurlan, M.A., Eremin, O., et al. (1992). Stimulation of human breast cancers by dietary L-arginine. *Clinical Science (London), 82,* 413–417.

Peteet, J.R., Medeiros, C., Slavin, L., & Walsh-Burke, K. (1981). Psychological aspects of artificial feeding in cancer patients. *Journal of Parenteral and Enteral Nutrition, 5,* 138–140.

Price, S.A., & Tisdale, M.J. (1998). Mechanism of inhibition of a tumor lipid-mobilizing factor by eicosapentaenoic acid. *Cancer Research, 58,* 4827–4831.

Riso, S., Aluffi, P., Brugnani, M., Farinetti, F., Pia, F., & D'Andrea, F. (2000). Postoperative enteral immunonutrition in head and neck cancer patients. *Clinical Nutrition, 19,* 407–412.

Robinson, L.E., Bussiere, F.I., Le Boucher, J., Farges, M.C., Cynober, L.A., Field, C.J., et al. (1999). Amino acid nutrition and immune function in tumour-bearing rats: A comparison of glutamine-, arginine- and ornithine 2-oxoglutarate-supplemented diets. *Clinical Science (London), 97,* 657–669.

Rose, D.P., Connolly, J.M., & Coleman, M. (1996). Effect of omega-3 fatty acids on the progression of metastases after the surgical excision of human breast cancer cell solid tumors growing in nude mice. *Clinical Cancer Research, 2,* 1751–1756.

Rouse, K., Nwokedi, E., Woodliff, J.E., Epstein, J., & Klimberg, V.S. (1995). Glutamine enhances selectivity of chemotherapy through changes in glutathione metabolism. *Annals of Surgery, 221,* 420–426.

Sacks, G.S., Genton, L., & Kudsk, K.A. (2003). Controversy of immunonutrition for surgical critical-illness patients. *Current Opinion in Critical Care, 9,* 300–305.

Salvalaggio, P.R., & Campos, A.C. (2002). Bacterial translocation and glutamine. *Nutrition, 18,* 435–437.

Salvalaggio, P.R., Neto, C.Z., Tolazzi, A.R., Gasparetto, E.L., Coelho, J.C., & Campos, A.C. (2002). Oral glutamine does not prevent bacterial translocation in rats subjected to intestinal obstruction and Escherichia coli challenge but reduces systemic bacteria spread. *Nutrition, 18,* 334–337.

Savarese, D., Al-Zoubi, A., & Boucher, J. (2000). Glutamine for irinotecan diarrhea. *Journal of Clinical Oncology, 18,* 450–451.

Savarese, D.M., Savy, G., Vahdat, L., Wischmeyer, P.E., & Corey, B. (2003). Prevention of chemotherapy and radiation toxicity with glutamine. *Cancer Treatment Reviews, 29,* 501–513.

Scott, H.R., McMillan, D.C., Brown, D.J., Forrest, L.M., McArdle, C.S., & Milroy, R. (2003). A prospective study of the impact of weight loss and the systemic inflammatory response on quality of life in patients with inoperable non-small cell lung cancer. *Lung Cancer, 40,* 295–299.

Scott, H.R., McMillan, D.C., Forrest, L.M., Brown, D.J., McArdle, C.S., & Milroy, R. (2002). The systemic inflammatory response, weight loss, performance status and survival in patients with inoperable non-small cell lung cancer. *British Journal of Cancer, 87,* 264–267.

Senkal, M., Zumtobel, V., Bauer, K.H., Marpe, B., Wolfram, G., Frei, A., et al. (1999). Outcome and cost-effectiveness of perioperative enteral immunonutrition in patients undergoing elective upper GI tract surgery: A prospective randomized study. *Archives of Surgery, 134,* 1309–1316.

Shewchuk, L.D., Baracos, V.E., & Field, C.J. (1997). Dietary L-glutamine supplementation reduces the growth of the Morris Hepatoma 7777 in exercise-trained and sedentary rats. *Journal of Nutrition, 127,* 158–166.

Shils, M.E. (1994). Nutrition and diet in cancer management. In M.E. Shils, J.A. Olson, & M. Shike (Eds.), *Modern nutrition in health and disease* (8th ed., pp. 1319–1342). Philadelphia: Lea & Febiger.

Smith, H.J., Lorite, M.J., & Tisdale, M.J. (1999). Effect of a cancer cachectic factor on protein synthesis/degradation in murine C2C12 myoblasts: Modulation by eicosapentaenoic acid. *Cancer Research, 59,* 5507–5513.

Stolina, M., Sharma, S., Lin, Y., Dohadwala, M., Gardner, B., Luo, J., et al. (2000). Specific inhibition of cyclooxygenase 2 restores antitumor reactivity by altering the balance of IL-10 and IL-12 synthesis. *Journal of Immunology, 164,* 361–370.

Swails, W.S., Kenler, A.S., Driscoll, D.F., DeMichele, S.J., Babineau, T.J., Utsunamiya, T., et al. (1997). Effect of a fish oil structured lipid-based diet on prostaglandin release from mononuclear cells in cancer patients after surgery. *Journal of Parenteral and Enteral Nutrition, 21,* 266–274.

Takagi, K., Yamamori, H., Furukawa, K., Miyazaki, M., & Tashiro, T. (2001). Perioperative supplementation of EPA reduces immunosuppression induced by postoperative chemoradiation therapy in patients with esophageal cancer. *Nutrition, 17,* 478–479.

Tayek, J.A., Manglik, S., & Abemayor, E. (1997). Insulin secretion, glucose production, and insulin sensitivity in underweight and normal-weight volunteers, and in underweight and normal-weight cancer patients: A Clinical Research Center study. *Metabolism, 46*(2), 140–145.

Tchekmedyian, N.S. (1998). Pharmacoeconomics of nutritional support in cancer. *Seminars in Oncology, 25*(2 Suppl. 6), 62–69.

Terry, P.D., Rohan, T.E., & Wolk, A. (2003). Intakes of fish and marine fatty acids and the risks of cancers of the breast and prostate and of other hormone-related cancers: A review of the epidemiologic evidence. *American Journal of Clinical Nutrition, 77,* 532–543.

Tisdale, M.J. (2001). Cancer anorexia and cachexia. *Nutrition, 17,* 438–442.

Tisdale, M.J. (2002). Cachexia in cancer patients. *Nature Reviews. Cancer, 2,* 862–871.

Tisdale, M.J., & Beck, S.A. (1991). Inhibition of tumour-induced lipolysis in vitro and cachexia and tumour growth in vivo by eicosapentaenoic acid. *Biochemical Pharmacology, 41*(1), 103–107.

Vahdat, L., Papadopoulos, K., Lange, D., Leuin, S., Kaufman, E., Donovan, D., et al. (2001). Reduction of paclitaxel-induced peripheral neuropathy with glutamine. *Clinical Cancer Research, 7,* 1192–1197.

van Bokhorst-De Van Der Schueren, M.A., Quak, J.J., von Blomberg-van der Flier, B.M., Kuik, D.J., Langendoen, S.I., Snow, G.B., et al. (2001). Effect of perioperative nutrition, with and without arginine supplementation, on nutritional status, immune function, postoperative morbidity, and survival in severely malnourished head and neck cancer patients. *American Journal of Clinical Nutrition, 73,* 323–332.

Van Buren, C.T., & Rudolph, F. (1997). Dietary nucleotides: A conditional requirement. *Nutrition, 13,* 470–472.

Wallace, J.M. (2002). Nutritional and botanical modulation of the inflammatory cascade—eicosanoids, cyclooxygenases, and lipoxygenases—as an adjunct in cancer therapy. *Integrative Cancer Therapies, 1*(1), 7–37; discussion 37.

Whitehouse, A.S., & Tisdale, M.J. (2003). Increased expression of the ubiquitin-proteasome pathway in murine myotubes by proteolysis-inducing factor (PIF) is associated with activation of the transcription factor NF-kappaB. *British Journal of Cancer, 89,* 1116–1122.

Wigmore, S.J., Barber, M.D., Ross, J.A., Tisdale, M.J., & Fearon, K.C. (2000). Effect of oral eicosapentaenoic acid on weight loss in patients with pancreatic cancer. *Nutrition and Cancer, 36*(2), 177–184.

Wigmore, S.J., Plester, C.E., Richardson, R.A., & Fearon, K.C. (1997). Changes in nutritional status associated with unresectable pancreatic cancer. *British Journal of Cancer, 75*(1), 106–109.

Wigmore, S.J., Ross, J.A., Falconer, J.S., Plester, C.E., Tisdale, M.J., Carter, D.C., et al. (1996). The effect of polyunsaturated fatty acids on the progress of cachexia in patients with pancreatic cancer. *Nutrition, 12*(1 Suppl.), S27–S30.

Wigmore, S.J., Todorov, P.T., Barber, M.D., Ross, J.A., Tisdale, M.J., & Fearon, K.C. (2000). Characteristics of patients with pancreatic cancer expressing a novel cancer cachectic factor. *British Journal of Surgery, 87*(1), 53–58.

Williams, J.Z., Abumrad, N., & Barbul, A. (2002). Effect of a specialized amino acid mixture on human collagen deposition. *Annals of Surgery, 236*, 369–374.

Wischmeyer, P.E. (2002). Glutamine and heat shock protein expression. *Nutrition, 18*, 225–228.

Wischmeyer, P.E., Kahana, M., Wolfson, R., Ren, H., Musch, M.M., & Chang, E.B. (2001). Glutamine reduces cytokine release, organ damage, and mortality in a rat model of endotoxemia. *Shock, 16*, 398–402.

Yaqoob, P., & Calder, P.C. (1997). Glutamine requirement of proliferating T lymphocytes. *Nutrition, 13*, 646–651.

Yeatman, T.J., Risley, G.L., & Brunson, M.E. (1991). Depletion of dietary arginine inhibits growth of metastatic tumor. *Archives of Surgery, 126*, 1376–1381.

Yoshida, S., Matsui, M., Shirouzu, Y., Fujita, H., Yamana, H., & Shirouzu, K. (1998). Effects of glutamine supplements and radiochemotherapy on systemic immune and gut barrier function in patients with advanced esophageal cancer. *Annals of Surgery, 227*, 485–491.

Young, M.R. (1994). Eicosanoids and the immunology of cancer. *Cancer Metastasis Review, 13*, 337–348.

Zaloga, G.P., Siddiqui, R., Terry, C., & Marik, P.E. (2004). Arginine: Mediator or modulator of sepsis? *Nutrition in Clinical Practice, 19*, 201–215.

Ziegler, T.R., Bazargan, N., Leader, L.M., & Martindale, R.G. (2000). Glutamine and the GI tract. *Current Opinion in Clinical Nutrition and Metabolic Care, 3*, 355–362.

CHAPTER 19

Palliative Care and Hospice

Clara Schneider, MS, RD, RN, LD, CDE

Overview

Palliative care and hospice are treatment options one may choose toward the end of life. Healthcare professionals should know the philosophy and benefits of the treatment choices to help their patients to make educated decisions. Nutritional care differs with older adults. Current thoughts on cachexia, anorexia, stomatitis, hydration, enteral and parenteral nutrition, nausea, constipation, as well as the ethics of end-of-life care are included in this chapter.

Palliative Care and Hospice Definitions

Palliative care refers to therapies that help to relieve symptoms without curing the disease (American Heritage Dictionary of the English Language, 2000). The World Health Organization (WHO, 2003) described palliative care as

> an approach that improves the quality of life of patients and their families facing the problems associated with life-threatening illness, through the prevention and relief of suffering by means of early identification and impeccable assessment and treatment of pain and other problems—physical, psychosocial, and spiritual.

Palliative care is not intended to hasten or postpone death; rather, the intent is to provide the patient with symptom control, especially from pain. By integrating psychological and spiritual needs, it can offer patients and their families a support system that can help to improve quality of life and help families to cope with the illness. A team approach is vital, and early intervention is key. If a palliative care team approach is established early in the course of illness, distressing complications from chemotherapy and radiation therapy can be better managed and help to improve patients' overall quality of life.

Palliative care can transpire at any time during a life-threatening illness and may occur with or without hospice care (Williams, 2004). Hospice care is defined as "care and support for individuals in the last phase of an incurable disease so that they may live as fully and comfortably as possible" (National Hospice and Palliative Care Organization, 2002). A patient in the United States can elect to have hospice care, but regulations must be followed. Many private insurances, as well as Medicare, pay hospice benefits. Often, people who medically qualify for hospice are eligible for Medicare, so it is appropriate to review the hospice benefit.

What Is the Medicare Hospice Benefit?

According to the Centers for Medicare and Medicaid Services (2004), for coverage under the Medicare hospice benefit, a patient must meet the eligibility requirements for Medicare Part A, and his or her physician, along with the hospice director, must verify that the patient has six months or less to live because of terminal illness. In addition, a statement must be signed choosing hospice care, and a Medicare-approved hospice program must provide the care (U.S. Department of Health and Human Services, 2003).

Certification periods are required for patients to be financially covered for hospice. Coverage is available based on predetermined guidelines set forth by Medicare or private insurance.

The services of many different types of healthcare professionals are available with hospice. Doctors, nurses, clergy, social workers, psychologists, dietitians, therapists, and home health aides are part of the hospice team. Volunteers also are available in many hospices, with duties including going to a patient's house to deliver food, prepare meals, or provide company.

Hospice care usually takes place in one's own home with the help of a family member or friend. If needed, the care may occur in a hospital or hospice inpatient unit for a short period of time (U.S. Department of Health and Human Services, 2003). Residential hospices and some skilled nursing facilities may provide hospice care. These hospice programs may be available to patients during the last few weeks of life or for total patient care, as appropriate.

Nutritional care by a registered dietitian optimally will occur before the patient has elected palliative care or hospice. Both the patient and family will benefit from an ongoing relationship with the dietitian. Meetings with the dietitian to discuss appropriate changes will help the patient to be comfortable before, during, and after the transition to palliative care and/or hospice.

Treatment Modalities and Nutrition Assessment

Unlike one specific disease process, treatment for palliative care and hospice care are disease-process specific. One commonality among hospice patients is that comfort measures are the extent of treatment rendered. For the patient who chooses palliative care only, the treatment may be much broader but always should be individualized.

Nutrition assessment tools are available for palliative care and hospice patients. The Patient-Generated Subjective Global Assessment (PG-SGA) is a nutrition screening tool that has been validated in outpatient palliative care and hospice settings (see Appendix A). According to Small, Carrara, Danford, Logemann, and Cella (2002), "this tool provides a global assessment of the patient's nutritional status based on nutrition-related history and physical symptoms and can be used to evaluate nutritional quality of life" (p. 14) . For inpatient assessment, the healthcare professional should refer to the organization's approved assessment tools.

Issues Affecting Nutritional Status

By the time a person gets the news that he or she is terminally ill, many symptoms already may be present or may develop shortly thereafter. Common symptoms may include cancer cachexia and anorexia. Weakness, pain, nausea, and vomiting also may develop. Cachexia is defined as a syndrome that combines weight loss, lipolysis, loss of muscle and visceral protein, anorexia, chronic nausea, and weakness (Blacker, 2002; Bruera, 1997). In a workshop held at the National Institutes of Health in 1997, Dr. Neil MacDonald made the following comments about cachexia.

The emerging view is that cachexia is a result of the combined action of tumor products (in cancer) and host immune factors, particularly cytokines, that lead to poor appetite, muscle wasting, and altered metabolism. By identifying potential causative agents, this model suggests several targets for therapeutic interventions. A particular goal would be to identify agents that can increase protein synthesis and decrease proteolysis. Gemzar® (gemcitabine, Eli Lilly and Company, Indianapolis, IN), a chemotherapeutic drug, has been shown to have measurable clinical benefit in treating cachexia. Oncologists should take a broader look at agents that might modify the host immune response with benefits in terms of pain as well as cachexia. Corticosteroids interfere with cytokine production and give temporary relief from anorexia but not from cachexia. Progestin improves appetite and may be best combined with exercise. CNS agents, androgen, and growth factors are being tested but are unproven. It may be possible to modify diet, but this approach has not been successful so far. (National Institutes of Health, 1997)

Additional cachexia research is indicated when combining appetite stimulants and ibuprofen. Initial results suggest that in advanced gastrointestinal cancer, quality of life and weight loss may be stabilized. Fish oils and eicosapentaenoic acid also are being researched and show much promise (Barber & Rogers, 2002).

Counseling Suggestions

Lift diet restrictions when possible for the patient who is terminally ill. Offer favorite foods in smaller quantities, more frequently, and as desired. The timing of offering foods should correspond to when the patient has the greatest appetite. Many times, patients are hungriest in the morning. Soft foods such as casseroles and ground meats in gravy are good food choices, as they will tend to save the energy expended by chewing. As the day progresses, energy might dwindle; thus, offering nutritious beverages (milkshakes and high-caloric, high-protein canned commercial products) may be appropriate. To maximize food intake, it may be better to offer fluids and ice chips after meals so that the patient does not consume less calories because he or she is filling up on fluids. Another good hint is to consult with the doctor to see if a glass of wine is appropriate to stimulate appetite (Barber & Rogers, 2002).

The National Cancer Institute (2005) and the American Institute for Cancer Research (2003) offer tips for feeding difficulties (see Appendix C). If patients have a metallic taste in their mouth, they should try using plastic utensils or suck on sugar-free lemon drops. For red meat taste changes, they should eat meat with a sweet fruit or food like cranberry sauce, jelly, or applesauce (National Cancer Institute). For symptoms of nausea, suggestions include eating small amounts of food often and slowly by offering the patient six or more small meals during the day rather than three large meals. Meals should be provided in a well-ventilated room because some patients find that the odors of some foods may produce nausea. Offer foods at room temperature or cooler because hot foods can exacerbate nausea. Do not offer favorite foods at this time as this may cause a permanent aversion to the food. A person experiencing nausea should try to eat sitting up and to rest sitting up or reclined with the head raised for about an hour after eating. If nauseated while resting, the patient should keep crackers at the bedside to nibble on before getting up. It may be helpful to keep food out of sight until it is time to eat (American Institute for Cancer Research).

Patients experiencing vomiting should avoid food or drink until the vomiting is under control. Once vomiting is under control, they should try drinking small amounts of clear liquids such as cool broth or flat soft drinks (carbonated beverages may cause burping, which can stimulate vomiting in some people). When patients are able to keep down clear liquids, they should try eating small amounts of soft foods such as warm cereal, pudding, frozen yogurt, or gelatin.

Once they can tolerate soft foods, they can gradually work their way back to a regular diet (American Institute for Cancer Research, 2003).

Biochemical disorders such as uremia, medications such as opioids, or toxins such as tumor-producing peptides may cause nausea and vomiting (Williams, 2004). It is helpful to have a pharmacist and physician evaluate the cause of nausea and choose an appropriate medication to decrease symptoms.

Constipation is another major problem in palliative and hospice care. It is especially common when narcotics are used. Many physicians will order laxatives (Peri-Colace® [docusate sodium/senna, Purdue Pharma, Stamford, CT]) or Senokot® (senna, Purdue Pharma) when ordering narcotics to help to prevent constipation. If constipation goes untreated, it may develop into an intestinal blockage or impaction. This may contribute to lack of appetite or nausea and vomiting. If this occurs, the physician may order phosphate enemas, mineral oil enemas, or other treatments as needed (Hospice Patients Alliance, 2004). Ask about stool frequency, and counsel the patient to inform his or her heathcare provider if stool is not passed every two to three days. Establish a bowel program with the patient based on individual needs. Constipation management may include increasing fiber or psyllium. Use caution with this recommendation because it may increase constipation if dehydration or poor motility is present (Hill, 2004). Poor hydration also can contribute to constipation, and with heart failure and kidney problems, fluid may be restricted. If there are no restrictions, increasing fluids and adding sorbitol may be of assistance. Juices such as prune, apple, and grape help with motility. Glycerin suppositories may aid intestinal lubrication (Hill).

With the patient who is terminally ill, the focus should be on quality of life. Help the patient by making suggestions of things he or she might enjoy. Remember that preferences are not always the same. Do not force your own wishes on the patient (Maillet, Potter, & Heller, 2002).

Hydration and Enteral and Parenteral Nutrition

When a patient is no longer able to eat or drink because of advancing cancer, the patient, family, or loved ones may raise the question of nutritional support, if it has not been addressed in an advance directive. Family members frequently question the use of nutrients with patients. Explaining this type of nutrition and its uses and shortcomings helps the family to make educated decisions. The American Society for Parenteral and Enteral Nutrition (2000) listed definitions that may help the healthcare professional to explain parenteral nutrition and enteral nutrition to the patient and his or her family.

Parenteral nutrition is one of the ways people receive food when they cannot eat. It is a special liquid food mixture given into the blood with a needle through a vein. The mixture contains all the protein, sugars, fat, vitamins, minerals, and other nutrients needed to sustain life. It is sometimes called total parenteral nutrition (TPN) or hyperalimentation.

Enteral nutrition is another way people can receive the nutrients they need to sustain life. Also called "tube feedings," it is thicker than parenteral nutrition and sometimes looks like a milkshake. It is given through a tube in the stomach or small intestine.

The term "hydration support" usually is thought of as fluids delivered into the body by nonoral methods: IV, subcutaneous (also called hypodermoclysis), and rectally (proctoclysis) or enteral (Ersek, 2003).

In patients with cancer who are terminally ill, enteral feeding and TPN have not been linked with increased survival time (Borum et al., 2000; Bruera, 1997). Barber and Rogers (2002) reviewed parenteral nutrition in cancer studies and found that it did not improve outcome but was associated with increased complications, increased infections, and a trend toward shorter survival time. These authors concluded that weight gain was blocked because of metabolic changes. The dietitian and medical team should assess each case individually. Sometimes enteral nutrition or hydration therapy is used early in palliative care. The focus should be to address patients' needs and find ways to possibly improve anorexia and weakness.

Patient and family satisfaction should be paramount in the nutritional plan (Bruera, 1997). If a patient wants enteral or parenteral nutrition, these options should be discussed and fully explained. Complications need to be addressed so the patient and his or her family know the risks as well as the possible benefits. Hospice Patients Alliance (2004) defined the catabolic state of metabolism as when food is not absorbed, whether or not nutrition is taken in. When the body is in the catabolic state, enteral feedings or TPN will not stop this process. When a person is near death, dehydration can have beneficial effects. When the body does not have optimal fluids, hemoconcentration and hyperosmolality occur. Azotemia and hypernatremia will develop, which can produce a tranquilizing result on the brain just before death (Hospice Patients Alliance). Coughing from pulmonary congestion, excess oral secretions, and frequent urination can be alarming to the family and patient. These occurrences are very uncomfortable as death approaches. These conditions can be minimized when hydration is not forced (Maillet et al., 2002). Enteral and parenteral nutrition do not help the patient at this time (Abrahm, 2000). Many medical organizations have position statements regarding the use of nutrition and hydration at the end of life. It is important to know what they have concluded in regard to these important issues. Often a professional, as well as the patient and his or her family, will have conflicting thoughts regarding feeding or withholding nutrition. Knowledge of the position statements provides guidance.

The American Academy of Hospice and Palliative Medicines (AAHPM, 2001) statement indicated the following.

> Hydration and nutrition are traditionally considered useful and necessary components of good medical care. They are provided with the

primary intention of benefiting the patient. However, when a person is approaching death, the provision of artificial hydration and nutrition is potentially harmful and may provide little or no benefit to the patient and at times may make the period of dying more uncomfortable for both patient and family. For this reason, the AAHPM believes that the withholding of artificial hydration and nutrition near the end of life may be appropriate and beneficial medical care.

Several of the goals of the Hospice and Palliative Nurses Association (2003) for artificial nutrition and hydration during end-of-life care are listed.

- Promote the education of healthcare providers to ensure that they understand the clinical, legal, and ethical issues regarding the use of artificial nutrition and hydration (ANH).
- Support education of patient, family, and other caregivers about the dying process and its effects on nutrition and fluid status.
- Teach caregivers to enhance the patient's comfort by providing frequent oral and skin care, effective and timely symptom management, and psycho-spiritual support. Support caregivers in coping with feelings of helplessness, loss, and fear.
- Recognize that in specific situations, ANH may be clinically beneficial. ANH also may be initiated or continued to honor the beliefs and values of some cultural and religious groups.
- Encourage nurses to collaborate with speech therapists, dietitians, and other healthcare providers to identify and implement strategies that enable caregivers to provide oral nutrition and fluids safely and effectively, as an alternative to ANH.
- Promote the use of a decision-making process that examines the benefits and burdens of ANH and includes the patient's clinical condition, goals, and values.
- Acknowledge and support the established legal and moral right of competent patients to refuse unwanted treatment, including ANH.
- Acknowledge and support the family's or other surrogate's role as decision-maker in cases where a patient is unable to make his or her wishes known or is unable to evaluate the benefits and burdens of artificial nutrition or hydration.
- Promote the use of advance directives such as living wills or the legal assignment of durable power of attorney for health care to document choices and values that should guide care at the end of life in the event that decision-making capacity is lost.
- Promote early discussions about the goals of care and treatment choices, including the expected benefits and burdens of possible end-of-life interventions (including ANH) prior to treatment initiation, refusal, or withdrawal.
- Encourage policies that guide a decision-making process for resolving disagreements about care among patients, families, surrogates, and healthcare team members.

- Support research on the outcomes of ANH in diverse groups of hospice and palliative care patients.

Feeding should start immediately with patients once they are medically stable and continue until the treatment is futile or until research has shown the futility of feeding (Maillet et al., 2002). Try to provide adequate nutrients and fluids to maintain or achieve a reasonable weight, maintain muscle mass, and achieve hydration. Feeding should only be stopped based on patient wishes, if feeding is medically contraindicated, or after the patient is diagnosed as persistently unconscious and the team has evidence of the patient's wish to stop nutrition and hydration (Maillet et al.). The healthcare professional must apply clinical judgment and skill in the assessment of each situation. This is especially critical when the discussion of therapy could lead to ANH (AAHPM, 2001).

Complementary Therapies in Palliative Care and Hospice

Use of complementary therapies may be beneficial in caring for patients at the end of life. Sensory therapies such as aromatherapy, reflexology, massage, Reiki, and acupuncture are options to consider. Other therapies such as homeopathy or the use of oral supplements such as vitamins, minerals, and herbs may be meaningful for some patients. Research should be performed to keep up with the current scientific knowledge base and to help patients make informed decisions. Two useful sources of information that include drug-medication interactions and side effects are the National Center for Complementary and Alternative Medicine (http://nccam.nih.gov) and the Complementary Medical Association (www.the-cma.org.uk).

Ethical Issues Related to End-of-Life Care

The patient's needs, wants, and desires must be the focus for ethical issues at the end of life. Constantly returning to the perspective of the patient and asking what is in the patient's best interest is the most reliable guide to good ethical deliberation (Maillet et al., 2002).

Decision-making issues surrounding the dying process are much easier when the decisions are made in advance. It is advantageous for the patient, family, and healthcare professionals to address wishes regarding hydration and artificial nutrition and for the patient to be informed and educated (Blacker, 2002). A registered dietitian should provide the patient with information on nutritional choices and consequences for the end-of-life stage and answer questions without any personal bias (Langdon, Hunt, Pope, & Hackes, 2002; Maillet et al., 2002).

Advance directives clearly outline a patient's wishes for health care should the patient be unable to communicate. Not all states regulate advance directives in the same manner (Hospice Net, 2004). Two different types of advance directives are a living will and medical power of attorney (POA). A living will allows the patient to decide and memorialize what types of medical treatment he or she desires at the end of life. A medical POA designates another person to make healthcare decisions on the patient's behalf if he or she is not able to make them (Hospice Net). In the absence of an advance directive, families often are left to argue over whether enteral or parenteral nutrition or hydration is appropriate without the benefit of the patient's input. By having an advance directive, this matter has been decided or the appropriate decision-making person has been named. It is paramount that education occurs for all family and staff who are involved in the patient's care so that they are aware of the requirements of the advance directive. Advance directives can differ by culture, and in some cultures, the patient may want the family to make all decisions. A patient should be asked if he or she wants to participate in decision making or if he or she would prefer that family members handle matters. Sometimes a patient may turn over the responsibility of decision making to the family and tell the team that he or she does not want to be informed of the decisions (Hospice Patients Alliance, 2004). Palliative care patients not in hospice should ask their medical care team for help in this area. Hospices have social workers available for help. For assistance in ethical deliberation, contact the American Society for Bioethics and Humanities (www.asbh.org).

Summary

When providing nutrition to patients undergoing palliative or hospice care, focus on individualized care, prevention, and the relief of suffering and distressing symptoms. The patient, early in the course of palliative care, should make nutrition decisions for end-of-life care. The dietitian should bring up the potential issues of hydration and enteral nutrition, as these issues need to be addressed regarding the patient's desires in advance of the need for the therapy. Hospice and palliative care consist of a team approach, and the viewpoints should be known and respected among disciplines. Early and frequent visits by the registered dietitian can be especially meaningful in the delivery of quality patient care. Nutrition-related issues must be addressed frequently. Ethics plays a critical role in caring for the patient who is at the end of life. Be aware of the importance of not imposing one's values onto the patient, instead being respectful at all times of the patient's wishes.

References

Abrahm, J. (2000). *A physician's guide to pain and symptom management in cancer patients.* Baltimore: The Johns Hopkins University Press.

American Academy of Hospice and Palliative Medicine. (2001, November). *Statement on the use of nutrition and hydration.* Retrieved January 23, 2004, from http://www.aahpm.org /positions/nutrition.html

American Heritage Dictionary of the English Language. (2000). *Palliative care.* Retrieved April 6, 2004, from http://www.bartleby.com/61/

American Institute for Cancer Research. (2003). *Nutrition of the cancer patient.* Retrieved March 28, 2004, from http://www.aicr.org/publications/brochures/online/ np.pdf

American Society for Parenteral and Enteral Nutrition. (2000). *What is PEN?* Retrieved March 14, 2004, from http://www.nutritioncare.org/pen/pen.html

Barber, M., & Rogers, B. (2002, August). *Advances in the management of tumor-induced weight loss.* Retrieved March 13, 2004, from http://www.medscape.com/viewpro-gram/2008

Blacker, S. (2002). Nutritional problems and the cancer patient: Psychosocial consid-erations. *Oncology Issues, 17*(2), 41–44.

Borum, M.L., Lynn, J., Zhong, Z., Roth, K., Connors, A.F., Jr., Desbiens, N.A., et al. (2000). The effect of nutritional supplementation on survival in seriously ill hospitalized adults: An evaluation of the SUPPORT data. Study to Understand Prognoses and Preferences for Outcomes and Risks of Treatments. *Journal of the American Geriatrics Society, 48*(Suppl. 5), S33–S38.

Bruera, E. (1997). ABC of palliative care: Anorexia, cachexia, and nutrition. *BMJ, 315,* 1219–1222.

Centers for Medicare and Medicaid Services. (2004). *Medicare Learning Network (Medlearn) hospice—educational resource web guide.* Retrieved July 8, 2004, from http://www.cms. hhs.gov/medlearn/refhospice.asp

Ersek, M. (2003). Artificial nutrition and hydration: Clinical issues. *Journal of Hospice and Palliative Nursing, 5*(4), 221–230.

Hill, T. (2004). *Managing symptoms and suffering at end of life.* California Coalition for Compassionate Care. Retrieved July 7, 2004, from http://www.finalchoices.calhealth. org

Hospice and Palliative Nurses Association. (2003). *Position statement on artificial nutrition and hydration in end-of-life care.* Retrieved March 27, 2004, from http://www.hpna. org/pdf/Artifical_Nutrition_and_Hydration_PDF.pdf

Hospice Net. (2004). *Advance directives.* Retrieved March 16, 2004, from http://www .hospicenet.org/html/directives.html

Hospice Patients Alliance. (2004). *Food, nutrition, artificial feeding methods, constipation and quality of life issues.* Retrieved February 8, 2004, from http://hospicepatients.org /hospic28.html

Langdon, D., Hunt, A., Pope, J., & Hackes, B. (2002). Nutrition support at the end of life: Opinions of Louisiana dietitians. *Journal of the American Dietetic Association, 102,* 837–840.

Maillet, J.O., Potter, R.L., & Heller, L. (2002). Ethical and legal issues in nutrition, hydration and feeding. *Journal of the American Dietetic Association, 102,* 716–726.

National Cancer Institute. (2005). *Nutrition in cancer care.* Retrieved February 2, 2005, from http://www.nci.nih.gov/cancertopics/pdq/supportivecare/nutrition/ patient

National Hospice and Palliative Care Organization. (2002). *Definition of hospice.* Retrieved July 7, 2004, from http://64.85.16.230/educate/content/elements/nhpcodefinition. html

National Institutes of Health. (1997, September). *Symptoms in terminal illness: A research workshop.* Retrieved March 15, 2004, from http://www.nih.gov/ninr/end-of-life. htm

Small, W., Carrara, R., Danford, L., Logemann, J., & Cella, D. (2002, March/April). *Quality of life and nutrition in the patient with cancer. Integrating nutrition into your cancer program.* Retrieved February 3, 2005, from http://www.accc-cancer.org/publications/Qualitylife.pdf

U.S. Department of Health and Human Services. (2003, July). *Medicare hospice benefits* [Publication No. CMS 02154]. Baltimore: Author.

Williams, C. (2004). *End of life care.* Retrieved July 7, 2004, from http://www.soros.org/initiatives/pdia/news/nursing

World Health Organization. (2003). *WHO definition of palliative care.* Retrieved April 2004, from http://www.who.int/cancer/palliative/definition

CHAPTER 20

Resources and References

Joyce G. Diacopoulos, RD, LDN, CNSD
Carolyn D. Nunnally, RN, MN

Evaluations of Internet Health Information

Nutrition information on cancer prevention, treatment, and survivorship abounds in the print media, Internet, and busy cancer center waiting rooms. The professional, whether a dietitian, nurse, or physician's assistant, is faced with numerous questions by other professionals and patients about nutritional concerns during cancer therapy as well as at the completion of therapy. The resources are overwhelming, and navigating through the most up-to-date, reliable, accurate information is time consuming when information is needed immediately.

The Internet is a vast source of information; it can be overwhelming to patients and professionals alike. The National Cancer Institute (www.cancer.gov) outlines 10 steps to evaluating medical resources on the Internet.

Who runs the Web site?	A reliable health-related Web site should make it easy to learn who is responsible for the site and the information presented.
Who pays for the site?	Funding for the site should be clearly stated. Sites/addresses ending in ".gov" denote a federal government–sponsored site. A drug company–sponsored Web site may have restrictions on content and how information is presented.
What is the purpose of the Web site?	Checking the "About this Site" link, which appears on many sites, will provide information about who runs and pays for the site, as well as the purpose of the site.

What is the source of the information?	Many health and medical Web sites post information collected from other Web sites or sources. The original source of the information should be clearly stated.
What is the basis of the information?	The site should identify who wrote the material, state the evidence the material is based on, and provide references for facts and figures. Opinions or advice should be set apart from information that is evidence-based.
How is the information selected?	Is there an editorial board? Are the qualifications of the reviewers of the material stated?
How current is the information?	It is important that medical information be reviewed and updated on a regular basis. The most recent update or review date should be clearly posted. Even if the information remains unchanged, the site should indicate that the material was reviewed recently and remains current.
How does the site choose to link to other sites?	Web sites usually have a policy about how they establish links to other sites. Some link to any site that asks or pays for a link; others only link to sites that have met certain criteria.
What information does the site collect about you and why?	Web sites routinely track the paths visitors take to their Web site. However, many ask you to subscribe or become a member sometimes for the purpose of collecting a user fee or selecting information for you that is relevant to your interests. In all cases, this will give the site personal information about you. The site requesting this information should tell you exactly what they will or will not do with this information. Be certain you read and understand any privacy policy. Do not sign up for anything you do not understand.
How does the site manage interactions with visitors?	There should always be a way for you to contact the site administrator with problems, feedback, or questions. If chat rooms or online discussion areas are part of the site, it should tell visitors what the terms of the service are. Are chat rooms moderated and, if so, by whom and why?

The following tips can aid in searching for nutrition-related information from the Internet.

1. Go to a Web site that is accredited and sponsored by a professional medical association. See Table 20-1 for information on selected Web sites that contain information on health and nutrition topics. Table 20-2 lists cancer- and nutrition-related publications.

2. Use a search engine. Different methods are used to compile lists of Web addresses, and by searching for the same terms on several different engines, you can get a broader picture of the topic you are investigating.

Table 20-1. Select Web Sites for Cancer and Nutrition Information

Resource	Web Address	General Information
ALCASE 800-298-2436	www.alcase.org	General information to patients and caregivers on all aspects of lung cancer. Education section provides nutrition information on symptom management of lung cancer and treatments.
American Botanical Council 512-926-4900	www.herbalgram.org	Information is provided on herbal medicine, Commission E monographs, and events.
American Brain Tumor Association 800-886-2282	www.abta.org	General information about brain tumors, treatment, clinical trials, and living with a brain tumor. Nutrition information is located under side effects and symptom management.
American Cancer Society 800-ACS-2345 (277-2345)	www.cancer.org	Site features information on specific cancers, treatments, symptom management guidelines, and nutritional impact of disease and/or treatment. A comprehensive, updated list of events and services is provided.
American Dietetic Association 800-877-1600	www.eatright.org	Official organization of food and nutrition professionals. General, current nutrition information is provided on a variety of topics.
American Institute for Cancer Research 800-843-8114 202-328-7744 (in Washington, DC)	www.AICR.org	Current information on nutrition, diet, and cancer with a focus on cancer prevention. Recipes and educational pamphlets are available as well as a free quarterly newsletter.

(Continued on next page)

Table 20-1. Select Web Sites for Cancer and Nutrition Information *(Continued)*

Resource	Web Address	General Information
American Society of Clinical Oncology 888-282-2552	www.ASCO.org	News and updates on cancer treatments and therapies, list of educational meetings, and clinical practice guidelines for physicians. Site includes links to People Living with Cancer Web site (www.plwc.org). Information on cancer, clinical trials, treatments, and symptom management, including nutrition.
American Society for Parenteral and Enteral Nutrition	www.nutritioncare.org	Site is geared toward practitioners in the field of nutritional support.
Cancer Care 800-813-HOPE (4673)	www.cancercare.org	Focus is assisting patients/ families in cancer diagnosis, treatments, and counseling. General and nutrition-related educational programs for professionals and patients via teleconferences and online. Section on symptom management includes nutritional issues.
Cancer Research and Prevention Foundation 800-227-2732	www.preventcancer.org	Promotes prevention and early detection of cancer through scientific research and education. Materials can be previewed online. Information is available in Spanish.
Cancer Nutrition Information Suzanne Dixon, MS, MPH, RD	www.cancernutritioninfo.com	Provides reviews of the latest cancer nutrition research for professionals and the public. A minimal fee is charged for the full site.
CancerSource 866-234-5025	www.cancersource.com	Up-to-date, complete, and current cancer information for consumers and professionals. Section on nutrition focuses on herbal products and complementary therapies.

(Continued on next page)

Table 20-1. Select Web Sites for Cancer and Nutrition Information
(Continued)

Resource	Web Address	General Information
Cancerfacts.com 877-422-3228	http://cancerfacts.com	Resource for patients with cancer, families, and healthcare professionals. Information regarding treatment decisions. Contains numerous links to other resources.
Candlelighters Childhood Cancer Foundation 800-366-CCCF	www.candlelighters.org	Site contains information on cancer and children, new therapies, survivorship, and support groups.
Center for Nutrition Policy and Promotion (Part of U.S. Department of Agriculture)	www.usda.gov/cnpp/contact. html	Focus is evaluation of scientific research linked to nutritional needs of the public.
Centers for Disease Control and Prevention 800-311-3435	www.cdc.gov/netinfo.htm	Site provides information on disease prevention, health promotion, and education. Section on health promotion includes an area on nutrition and cancer and stem cell transplantation.
Chemocare.com by Scott Hamilton	www.chemocare.com	Information on care during chemotherapy and beyond; includes section on eating well during and after chemotherapy.
Consumer Lab 201-261-5616	http://consumerlab.com	Information on nutritional products and purchasing, recalls, and warnings. Includes an encyclopedia of science-based health information and natural remedies; drug interactions. A fee is required for use of full site.
A Dietitian's Cancer Story Diana Dyer, MS, RD 734-946-9260	www.cancerrd.com	Provides information, recipes, and tips to cancer survivors regarding nutritional and lifestyle choices.

(Continued on next page)

Table 20-1. Select Web Sites for Cancer and Nutrition Information
(Continued)

Resource	Web Address	General Information
Food and Nutrition Information Center, Sponsored by the National Agricultural Library 301-504-5719	www.nal.usda.gov/fnic	Site provides credible and accurate nutrition resources for consumers and healthcare professionals.
Healthfinder	www.healthfinder.gov	Site provides information with links to other cancer and nutrition Web sites.
Hospice Education Institute/Hospicelink 800-331-1620 207-255-8800	www.hospiceworld.org	Books and pamphlets are available from the Hospice Education Institute on hospice-related subjects. Toll-free "Hospicelink" line provides callers with names and addresses of hospice and palliative care programs throughout the United States.
Institute of Medicine 202-334-2352	www.iom.edu/topics.asp	Information is provided on 17 topic areas, including food and nutrition, dietary references, intakes, and a guide for vitamin and mineral use.
International Myeloma Foundation 800-452-CURE	www.myeloma.org	Treatment and management of multiple myeloma. Provides information on family seminars and clinical conferences. Books and audio tapes are available for purchase. Available in several languages. Free newsletter.
Leukemia and Lymphoma Society 800-955-4572	www.leukemia-lymphoma. org/hm_lls	Nutrition for control of fatigue. Publications are free and available on the Web. Information is available in Spanish.

(Continued on next page)

Table 20-1. Select Web Sites for Cancer and Nutrition Information
(Continued)

Resource	Web Address	General Information
Living With It	www.livingwithit.org	Designed as a support program for women with breast cancer and provides education, diet, and exercise tips, personal stories, financial advice, and more.
Lung Cancer (A CancerCare Web site) 800-646-LUNG (5864)	www.lungcancer.org	Sections for patients, caregivers, and healthcare professionals. Very little nutrition information is provided. Contents are available in Spanish.
Multiple Myeloma Research Foundation 203-972-1250	www.multiplemyeloma.org	Information about multiple myeloma. Focus is on multiple myeloma research.
National Bone Marrow Transplant Link 800-LINK-BMT (546-5268)	www.nbmtlink.org	Publications are available on marrow and stem cell transplantation. Web site contains links to other sites.
National Brain Tumor Foundation 800-934-CURE (2873)	www.braintumor.org	General information about brain tumor treatment, support groups, and alternative therapies. Link to fact sheet that provides general nutrition tips for patients with brain tumors.
National Cancer Institute 800-4-CANCER	www.nci.nih.gov/cancerinfo/	Information on clinical trials, types of cancer, support, and coping. Provides nutritional support during cancer treatment as well as healthy eating for prevention of cancer.
National Center for Complementary and Alternative Medicine 888-644-6226	www.nccam.nih.gov	Authoritative information on complementary and alternative medicines and products.
National Childhood Cancer Foundation 800-458-6223 (U.S. and Canada)	www.nccf.org	Provides timely information on the search for cure in childhood cancers. Free newsletter.

(Continued on next page)

Table 20-1. Select Web Sites for Cancer and Nutrition Information *(Continued)*

Resource	Web Address	General Information
National Coalition for Cancer Survivorship 877-NCC-YES 877-662-7937	www.canceradvocacy.org	Cancer resources and treatments. Site has updates on new drugs and links to numerous nutrition Web sites and publications.
Nutrition Data Nutrition Facts Calorie Counter	www.nutritiondata.com	Provides nutrition facts, calorie counts, and nutrient data for foods and recipes.
Nutrition Navigator	http://navigator.tufts.edu	First online rating and review guide to nutrition Web sites. Site offers a variety of health topics, including cancer.
Office of Dietary Supplements (National Institutes of Health) 301-435-2920	http://dietary-supplements.info.nih.gov	Health information on all types of dietary supplements. Health information section lists extensive dietary supplement and vitamin and mineral fact sheets, which are specific to adequate dietary intakes.
Oley Foundation 800-766-OLEY	http://c4isr.com/oley/	Home parenteral and enteral nutrition. Site provides information, outreach, support, and activities for consumers, patients, caregivers, and professionals.
OncoLink Fax: 215-349-5445	www.oncolink.org	An educational site for consumers and healthcare professionals. Focus is on accurate cancer information—diagnosis, treatment, and research.
Oncology Nursing Society 866-257-4ONS (4667)	www.ons.org	Information for oncology nurses, healthcare providers, patients, and their families. Clinical practice section contains discussion of anorexia, evaluation of nutritional status, and an extensive reference list. Foreign languages available.

(Continued on next page)

Table 20-1. Select Web Sites for Cancer and Nutrition Information
(Continued)

Resource	Web Address	General Information
Oncology Nutrition Dietetic Practice Group, A dietetic practice group of the American Dietetic Association	www.oncologynutrition.org	Premier Web site provides information on oncology nutrition practices, research, prevention, treatment, recovery, and palliative care.
OvCa Ovarian Cancer Johns Hopkins University	http://ovariancancer.jhmi.edu/resources.cfm	General information is provided on resources, clinical trials, and nutrition tips for specific patients with ovarian cancer and survivors.
Pancreatic Cancer Action Network 877-272-6226	www.pancan.org	Provides information on nutritional issues related to pancreatic cancer risk and treatment. Link to diet and nutrition information for patients with pancreatic cancer. Services to patients, families, and healthcare professionals are provided at no cost.
Prostate Cancer Foundation 800-757-CURE	www.prostatecancerfoundation.org	Supports nutrition studies to explore new dietary and lifestyle strategies that impact the development and progression of prostate cancer. Publishes "Nutrition and Prostate Cancer," a monograph from the CaP CURE Nutrition Project.
Prosure® 800-986-8502	www.prosure.com	Specialized therapeutic nutritional supplement for people with cancer. Web site has links to research, recipes, and understanding weight loss and cancer.
Quackwatch Steven Barrett, MD 610-437-1795	www.quackwatch.org	Guide to health fraud, quackery, and unproven therapies. Available in several languages.

(Continued on next page)

Table 20-1. Select Web Sites for Cancer and Nutrition Information
(Continued)

Resource	Web Address	General Information
Support for People with Oral and Head and Neck Cancer 800-377-0928	www.spohnc.org	Product directory for nutritional supplements, xerostomia, and oral hygiene. Lists abstracts from the SPOHNC newsletter containing nutrition information for patients with oral and head and neck cancers.
Susan G. Komen Breast Cancer Foundation 800-I'M AWARE	www.komen.org	"Facts for Life" patient education sheet with tips for diet and nutrition during treatment. Enter "nutrition" in "site search" block to reach this information.
United Ostomy Association, Inc. 800-826-0826	www.uoa.org	Lists available brochures, books, and nutrition guides for patients with ostomies. Nominal fee for publications; members receive a discount.
U.S. Food and Drug Administration 888-463-6332	www.cfsan.fda.gov/~dms/supplmnt.html	Links to dietary supplements and adverse event reporting. Provides warnings and safety information.
US TOO—Prostate Education and Support 800-80-US-TOO 800-808-7866	www.ustoo.com	Nonprofit organization for men with prostate cancer and their families. Site contains education, support, and monthly "Hot Sheet" newsletter, which may contain nutrition topics.
Web Whispers	www.webwhispers.org	Dedicated to patients and survivors diagnosed with laryngeal cancer. Includes nutrition tips and recipes.
The Wellness Community	www.wellness-community.org	Free emotional support, education, and hope for people with cancer and their caregivers. Site has a section on maximizing nutrition and managing nutritional symptoms.

Table 20-2. Nutrition and Cancer Publications for Patients With Cancer, Survivors, Caregivers, and Healthcare Professionals

Resource	Web Address	General Information
AICR American Institute for Cancer Research newsletter 202-328-7744 800-843-8114	www.aicr.org	Free quarterly newsletter. Focus is on nutrition and cancer prevention. Seasonal recipes and nutrition-related issues in cancer
"Diet and Nutrition Nutritional Concerns With Pancreatic Cancer" Pancreatic Cancer Action Network, Inc. 877-272-6226	www.pancan.org	Specific to patients with pancreatic cancer and their nutritional issues
"Eating Hints for Patients With Cancer Before, During, and After Treatment" NIH/National Cancer Institute 800-4-CANCER	www.cancer.gov	Free nutrition information on eating problems during and after treatment. Specific recommendations for special issues: fatigue, depression, and neutropenia. Recipes and snack ideas are included. English and Spanish editions are available.
Food and Fitness Advisor by Weill Medical College of Cornell University 800-829-2505	www.foodandfitnessadvisor .com	By subscription/monthly. Accurate, timely medical news and information, including topics such as cancer
"Living Smart, The American Cancer Society's Guide to Eating Healthy and Being Active" 800-ACS-2345	www.cancer.org	Guidelines for nutrition and physical fitness for patients and survivors. Free
Nutrition Action Health Letter from Center for Science in the Public Interest 202-332-9110	www.cspinet.org	By subscription/monthly. Nutrition information on a variety of topics, including cancer

(Continued on next page)

Table 20-2. Nutrition and Cancer Publications for Patients With Cancer, Survivors, Caregivers, and Healthcare Professionals *(Continued)*

Resource	Web Address	General Information
"Nutrition Intervention for Adults with Cancer" Novartis Medical Nutrition 800-333-3785	www.novartisnutrition. com	Nutrition-related issues with management suggestions. Table with nutritional risk considerations. The current role of nutrition in patients with cancer by Novartis Medical Nutrition. Free 46-page monograph written for the healthcare professional involved in the treatment of cancer.
"Nutrition for the Person With Cancer" 800-ACS-2345	www.cancer.org	Free booklet with tips for nutrition symptom management during and after treatment. Contains recipes and cancer-related resources. English and Spanish editions are available.
"Time to Take Five: Eat Five Fruits and Vegetables a Day" National Cancer Institute 800-4-CANCER	www.cancer.gov	Provides tips on how to obtain five servings of fruits and vegetables. Includes recipes. Free
Tufts University Health & Nutrition Letter 800-274-7581	www.healthletter.tufts. edu	By subscription/monthly. Medical news, hot nutrition topics, drugs, and therapies

Appendices

Appendix A. Scored Patient-Generated Subjective Global Assessment (PG-SGA)

Scored Patient-Generated Subjective Global Assessment (PG-SGA)

Patient ID Information

History (Boxes 1-4 are designed to be completed by the patient.)

1. Weight (*See Worksheet 1*)

In summary of my current and recent weight:

I currently weigh about _____ pounds
I am about _____ feet _____ tall

One month ago I weighed about _____ pounds
Six months ago I weighed about _____ pounds

During the past two weeks my weight has:
□ decreased (1) □ not changed (0) □ increased (0)

Box 1 □

2. Food Intake: As compared to my normal intake, I would rate my food intake during the past month as:

□ unchanged (0)
□ more than usual (0)
□ less than usual (1)

I am now taking:
□ *normal food* but less than normal amount (1)
□ little solid food (2)
□ only liquids (3)
□ only nutritional supplements (3)
□ very little of anything (4)
□ only tube feedings or only nutrition by vein (0)

Box 2 □

3. Symptoms: I have had the following problems that have kept me from eating enough during the past two weeks (check all that apply):

□ no problems eating (0)
□ no appetite, just did not feel like eating (3)
□ nausea (1)   □ vomiting (3)
□ constipation (1)   □ diarrhea (3)
□ mouth sores (2)   □ dry mouth (1)
□ things taste funny or have no taste (1)   □ smells bother me (1)
□ problems swallowing (2)   □ feel full quickly (1)
□ pain; where? _____ (3)   □ fatigue (1)
□ other** _____ (1)
** Examples: depression, money, or dental problems

Box 3 □

4. Activities and Function: Over the past month, I would generally rate my activity as:

□ normal with no limitations (0)
□ not my normal self, but able to be up and about with fairly normal activities (1)
□ not feeling up to most things, but in bed or chair less than half the day (2)
□ able to do little activity and spend most of the day in bed or chair (3)
□ pretty much bedridden, rarely out of bed (3)

Box 4 □

Additive Score of the Boxes 1-4 □ A

(Continued on next page)

Appendix A. Scored Patient-Generated Subjective Global Assessment (PG-SGA) *(Continued)*

Scored Patient-Generated Subjective Global Assessment (PG-SGA)

The remainder of this form will be completed by your doctor, nurse, or therapist. Thank you.

5. Disease and its relation to nutritional requirements *(See Worksheet 2)*

Additive Score of the Boxes 1-4 ☐ **A**
(See Side 1)

All relevant diagnoses (specify) _____

One point each : ☐ Cancer ☐ AIDS ☐ Pulmonary or cardiac cachexia ☐ Presence of decubitus, open wound, or fistula
☐ Presence of trauma ☐ Age greater than 65 years ☐ Chronic renal insufficiency

Primary disease stage (circle if known or appropriate) I II III IV Other _____

Age _____ Numerical score from Worksheet 2 ☐ **B**

6. Metabolic Demand *(See Worksheet 3)*

Score for metabolic stress is determined by a number of variables known to increase protein & calorie needs. The score is additive so that a patient who has a fever of > 102 degrees (3 points) and is on 10 mg of prednisone chronically (2 points) would have an additive score for this section of 5 points.

Stress	none (0)	low (1)	moderate (2)	high (3)
Fever	no fever	>99 and <101	≥101 and <102	≥102
Fever duration	no fever	<72 hrs	72 hrs	> 72 hrs
Corticosteroids	no corticosteroids	low dose (<10mg prednisone equivalents/day)	moderate dose (≥10 and <30mg prednisone equivalents/day)	high dose steroids (≥30mg prednisone equivalents/day)

Numerical score from Worksheet 3 ☐ **C**

7. Physical *(See Worksheet 4)*

Physical exam includes a subjective evaluation of 3 aspects of body composition: fat, muscle, & fluid status. Since this is subjective, each aspect of the exam is rated for degree of deficit. Muscle deficit impacts point score more than fat deficit. Definition of categories: 0 = no deficit, 1+ = mild deficit, 2+ = moderate deficit, 3+ = severe deficit.

Muscle Status:					Fat Stores:				
temples (temporalis muscle)	0	1+	2+	3+	orbital fat pads	0	1+	2+	3+
clavicles (pectoralis & deltoids)	0	1+	2+	3+	triceps skin fold	0	1+	2+	3+
shoulders (deltoids)	0	1+	2+	3+	fat overlying lower ribs	0	1+	2+	3+
interosseous muscles	0	1+	2+	3+	**Global fat deficit rating**	**0**	**1+**	**2+**	**3+**
Scapula (latissimus dorsi, trapezius, deltoids)	0	1+	2+	3+					
thigh (quadriceps)	0	1+	2+	3+					
calf (gastrocnemius)	0	1+	2+	3+					
Global muscle status rating	**0**	**1+**	**2+**	**3+**					

Fluid Status:				
ankle edema	0	1+	2+	3+
sacral edema	0	1+	2+	3+
ascites	0	1+	2+	3+
Global fluid status rating	**0**	**1+**	**2+**	**3+**

Numerical score from Worksheet 4 ☐ **D**

Total PG-SGA score ☐
(Total numerical score of A+B+C+D above)
(See triage recommendations below)

Clinician Signature _____ RD RN PA MD DO Other _____ Date _____

Nutritional Triage Recommendations: Additive score is used to define specific nutritional interventions including patient & family education, symptom management including pharmacologic intervention, and appropriate nutrient intervention (food, nutritional supplements, enteral, or parenteral triage). First line nutrition intervention includes optimal symptom management.

0-1   No intervention required at this time. Re-assessment on routine and regular basis during treatment.
2-3   Patient & family education by dietitian, nurse, or other clinician with pharmacologic intervention as indicated by symptom survey (Box 3) and lab values as appropriate.
4-8   Requires intervention by dietitian, in conjunction with nurse or physician as indicated by symptoms survey (Box 3).
≥9   Indicates a critical need for improved symptom management and/or nutrient intervention options.

©FD Ottery, 2005 email: fdottery@savientpharma.com or noatpres1@aol.com

Appendix A. Scored Patient-Generated Subjective Global Assessment (PG-SGA) *(Continued)*

Worksheets for PG-SGA Scoring

© FD Ottery, 2001

Boxes 1-4 of the PG-SGA are designed to be completed by the patient. The PG-SGA numerical score is determined using 1) the parenthetical points noted in boxes 1-4 and 2) the worksheets below for items not marked with parenthetical points. Scores for boxes 1 and 3 are additive within each box and scores for boxes 2 and 4 are based on the highest scored item checked off by the patient.

Worksheet 1 - Scoring Weight (Wt) Loss

To determine score, use 1 month weight data if available. Use 6 month data only if there is no 1 month weight data. Use points below to score weight change and add one extra point if patient has lost weight during the past 2 weeks. Enter total point score in Box 1 of the PG-SGA.

Wt loss in 1 month	Points	Wt loss in 6 months
10% or greater	4	20% or greater
5-9.9%	3	10 -19.9%
3-4.9%	2	6 - 9.9%
2-2.9%	1	2 - 5.9%
0-1.9%	0	0 - 1.9%

Score for Worksheet 1 [ ]
Record in Box 1

Worksheet 2 - Scoring Criteria for Condition

Score is derived by adding 1 point for each of the conditions listed below that pertain to the patient.

Category	Points
Cancer	1
AIDS	1
Pulmonary or cardiac cachexia	1
Presence of decubitus, open wound, or fistula	1
Presence of trauma	1
Age greater than 65 years	1

Score for Worksheet 2 = [ ]
Record in Box B

Worksheet 3 - Scoring Metabolic Stress

Score for metabolic stress is determined by a number of variables known to increase protein & caloric needs. The score is additive so that a patient who has a fever of > 102 degrees (3 points) and is on 10 mg of prednisone chronically (2 points) would have an additive score for this section of 5 points.

Stress	none (0)	low (1)	moderate (2)	high (3)
Fever	no fever	>99 and <101	≥101 and <102	≥102
Fever duration	no fever	<72 hrs	72 hrs	> 72 hrs
Corticosteroids	no corticosteroids	low dose (<10mg prednisone equivalents/day)	moderate dose (≥10 and <30mg prednisone equivalents/day)	high dose steroids (≥30mg prednisone equivalents/day)

Score for Worksheet 3 = [ ]
Record in Box C

Worksheet 4 - Physical Examination

Physical exam includes a subjective evaluation of 3 aspects of body composition: fat, muscle, & fluid status. Since this is subjective, each aspect of the exam is rated for degree of deficit. Muscle deficit impacts point score more than fat deficit. Definition of categories: 0 = no deficit, 1+ = mild deficit, 2+ = moderate deficit, 3+ = severe deficit. Rating of deficit in these categories are *not* additive but are used to clinically assess the degree of deficit (or presence of excess fluid).

Fat Stores:

orbital fat pads	0	1+	2+	3+
triceps skin fold	0	1+	2+	3+
fat overlying lower ribs	0	1+	2+	3+
Global fat deficit rating	**0**	**1+**	**2+**	**3+**

Muscle Status:

temples (temporalis muscle)	0	1+	2+	3+
clavicles (pectoralis & deltoids)	0	1+	2+	3+
shoulders (deltoids)	0	1+	2+	3+
interosseous muscles	0	1+	2+	3+
scapula (latissimus dorsi, trapezius, deltoids)	0	1+	2+	3+
thigh (quadriceps)	0	1+	2+	3+
calf (gastrocnemius)	0	1+	2+	3+
Global muscle status rating	**0**	**1+**	**2+**	**3+**

Fluid Status:

ankle edema	0	1+	2+	3+
sacral edema	0	1+	2+	3+
ascites	0	1+	2+	3+
Global fluid status rating	**0**	**1+**	**2+**	**3+**

Point score for the physical exam is determined by the overall subjective rating of total body deficit.

No deficit	score = 0 points
Mild deficit	score = 1 point
Moderate deficit	score = 2 points
Severe deficit	score = 3 points

Score for Worksheet 4 = [ ]
Record in Box D

Worksheet 5 - PG-SGA Global Assessment Categories

Category	Stage A Well-nourished	Stage B Moderately malnourished or suspected malnutrition	Stage C Severely malnourished
Weight	No wt loss **OR** Recent non-fluid wt gain	~5% wt loss within 1 month (or 10% in 6 months) **OR** No wt stabilization or wt gain (i.e., continued wt loss)	> 5% wt loss in 1 month (or >10% in 6 months) **OR** No wt stabilization or wt gain (i.e., continued wt loss)
Nutrient Intake	No deficit **OR** Significant recent improvement	Definite decrease in intake	Severe deficit in intake
Nutrition Impact Symptoms	None **OR** Significant recent improvement allowing adequate intake	Presence of nutrition impact symptoms (Box 3 of PG-SGA)	Presence of nutrition impact symptoms (Box 3 of PG-SGA)
Functioning	No deficit **OR** Significant recent improvement	Moderate functional deficit **OR** Recent deterioration	Severe functional deficit **OR** recent significant deterioration
Physical Exam	No deficit **OR** Chronic deficit but with recent clinical improvement	Evidence of mild to moderate loss of SQ fat &/or muscle mass &/or muscle tone on palpation	Obvious signs of malnutrition (e.g., severe loss of SQ tissues, possible edema)

Global PG-SGA rating (A, B, or C) = [ ]

Appendix B. Body Mass Index (also known as Quetelet's Index)

Weight (kg)

Body mass index = Height (m²)

Body Mass Index	Classification
≥ 40	Obesity grade III
35–39.9	Obesity grade II
30–34.9	Obesity grade I
25–29.9	Overweight
18.5–25	Normal
17–18.4	Protein-energy malnutrition grade I
16–16.9	Protein-energy malnutrition grade II
< 16.0	Protein-energy malnutrition grade III

Note. Based on information from Charney & Malone, 2004.

Appendix C. Nutrition Impact Symptoms and Interventions

Anorexia
- Determine specific factors contributing to symptom, such as pain, constipation, and gastrointestinal symptoms, and treat appropriately.
- Encourage small, frequent feedings.
- Encourage nutrient-dense foods, and add protein and calories to favorite foods by using extra butter, margarine, cheese, and non-fat dry milk powder.
- Evaluate anorexic effects of other medications.
- Drink nutrient-dense beverages between meals to avoid feeling too full with meals.
- Consider pharmacologic therapy with appetite-enhancing medications.

Taste alterations
- Identify specific taste sensations altered, and correlate findings with specific selections, such as adding seasonings/flavorings or substituting specific food group with items of comparable nutrient content (e.g., fish, poultry, legumes in place of meats) and avoid offending foods.
- Clear palate prior to meals by brushing teeth, gums, and oral cavity and rinsing with baking soda and salt water.
- Use plastic utensils to decrease metallic taste.
- Include foods that have a pleasing taste.
- Avoid cigarette smoking.
- Suck on fruit-flavored candies, or chew gum between meals.
- Eat tart foods such as sherbet, Italian ices, and sorbet, as they may be better tolerated than sweet foods.

(Continued on next page)

Appendix C. Nutrition Impact Symptoms and Interventions *(Continued)*

Taste alterations *(cont.)*	• Add lemon, lime, vinegar, or salt to foods that are too sweet. • Try marinades and spices to mask strange tastes. • Avoid canned food products if metallic taste is problematic. • Eat foods that do not need to be heated up, as they are better tolerated than cooked foods with more prominent odors and flavors. Try eating cold foods such as sandwiches, cottage cheese, and yogurt.
Mucositis	• Prevention is key—good oral hygiene with frequent mouth rinses is important (avoid alcohol-based products). • Treat oral lesions pharmacologically as appropriate (antifungal meds if needed). • Consider using oral topical agents and anesthetics, such as viscous lidocaine and institution-specific mouth rinses, that are combinations of nystatin, Maalox® (Novartis, Parsippany, NJ), diphenhydramine, hydrocortisone, and viscous lidocaine. • Adjust texture and temperature as tolerated. • Avoid carbonated beverages. • Avoid caffeine, alcohol, and tobacco products. • Avoid other irritants (e.g., acidic, spicy foods). • Try ice chips prior to and during bolus infusion of 5-FU, as this causes vasoconstriction in oral mucosa and may minimize mucosal damage. • Try oral glutamine supplementation—optimal dose is 10 g tid. • Consider feeding tube if unable to obtain adequate nourishment orally.
Nausea/vomiting	• Provide optimal antiemetic medication for planned therapy. • Use relaxation techniques for anticipatory vomiting. • Evaluate other factors possibly contributing to vomiting, such as constipation, brain metastasis, and other medications. • Eat small, frequent, low-fat meals with minimal odors. • Try dry, starchy, and/or salty foods, such as pretzels, saltines, potatoes, noodles, and cereals. • Try foods at cold or room temperature. • Sip on ginger ale, tea, or candied dried ginger. • Avoid favorite foods until symptoms resolve. • Consume clear liquids such as broth, gelatin, or juice drinks on chemotherapy days, as these may be better tolerated than solid food.
Diarrhea	• Assess severity, including hydration status and associated symptoms. • Consider diagnostic evaluation, including stool analysis if diarrhea is not treatment-related to ensure appropriate management. • Verify that diarrhea is not related to impaction, especially in patients on narcotic medications. • Try prophylactic glutamine supplementation—optimal dose 10 g tid. • Drink adequate fluid intake—at least one cup of fluid for each loose bowel movement added to usual intake.

(Continued on next page)

Appendix C. Nutrition Impact Symptoms and Interventions *(Continued)*

Diarrhea *(cont.)*	• Replace fluid with sodium- and potassium-containing fluids, such as broth and sports drinks with less than 15 g of carbohydrate per serving. • Drink clear liquids or follow BRAT (bananas, rice, applesauce, toast) diet for 24–48 hours until symptoms improve. • Practice minimum- to low-residue diet for maintenance to control frequency, with increased intake of foods high in soluble fiber (bananas, oatmeal, white rice, applesauce, and noodles). • Restrict lactose if enteritis or small bowel is in radiation therapy field. • Ensure that adequate pharmacologic treatment is being used.
Fatigue	• Recognize that the person experiencing fatigue defines it. • Assess for treatable causes of fatigue such as anemia, infection, pain, neutropenia, depression, and medication side effects, and manage appropriately. • Educate patient as to potential side effects of treatment and how to manage them appropriately. • Maintain optimal nutritional status. • Encourage light exercise unless contraindicated by medical condition. • Encourage assistance with housework and meal preparation.
Xerostomia	• Try tart foods to stimulate saliva. • Sip on liquids or suck on ice chips throughout the day. • Avoid caffeine, alcohol, and tobacco products. • Try using a cool mist humidifier at bedtime. • Try drinking through a straw. • Rinse mouth frequently with mild saline solution. • Add extra sauces and gravies to foods.
Lactose intolerance	• Use a lactase enzyme supplement to help to digest dairy products or use dairy products already treated with lactase enzyme. • Substitute milk with nondairy beverage, soy, or rice milk.
Early satiety	• Eat small, frequent, nutrient-dense meals and snacks. • Add protein and calories to favorite foods using extra butter, margarine, cheese, and nonfat dry milk powder. • Try high-calorie/high-protein liquid drinks, which may be better tolerated than solid foods. • Keep nutrient-dense snacks available, and snack frequently. • Capitalize on the times when feeling the best. • Try pharmacologic treatment with medications that increase digestive motility.
Constipation	• Eat at regular intervals throughout the day. • Increase fluid intake. • Increase dietary fiber. • Try hot beverages as a bowel stimulant. • Increase physical activity as tolerated. • Establish an appropriate bowel program, including the regular use of pharmacologic agents.

(Continued on next page)

Appendix C. Nutrition Impact Symptoms and Interventions *(Continued)*

Dysphagia	• Modify diet consistency and follow swallowing techniques provided by the speech pathologist. • Eat softer, moist, or pureed foods. • Use commercially available food thickeners, tapioca, instant mashed potatoes, or infant rice cereal to thicken liquids. • Avoid breads, cakes, dry cookies, and crackers unless taken with plenty of liquids. • Consider feeding tube if unable to obtain adequate nourishment orally.
Esophagitis	• Eat soft, moist foods with extra sauce, dressings, and gravies. • Avoid acidic foods such as tomatoes, citrus foods, carbonated beverages, and alcohol. • Avoid spicy foods. • Avoid dry, coarse, or rough foods. • Rinse mouth and gargle frequently with mild saline solution. • Avoid alcohol-based mouthwashes. • Try pharmacologic treatment to coat or numb esophagus prior to eating. • Consider feeding tube if unable to obtain adequate nourishment orally.

Note. Based on information from American Cancer Society, 2002; Eldridge & Hamilton, 2004; National Cancer Institute, 2003, 2004.

Appendix D. Nutrition Sequelae of Radiation Therapy and Suggested Nutritional Interventions

Site of Radiation	Acute Side Effects	Chronic Side Effects	Intervention
Tongue, soft and hard palate, tonsils, pharynx, nasopharynx, mandible	Mucositis	Oropharyngeal ulcers	Oral anesthetics, good oral care, avoid temperature extremes and irritants
	Xerostomia	Xerostomia	Moist foods, artificial saliva, extra fluids with meals
	Dysgeusia	Dysgeusia	Determine specific aberrations and use of acceptable seasonings and flavors.
	Dental caries	Dental caries	Good oral care, topical fluoride, avoid sticky, sugary foods

(Continued on next page)

Appendix D. Nutrition Sequelae of Radiation Therapy and Suggested Nutritional Interventions *(Continued)*

Site of Radiation	Acute Side Effects	Chronic Side Effects	Intervention
	Viscous saliva		Pureed or liquid diet, limit milk products, avoid oily, greasy, and dry foods
		Osteoradi-onecrosis	Pureed/liquid diet if able to tolerate; total parenteral nutrition (TPN) or tube feedings
		Fistula	Depending on location, may need tube feeding until healed or surgery
		Trismus	Depends on severity—liquids or tube feeding
Esophagus, thorax, thyroid, thoracic and cervical spine	Esophagitis, dysphagia	Esophagitis, esophageal stricture, fibrosis	Adjust texture, avoid irritants; adjust liquids as needed for dysphagia; dilatation for stricture, tube feeding for dysphagia
Bladder, prostate, colon, rectum, male and female sexual organs	Colitis, cystitis, diarrhea	Chronic colitis, proctitis	Low-residue, low-lactose diet and avoid irritants, if small bowel is in field
		Radiation enteritis	Low-residue, lactose-reduced, low-fat diet; may need bowel rest with elemental formula or TPN
Stomach, liver, pancreas, bile duct, small intestine	Nausea, vomiting	Gastrointestinal ulceration, perforation	Antiemetic medications prior to meals, small feedings, avoid foods with strong odor, use liquids between meals; try low-fat diet
	Enteritis, malabsorption	Intestinal fistula, fibrosis, necrosis, obstruction	Pancreatic enzymes, low-fat, low-residue, low-lactose diet may be needed; tube feeding with elemental formula or TPN if high output from fistula

Note. Based on information from Eldridge & Hamilton, 2004; National Cancer Institute, 2004.

Appendix E. Components of a Comprehensive Nutrition Assessment

Diet history
- Food intolerances/preferences
- Food allergies
- Appetite changes
- Alcohol intake

Demographic data

Medical history
- Tumor burden
- Comorbid conditions
- Cancer treatment plan

Weight history
- Pre-illness weight
- Weight changes
- Percent weight change over time

Medications
- Narcotic medications
- Medications with potential to impact nutritional status

Bowel pattern

Vitamin/herb/nutritional supplement intake

Presence of nutrition impact symptoms
- Nausea/vomiting
- Constipation/diarrhea
- Xerostomia
- Dysgeusia
- Dysosmia
- Early satiety
- Dysphagia
- Mucositis
- Pain

Social data
- Caregiver support
- Ability to shop and prepare meals
- Financial concerns
- Religious, cultural, and lifestyle factors influencing intake
- Literacy level

Performance status

Biochemistries
- Serum albumin and prealbumin
- Liver function studies
- Serum sodium, potassium, and phosphorus
- Glucose
- BUN and creatinine
- Calcium
- Hematologic parameters—absolute neutrophil count, white blood cell count, red blood cell count

Pertinent physical findings
- Presence of ascites
- Edema
- Condition of oral cavity
- Dentition
- Wounds
- Wasting
- Cachexia
- Skin turgor

Assessment of nutritional needs

Assessment of appropriate medical nutrition therapy, including route of nutritional support

Appendix F. Harris-Benedict Equation Used for Estimating Energy Expenditure

BEE (men) = 66.47 + 13.75 (wt in kg) + 5 (ht in cm) − 6.76 (age in years)

BEE (women) = 655.1 + 9.56 (wt in kg) + 1.85 (ht in cm) − 4.68 (age in years)

EEE = BEE x activity factor x stress factor
Activity factors: 1.2 = bed or 1.3 = ambulatory

Stress factors: 1.2–1.3 = minor surgery and/or cancer treatment, or 1.4 = major surgery or hypermetabolic

BEE—basal energy expenditure; EEE—estimated energy expenditure

Note. Based on information from Dempsey & Mullen, 1985; Merrick et al., 1998.

Appendix G. Protein Requirements for Adults

Condition Description	Protein Requirement
Dietary reference intake	0.8 grams/kilogram
Adult maintenance	0.8–1.9 g/kg
Cancer	1.0–1.2 g/kg
Cancer cachexia	1.2–1.5 g/kg
Obesity, stressed	1.5–2.0 g/kg
Critical illness	1.5–2.0 g/kg

Note. Based on information from Charney & Malone, 2004.

Appendix H. Hamwi Method for Determining Desirable Body Weight in Adults

Women = 100 pounds for the first 5 feet; 5 pounds for every inch thereafter

Men = 106 pounds for the first 5 feet; 6 pounds for every inch thereafter

For both calculations, in pounds or kilograms, 10% is added or subtracted to the final value for variations in body frame size.

Note. Based on information from Charney & Malone, 2004.

Appendix I. Guidelines for Assessing Calorie, Protein, and Fluid Needs for the Adult Patient With Cancer

Calorie Needs Estimation	Clinical Situation
25–30 kcal/kg	Maintenance
30–35 kcal/kg	Malnourished and/or high-stress treatment such as bone marrow transplant
35–45 kcal/kg	Severely depleted or hypermetabolic
Protein Needs	
0.8–1.0 g/kg	Recommended Dietary Allowance (RDA) for adults
1.0–1.5 g/kg	Most patients with cancer (adjust for visceral protein status, albumin levels)
1.5 g/kg	Bone marrow transplant recipients
1.5–2.0 g/kg	Severely depleted patient with cancer
Fluid Needs (choose one of two methods)	
A. RDA/calorie based	1 ml/kcal
B. Age-based • < 55 yrs of age • 55–65 yrs of age • > 65 yrs of age	• 30–40 ml/kg • 30 ml/kg • 25 ml/kg

Note. Based on information from Dempsey & Mullen, 1985; Merrick et al., 1998.

Appendix J. Nutritional Risk Index

Risk = 1.59 x serum albumin (g/l) + 0.417 x (current weight/usual weight) x 100

Borderline malnutrition: 97.5–99
Mild malnutrition: 83.5–97.4
Severe malnutrition: < 83.5

Note. Based on information from Yeatman, 2000.

Appendix K. Food Safety Guidelines for Patients With Low Immune Function or Who Are Neutropenic

Safe food handling can help to decrease a person's risk of food-borne illness. People with weakened immune systems must take extra caution to avoid putting themselves at risk to become infected by a food-borne pathogen. It is important to handle food safely, starting with the buying process, through to eating, and on to storing leftovers.

Shopping
- Shop for groceries when you can take food home right away; do not leave food sitting in the car.
- Avoid cans of food that are dented, leaking, or bulging.
- Do not purchase food in cracked glass jars.
- Ensure that safety buttons on metal lids are down and do not make a clicking noise when pushed. Make sure that tamper-resistant safety seals are intact.
- Avoid food in torn or punctured packaging.
- Pick up perishable foods (e.g., meat, eggs, milk) last.
- Place packaged meat, poultry, or fish in separate plastic bags to prevent meat juices from dripping onto other groceries or other meats.
- Make sure the "sell by" or "use by" date has not passed.
- Do not buy any food that has been displayed in any unclean or unsafe manner (e.g., meat allowed to sit outside of refrigeration, cooked shrimp displayed next to raw shrimp).
- When ordering in the deli department, make sure the clerk washes his or her hands between handling raw food and cooked food.

Storage
- Keep your refrigerator and freezer clean.
- Use a refrigerator thermometer to make sure the temperature inside is 40°F or below.
- Make sure the temperature inside the freezer is 0°F.
- Upon arriving home from the store, immediately refrigerate and freeze appropriate foods.
- Leave eggs in their carton; do not place in refrigerator door.
- Store raw meat, poultry, and fish on the bottom shelf of the refrigerator to avoid their juices dripping onto other foods. Raw ground meat, poultry, and fish may be stored for one to two days; other red meat may be stored for three to five days.
- Store canned foods and other shelf-stable products in a cool, dry place. Avoid hot garages and damp basements.

Preparation
- Wash hands before, during, and after food preparation and service.
- Use plastic or glass surfaces for cutting raw meat and poultry. Use a separate cutting board for preparing other foods, such as fruits, vegetables, and bread.
- Wash cutting boards with hot, soapy water after each use. Cutting boards (except those that are made with laminated wood) can all be washed in the dishwasher.
- After handling raw meat, poultry, and fish, wash hands, work surfaces, and utensils with hot soapy water.
- Wash all fruits and vegetables before cutting, cooking, or eating them raw.
- Defrost frozen food on a plate in the refrigerator or in the microwave. Cook food immediately after thawing.
- Use different utensils and dishes for cooked foods than you used for raw foods.
- Wash kitchen towels and clothes often in hot water in a washing machine.

(Continued on next page)

Appendix K. Food Safety Guidelines for Patients With Low Immune Function or Who Are Neutropenic *(Continued)*

- A sanitizing solution can be made with one teaspoon of liquid chlorine bleach mixed with one quart of water. Use solution on countertops and other work surfaces. Do not rinse. Allow surfaces to air dry.

Cooking
- Keep hot foods hot at 140°F or higher and cold foods cold at 40°F or lower.
- Do not leave perishable foods out for more than two hours.
- Promptly refrigerate or freeze leftovers in shallow containers or wrapped tightly in bags.
- Use leftovers within three to four days.
- When reheating foods in the microwave, cover and rotate or stir foods once or twice during cooking. The food should be steaming hot.
- Do not eat foods past their expiration date.
- Follow the handling and preparation instructions on product labels to ensure top quality and safety.

Meat, Poultry, and Fish
- Do not eat raw or undercooked meat.
- Cook all meat and poultry until it is no longer pink in the middle.
- Fish should be cooked until it is flakey, not rubbery.
- The temperature inside the meat should be more than 165°F.
- Cook poultry to an internal temperature of 180°–185°F.
- Cook fish to 160°F.
- Do not eat stuffing cooked inside poultry. Instead, cook separately to 165°F.
- Cook only shellfish that are closed. Discard any shellfish that do not open during cooking.

Dairy
- Eat or drink only pasteurized milk or dairy products.

Eggs
- Cook eggs until the yolk and white are solid, not runny.
- Do not eat foods that may contain raw eggs, such as Caesar salad dressing or cookie dough.
- If eating fried eggs, be sure eggs are fried on both sides.

Fruits and Vegetables
- Raw fruits and vegetables are safe to eat if washed carefully first.
- Discard any fruits or vegetables with mold.
- Wash fruits and vegetables well under cool running water.
- Do not let cut fruits or vegetables sit unrefrigerated.
- Discard the outermost leaves of a head of lettuce or cabbage.

Water
- Do not drink water straight from lakes, rivers, streams, or springs.
- Always check with your local health department and water company to learn if they have issued any special notices for people with weakened immune systems.
- Water bottles and ice trays should be cleaned with soap and water before use.

(Continued on next page)

Appendix K. Food Safety Guidelines for Patients With Low Immune Function or Who Are Neutropenic *(Continued)*

Other
- Home canned foods: Use within one year of canning. Cook food for 10 minutes before eating.
- Commercially canned foods: Safe to eat without any further cooking.
- Condiments: Use a clean utensil when dipping into jars. Keep jars refrigerated. Do not use homemade mayonnaise.
- Baby food: Use a clean utensil to remove amount needed from jar. Store open jars in the refrigerator.

Eating Out
- Avoid the same foods when eating out as you would at home (e.g., raw meats, undercooked eggs).
- If the food arrives undercooked, send it back.
- Avoid foods that may contain raw eggs, such as Caesar salad dressing or hollandaise sauce.
- If you are not sure about the ingredients in a dish, ask your waiter before you order.
- Do not order any raw or lightly steamed fish or shellfish, such as oysters, clams, mussels, sushi, or sashimi.

Traveling
- Do not eat uncooked fruits and vegetables unless you can peel them.
- Avoid salads.
- Eat cooked foods while they are still hot.
- Boil all water before drinking it.
- Use only ice made from boiled water.
- Drink only canned or bottled drinks or beverages made with boiled water.
- Steaming hot foods, fruits you peel yourself, bottled and canned processed drinks, and hot coffee or tea should be safe.
- Talk with your healthcare provider about other advice on travel abroad.

Note. Based on information from Centers for Disease Control and Prevention, 2003a, 2003b, 2003c; United States Department of Agriculture, 2004.

References

American Cancer Society. (2002). *Nutrition for the person with cancer: A guide for patients and families.* Atlanta, GA: Author.

Centers for Disease Control and Prevention. (2003a). *An ounce of prevention: Keeps the germs away.* Retrieved March 13, 2004, from http://www.cdc.gov/ncidod/op/food.htm

Centers for Disease Control and Prevention. (2003b). *Safe food and water: A guide for people with HIV infection.* Retrieved March 13, 2004, from http://www.cdc.gov/hiv/pubs/brochure/food.htm

Centers for Disease Control and Prevention. (2003c). *What can consumers do to protect themselves from foodborne illness?* Retrieved March 13, 2004, from http://www.cdc.gov/ncidod/dbmd/diseaseinfo/foodborneinfections_g.htm#consumersprotect

Charney, P., & Malone, A. (Eds.). (2004). *ADA pocket guide to nutrition assessment.* Chicago: American Dietetic Association.

Dempsey, D., & Mullen, J. (1985). Macronutrient requirements in the malnourished cancer patient: How much of what and why? *Cancer, 55,* 290–294.

Eldridge, B., & Hamilton, K.K. (2004). *Management of nutrition impact symptoms in cancer and educational handouts* (2nd ed.). Chicago: American Dietetic Association.

Merrick, H., Long, C.L., Grecos, G.P., Dennis, R.S., & Blakemore, W.S. (1998). Energy requirements for cancer patients and the late effect of total parenteral nutrition. *Journal of Parenteral and Enteral Nutrition, 12*(1), 8–14.

National Cancer Institute. (2003). *Eating hints for cancer patients before, during and after treatment.* Washington, DC: Author.

National Cancer Institute. (2004). *Nutrition in cancer care (PDQ®).* Retrieved August 30, 2004, from http://www.cancer.gov/cancerinfo/pdq/supportivecare/nutrition/healthprofessional

United States Department of Agriculture. (2004). *Food safety for persons with AIDS.* Retrieved March 13, 2004, from http://www.fsis.usda.gov/OA/pubs/aids.htm

Yeatman, T.J. (2000). Nutritional support for the oncology patient. *Cancer Control, 7,* 563–565.

Index

The letter f *after a page number indicates that relevant content appears in a figure; the letter* t, *in a table.*